THAI MASSAGE &
THAI HEALING ARTS

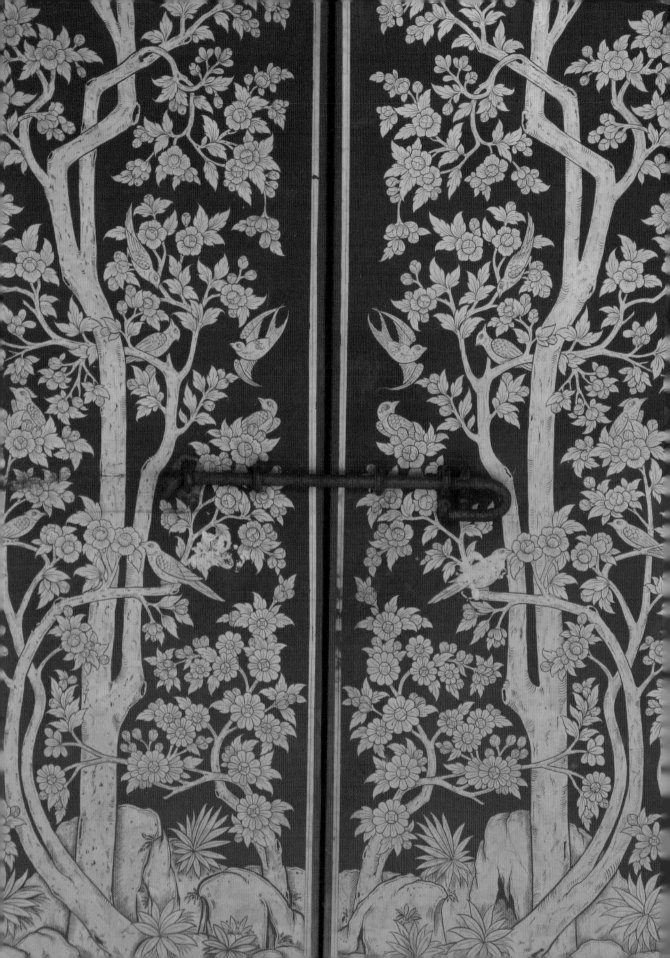

THAI MASSAGE & THAI HEALING ARTS

Practice, Culture and Spirituality

Bob Haddad

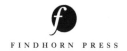

FINDHORN PRESS

© Bob Haddad 2013

The right of Bob Haddad to be identified as the author
of this work has been asserted by him in accordance
with the Copyright, Designs and Patents Act 1998.

Published in 2013 by Findhorn Press, Scotland

ISBN 978-1-84409-616-9

A CIP record for this title is available from the British Library.

Photo and illustration credits see page 318

Edited by Nicky Leach and Bob Haddad
Cover design by Bob Haddad and Thierry Bogliolo
Text design by Geoff Green Book Design, Cambridge
Printed and bound in China

Published by
Findhorn Press
117–121 High Street,
Forres IV36 1AB,
Scotland, UK
t +44 (0)1309 690582
f +44 (0)131 777 2711
e info@findhornpress.com
www.findhornpress.com

Acknowledgments

The process of writing, researching, compiling, and editing this book was long and sometimes arduous, but it was always extremely gratifying. Many people helped me to make it possible.

Thank you:
To my parents, who gave me life and sustained me, and to my life teachers, who offered me seeds of meaningful interconnectedness;

To my many Thai massage teachers, each of whom helped to shape my journey in *nuad boran* and Thai healing arts, especially my mentors Asokananda and Ajahn Pichest Boonthumme;

To the contributing writers in this anthology, for their individual perspectives, and for their acceptance of my direction, involvement, and editing;

To each of the photographers who have allowed photos to be reproduced in this book, and also to the models in the photos. To Celia Barenholtz, for her excellent photo editing;

To my colleagues and students for their acknowledgment, support, and enthusiasm, and to my clients for unknowingly being wonderful teachers. To the members and supporters of Thai Healing Alliance International (THAI), for working toward a higher level of awareness, practice, and study of traditional Thai massage around the world;

To Jivaka, for his presence, guidance, and intercession in my practice: *Om namo sirasa ahang;* To Ajahn Pichest, the spirit-guides, reusi, and all those who have helped me to become more aware of the nature, role, and importance of spiritual healing;

To Somananda Yogi, for his selfless guidance, advice, and support of this project;

To all my dear friends who have encouraged and supported me in my life;

To Findhorn Press, especially to Sabine and Thierry, for their care and interest in publishing this book.

Contents

Preface

Most Thai massage books available today are instruction manuals based on sequences, designed to teach students how to execute techniques that may be performed during a Thai massage. Printed materials all around the world and on the Internet may present volumes of information, but one cannot learn how to execute techniques, how to breathe and move organically, how to sense energy blockages, or how to effectively and holistically offer a Thai healing session by simply reading a book.

This book is different. There are no proposed sequences, and only a few detailed notes about specific Thai massage techniques appear in these pages. Rather than focusing on techniques and sequences, this anthology reflects the authors' cumulative experience in the world of traditional Thai healing arts. It suggests ways to refine and deepen personal and professional practice, and it offers a wealth of previously unavailable information on aspects of Thai culture and spirituality, and on the history and evolution of the powerful healing modality known today as traditional Thai massage.

Much of the information presented in this compendium has never before been available in print, but it is by no means exhaustive. For example, the book contains an essay on Thai element theory but not about the taste system used in Thai medicine. There is an article on *tok sen* (a folk healing tradition that uses a wooden hammer and chisel) but nothing about *yam khang*, another Lanna tradition that uses fire and hot oil as the vehicle for healing. The reason for these omissions is simple. Traditional healing arts in Thailand are so varied, and the actual practice of nuad boran is so deep, that it would be difficult and unrealistic to attempt to present everything in one book.

In writing, compiling, and editing the essays that comprise this book, I've tried to present Thai massage as a unique healing art that comes from, and exists within, a framework of Thai traditional medicine, and as something that is also deeply connected to Thai Buddhist spirituality and Thai culture.

Content

The book is divided into several sections, each containing entries by different authors of varying length:

Section 1 (Introduction) This section presents general information on the evolution, concepts, theory, myths, historical facts, and intent of traditional Thai massage.

Section 2 (Mastery of Practice) offers specific information about developing, refining, and maintaining a healthy Thai massage practice. It includes essays on breath and body mechanics, acupressure concepts and techniques, ways to use your feet creatively, herbal compress therapy, self-protection techniques, body language, and information about sen lines and Thai element theory.

Section 3 (Spiritual and Cultural Connections) presents articles on traditional Thai healers, magic and spirituality in Thai society, Jivaka Kumarabhacca, Buddhist influence in Thai massage, the reusi tradition, and accessory modalities such as *tok sen* (hammering therapy) and *reusi dat ton* (Thai hermit stretching exercises).

Section 4 (Thai Therapists Speak) features articles and accounts by individual Thai therapists and teachers around the world who offer unique perspectives on their study, experiences, and work in traditional Thai massage and Thai healing arts.

The final section features a glossary, a bibliography, photo and illustration credits, biographies of the contributing writers, and an index.

Throughout the book, I have used italics the first time each non-English word appears in a given essay. Afterward, those words remain in plain type for the rest of that essay. Please refer to the glossary as necessary when reading this book.

Never before has such wide-ranging and extensive information about Thai healing arts been compiled and presented in print. I feel honored to be offering this information, along with the contributions of my colleagues, as traditional Thai massage continues to touch and transform the lives of many more people around the world.

Bob Haddad

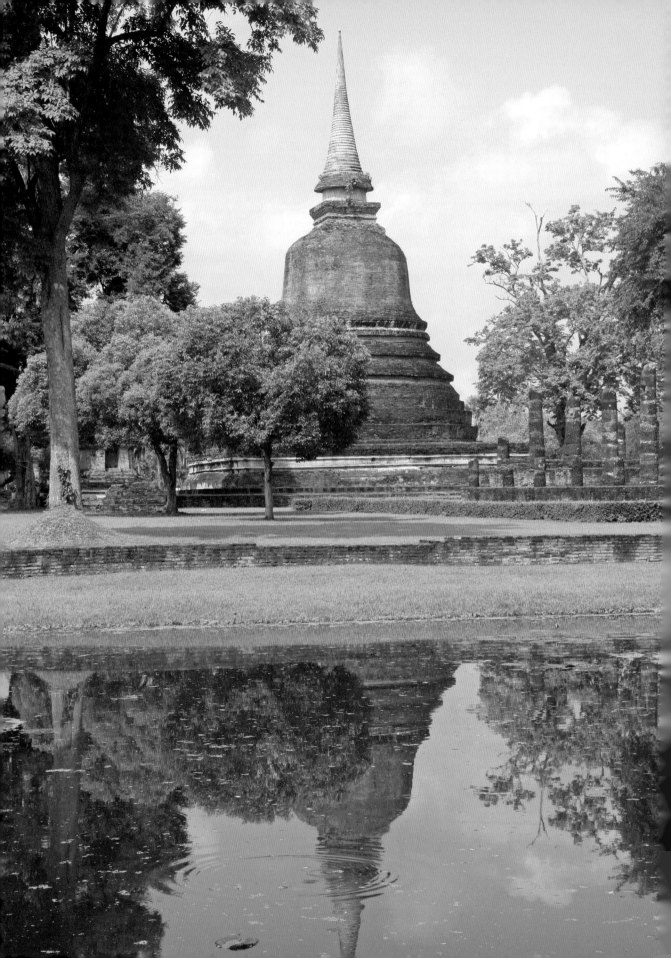

Section 1

Introduction

Practice, Culture, and Spirituality: Introduction

BOB HADDAD

The first time I experienced Thai massage, or *nuad phaen boran*, as it is known in the Thai language, I knew it was something very powerful. I was traveling with a friend who had recently taken an introductory course, and she wanted to practice some techniques on me. We moved the furniture in the room, put a blanket on top of the rug, and she began to work on me in supine position, based on a sequence she had learned from her teacher. I remember the sensation of palming on my feet and legs, and how nice it felt for my body to be opened and relaxed in that way.

I have no recollection of the other things she did that day, except for one brilliant move: a suspended spinal twist. While I was lying on my side, she braced her lower leg against my thigh, and she placed my right hand on my left shoulder. Then, while holding on to my left hand, she pulled my upper torso into the air, and my spine moved into a delicious twist. As I surrendered to that moment, suspended in space, my head dangling backward and my breath deep and long, I flashed back to earlier times in my life when I'd practiced yoga on a daily basis. I realized that the close connection I once had between my body and my spiritual center had become clouded, and that it needed to become clear again. There, while suspended in that pose, I knew that I wanted to learn more about this thing called "Thai massage."

When I returned home, I began to read about Thai massage. I reviewed on the Internet the very few courses of study that were available in Thailand at that time, I checked the price of airfare, and within a few weeks I was in Chiang Mai, beginning an introductory course with Chongkol Setthakorn, my first teacher. I stayed in Thailand for a month on that trip, and when I returned home, I began to practice on my friends in a spare room of my house.

With instruction books and a notebook at my side, I followed the sequence that was laid out in my books over and over again, and I asked as many friends as possible to allow me to work on them. Over time I got better. I listened to the feedback that my "victims" offered, and I tried to remember as much as possible about each person's likes and dislikes by writing notes in a book. I continued practicing those basic techniques for several months until I learned each sequence by memory. I began to take courses with other teachers in my own country, I returned to Thailand for additional study, and I continued to work on my friends for free until they began to leave donations as they left my practice room. "I'm leaving some money on the table for you," they would say.

After eighteen months of study, I had begun to accept donations, but I still didn't feel ready to practice professionally. I was following all the sequences I'd learned from various teachers, but something was still missing, and I didn't know what it was. The next few years of study would help me to understand more clearly. Profound experiences and special people I encountered along the way encouraged me to find in myself that missing link.

Lessons along the way

I knew that a German-born teacher named Asokananda lived in a Lahu tribal village north of Chiang Mai. I had bought a few of his books in Thailand, and I wanted to study with him. He was teaching in Europe at the time, so I registered for an advanced course that was being held in Spain. After I sent in my registration, the teacher contacted me and asked me to tell him about my study background. I briefly explained with whom I had studied, and for how long. He responded that based on my study and experience to date, he would not be able to accept me into his class. I wrote back immediately and told him that I truly wanted to study with him. I made a more complete list of all the workshops I had taken, and I told him that although I had been studying and practicing for almost two years, I felt that something was missing and I needed a guide to help me find it. After a few days, he e-mailed me again, and he gave me his permission to register for the weeklong course.

The first day of class was a revelation for me. Asoka, as some of his students affectionately called him, welcomed us, and then he asked us to choose a partner and to begin work. We asked him what he wanted us to do, and he simply said "just begin to work." I took a moment to focus and pray, and I began to work on my partner's feet – palming, twisting, compressing, stretching, pressing points on the soles, working the lines and the toes, pulling the feet, cracking the knuckles, rotating the ankles – many of the standard Thai techniques I had learned for the feet.

We all worked in silence as the teacher observed. Occasionally, he would come close and speak quietly to one of us. We continued working for several more minutes, each in our own way, and I got to the point where it was time to work on my partner's lower legs. I began to palm-walk on her feet, then on her calves in an alternating fashion – first palming one leg, then the other, and repeating this left-right pattern as I moved upward. All my previous teachers had taught me to palm-walk in this way. Asokananda approached me, and he said softly: "That is a perfectly legitimate and effective way to work the lower legs with your palms, but in this particular case, I wouldn't do it that way." He smiled at me, and then he turned and walked away.

"What does that mean?" I thought to myself, "and what should I do now?" I had absolutely no idea what to do, and I looked toward him, expecting him to instruct me, to tell me, to show me exactly what I should do, but he was already whispering to someone else at the end of the room. I glanced over to another student a few feet away, and I saw that she was palming both of her partner's legs simultaneously, not in alternating fashion as I had been working. I looked down at my practice partner and noticed that one of her feet was slightly more upright than the other. I opened her legs a little wider so I could get closer, and I began to palm simultaneously, leaning in with my body-weight, just as the other student was doing. A short time after making this modification, I felt my partner's more upright leg surrender slightly to my touch, and by the time I had finished palming simultaneously up and down her legs, both of her feet were equidistant to the mat. Surprised, I looked over to Asokananda at the end of the room. He saw me raise my head, and he looked at me and smiled.

This was the first turning point in my journey into the world of nuad boran. I was impressed that making such a slight adjustment in my technique and body mechanics could bring about a visible change for the receiver, but I was even more impressed with the teacher. He hadn't been judgmental at all when I was working in alternating fashion. In fact, before he offered his comment, he validated me first by saying that what I was doing was legitimate and perfectly acceptable. Then he smiled and left me to discover the adjustment I needed to make for myself, without ever telling me what to do. He gave me permission to break away from my methodical sequence, so that I could pay closer attention to the individual before me, yet all the while, he kept a watchful eye over me from across the room. I was so impressed and humbled by his teaching style that I immediately knew that I wanted to study further with him. This began a friendship with Asokananda that lasted until his untimely death.

A few years later, I was sitting at an outdoor restaurant in Chiang Mai with some friends, when a Thai massage colleague passed by. She came over to our table, and by the expression on her face, we all knew something was very wrong. She told us that Chaiyuth Priyasith, the great Thai massage teacher, had suddenly died that afternoon, and that she and other students were with him when it happened. We were shocked by the news of his passing, but even more surprised by the way it happened. Chaiyuth had collapsed and died during a ceremonial spirit dance while paying homage to Jivaka Kumarabhacca, the legendary Indian doctor revered throughout Thailand as the ancestral teacher of traditional medicine (see "Memorial for Chaiyuth" in this book). We consoled our friend, and I made plans to meet her the next morning to learn details of the funeral.

Two days later, I joined a large crowd of people at Wat Mahawan for the prayer, grieving, food, and music that are typical of a Thai funeral. Just as we began to take our seats, Asokananda arrived on a motorbike. He noticed me, and he invited me to sit with him. I could see that he was quite upset, yet he spoke softly. We sat with other mourners as a row of monks on an elevated platform chanted for the release of Chaiyuth's soul from his body. Occasionally during the ceremony, Asokananda told me about his experiences with Chaiyuth, and how he and Pichest Boonthumme were his most important teachers.

Attending the funeral of a Thai massage master made a lasting impression in my heart for two main reasons. First was the way in which Chaiyuth had died. At that point in my study, I was beginning to understand the important role that spirituality played in Thai healing arts, but the fact that Chaiyuth had died while apparently channeling the energy of Jivaka motivated me to move more deeply into the spiritual aspect of the work. Secondly, while I sat there at the funeral with my teacher, who was himself a student of the deceased, I couldn't have imagined that this would be one of the last times I would be sharing intimate moments with Asokananda. Though we corresponded regularly after Chaiyuth's death, Asokananda succumbed to cancer quickly, and he died the following year.

During that same trip to Thailand, I had begun to think about the need for a unified voice for traditional Thai massage. All around the world, and especially in Thailand, foreigners (*farang* in Thai language) were taking courses at schools that promised to make them proficient at Thai massage in just a few weeks or months of study. Some were offering "teacher training" programs that, I felt, provided inadequate training and gave students an inflated sense of ego. Time after time in my study with various teachers, I'd met students who believed that they were qualified Thai massage therapists. Yet just by observing their body mechanics and their straight-from-the-book sequences, I knew that they were far from being accomplished practitioners. I had spent a year and a half studying and practicing before I even accepted donations, and these young people were taking Thai massage classes for only a few weeks, returning to their countries with certifications that weren't legally binding, and immediately starting to practice professionally.

At this time I had already been studying with my second transformative teacher, Pichest Boonthumme. Those who regularly studied with him seemed to have "beginners' minds," diminished egos, and a deeper dedication to the practice. Students of all ages and levels of experience were in the same class. Some had been returning to study with him for many years, and several of us had become friends. One day I asked two of my classmates if I could brainstorm with them about the possibility of forming an organization that would propose basic standards of study and practice of traditional Thai massage. We met over dinner, discussed what each of us felt were important things to consider, and I scribbled some notes on a napkin. I worked on that list over the next few months, and with the help of colleagues and teachers, I developed a loose organizational structure for what would eventually become Thai Healing Alliance International (THAI). The guidelines we created became the first nonpartisan international standards for the study and practice of traditional Thai massage.

Ajahn Pichest (*ajahn* = teacher) was helping me to understand how important it was to be still, to meditate, and to use sensing, intuition, and good body mechanics as I worked. I was refining my ability to feel blockages in the human energy system with my hands, but I was in the presence of a master who sometimes didn't even have to touch someone in order to detect a blockage.

Later that same year I returned to Thailand a second time for more study. After a month of study with Pichest and other teachers, a friend joined me in Chiang Mai, as we had made plans to vacation together on the beautiful islands of southern Thailand over the end-of-year holidays. We had bought air tickets to fly to Krabi on the mainland, and from there we would take a ferry to Koh Phi Phi. I decided to visit Pichest on Friday for morning prayers and to say goodbye, and my friend asked if she could come along. After prayers, Pichest turned around to face the group, so he could begin his daily discourse. Within a few seconds, he looked straight at me, and asked me if I was leaving the next day for southern Thailand. I replied that no, I was leaving on Sunday. "Morning or afternoon?" he asked. "Morning" I said. He became visibly upset upon hearing my answer, and he quickly summoned me to his altar. As I knelt before the altar with my hands in prayer position (*wai*), he began to bless me and to recite prayers over me, while tying knotted string bracelets around my wrists. Every once in a while, he would look up at me and say "be careful when you go, be careful" and then he would return to the prayers.

I had received blessings from him before, but never in such a deep way or for such an extended period of time. He continued the prayers for another few minutes. When he finally stopped, he looked at me with great concern, and he told me once again that I needed to be careful. I thanked him, offered a wai to him and to the altar, and I slowly backed away. As I turned around, I made an eye signal to my friend that it was time for us to go. Consequently she bowed and stood up to leave the room. "Oh, you are with Bob? Come here," he said, as he motioned to her with his hand. My friend knelt at the altar, and he also began to bless her, saying every once in a while, "Be careful with Bob when you go. Be careful."

After his blessing, he took a white object from a box nearby, placed it in her open hand, then closed her hand around it and said a final prayer. He had given her a tiny statue of Jivaka Kumarabhacca. She offered a final wai, and we left the classroom to begin our journey back to Chiang Mai. My friend was elated at having been blessed by my teacher, but I was very worried about what had just happened. Why was he so concerned about my safety? What did all of those blessings mean? What should I be careful about?

We spent Christmas Day, a Saturday, preparing for our early departure the following day. The next day – December 26, 2004 – we took an early morning flight from Chiang Mai to Bangkok, where we would make a connecting flight. We got our boarding passes for the flight to Krabi, and we were standing in line, waiting to board the plane at 9:30 a.m., when all of a sudden pandemonium broke out. People began to run and scream all around the airport terminal. The noise level rose dramatically, and some people began to cry hysterically. Someone said, "Look at the television," so we rushed to a TV monitor in the departure lounge. What we saw would become forever etched in my mind. A massive tsunami had made a direct hit in southern Thailand. We stood with our mouths open, as we watched a live broadcast of rushing waves, and boats, homes and wreckage being swept to sea. Thousands of people were already feared dead in the region. On the bottom of the screen, Thai words, along with an English translation, described where the live broadcast was taking place. It was in Krabi.

I looked at the TV screen to read that word again, then I looked down at the boarding pass in my hand, and I read the very same word, Krabi. I was stunned. There was so much noise and commotion all around us that we decided to leave the boarding area and sit down in a quieter place to discuss what we would do. We went into a glass-enclosed restaurant, we ordered a coffee, and then suddenly we both realized that this was the reason that Pichest had been so worried. This was why he had told me to be so careful. He had sensed the danger zone that I was entering as I left the safety of the hills of northern Thailand. That realization was almost as shocking as the news of the tsunami.

Within a few seconds, I knew that I had to call him. If he had known that I was about to be in danger, then he surely would be worrying about me right now. I went to a public phone nearby and called him. "Ajahn Pichest, this is Bob." "Ah, Bob," he replied, "you OK?" I told him I was fine, and that we were just about to board the plane to Krabi when the tsunami struck. "Tsunami very strong energy," he replied. We spoke for only another few seconds, and I told him I would be in touch with him again soon.

My intimate experiences with Asokananda, Chaiyuth, and Pichest, as well as several other meaningful incidents that have taken place over the years, have been the building blocks of my study and practice in Thai healing arts. My path in life has been shaped by consequence, by the decisions I've made, and by those whom I've met along the way. I am fortunate to have been blessed, figuratively and literally, by teachers, colleagues, clients, and students who have helped me to discover the magic, spirituality, and great healing power of traditional Thai massage.

Understanding Nuad Boran

So what is Thai massage? Well, for one thing, it's not "massage" as we know it in the West. In fact, it is unfortunate that the term "Thai massage" has become so popular because that second word, massage, is misleading and inaccurate. Massage tables or oil aren't used, there is no rubbing on the skin or kneading of the muscles, and the receiver remains clothed. The goal is not to work muscles, fascia, tendons, ligaments, organs, and soft tissue, though these anatomical elements are positively affected by the work. Neither is its purpose to simply stretch and apply passive yoga to another person on a floor mat. At its essence, nuad boran is a balanced blend of physical, energetic, and spiritual healing techniques and concepts. It is the skilful combination of applying both broad and targeted acupressure, finding and dissolving blockages, stimulating energy lines (sen), opening and toning the body with yoga-like stretches, and last but not least, allowing and encouraging the receiver to engage in a process of self healing, deep relaxation, and renewal.

Unfortunately, the world is filled with people who teach or practice Thai massage without having adequate knowledge or study experience. Many students lack the discipline, humility, or personal development that is required in order to take a slow and comprehensive approach toward learning. The Western model of learning in "levels" complicates the situation even further. Some teachers and schools in Thailand and around the world respond to this by marketing their courses in levels, and by creating and promoting curricula that claim to certify students as practitioners or teachers in a short period of time. Some new practitioners may study only for a few weeks or months before beginning to charge money for their services. All too often, students who take a hurried approach to learning emerge as unaccomplished and unrefined practitioners. Mixing Thai massage with other established modalities such as western table massage and yoga is also common. These hybrid forms may include elements of nuad boran, but they shouldn't be confused with, or presented as traditional Thai massage.

Some practitioners and teachers, even after many years of practice, never understand or experience the deep spiritual and energy-based aspects of the work. These therapists apply acupressure and stretching techniques in a mechanical way, following sequences that they learned from their teachers, but without being sensitive and attentive to their clients' needs. They haven't yet understood how important it is to deviate from a sequence, to follow their intuition, to avoid working in certain areas, or to "listen" to the body of their client in order to understand how to best encourage and facilitate healing.

In my practice and study over many years, I've come to realize that certain perceptions and preconceptions about nuad boran are simply not true. I also believe that extremely important elements of this healing art are missing from many training programs around the world, including in Thailand. Instead, they remain either unspoken or unaddressed. What follows, in my opinion, are a few of these considerations:

Individualized treatments

Traditional Thai massage is not a sequence of techniques and movements that can be applied to all people. When we first learn Thai massage, it's important to study and memorize sequences for each of the major body positions: supine, seated, side, and prone. These basic sequences help us to become familiar with techniques, and they allow us to learn how to transition from one movement to the next. An effective Thai treatment, however, cannot be given by mechanically following a sequence, no matter whose sequence it is, or how long it has been practiced. Teachers and schools that train students to follow proprietary fixed sequences for all clients may be hindering students from growing into deeply sensitive therapists. Along the way, there must be adaptation, exploration, and experience with a wide variety of different people. Generally speaking, only after several years of practice and study can we develop the sensitivity and awareness that is needed to effectively work with each person in an individualized fashion.

Individualized holistic treatment is at the heart of Thai healing arts, and Thai massage should be administered in this way in order to be fully effective. An accomplished Thai therapist continually practices and studies, preferably with a variety of teachers, throughout his entire career. He "listens" to the body of each client as he works, learns to sense energy flow and blockages, and relies on intuition, sensitivity, and stillness to guide him through each treatment.

The importance of self-healing

Much of the healing that takes place during a session results from the combined efforts of both the practitioner and the receiver. The therapist is not always the one to whom all credit is due. In fact, most therapists are not the great healers that their clients, students, and they themselves may think they are. The client is constantly on his or her own path of self-exploration, self-love, spirituality, self-surrender, and self-healing while receiving Thai treatments. Skilled and accomplished Thai therapists are as much witnesses to this self-healing as they are therapists. Masterful Thai massage therapists facilitate and encourage healing in others through their sensitive touch, their application of *metta* (loving-kindness), and the atmosphere of safety, trust, and confidence that they establish and maintain in their practice.

Body mechanics and breathwork are essential

Though they are not taught in many workshops and training programs, good body mechanics and correct breathing play extremely important roles in Thai massage. An experienced Thai therapist works only within his immediate reach, and positions his body directly ahead of, or on top of, the area where he is working. The *hara*, the core area located slightly below the navel, is where all movement should originate. A therapist's back should be straight, the shoulders relaxed, the chest open, and in most cases, arms should be straight and locked at the elbows when applying pressure. Masterful Thai therapists utilize correct breathing patterns as they work, they remain observant of their client's breathing throughout each session, and they adjust their breathing to work most effectively with that of their client. More information on this topic may be found in the essay in this book entitled "Breath and Body Mechanics in Nuad Boran."

Distractions and ego get in the way

Thai massage is most powerful and effective when it is carried out, for the most part, in silence. The therapist needs to focus his energies, observe the body, hear the breath, and adapt his techniques to the needs of the individual before him. The receiver should ideally feel at peace and spiritually centered, with his nervous system in a parasympathetic (relaxed) state, since these conditions always encourage good results. Excessive talking during a session can be a distraction, and so can music, especially if it's not at a low volume. I've found it's best to not engage clients in conversation, to comment about their condition, or to offer excessive prompting or coaching. It's also extremely important to suppress one's ego during a Thai massage session. Don't execute certain techniques or postures because you think your clients want you to do them, or in order to impress them. Be humble, stay open to subtle energies, work slowly and in a meditative way, and try to encourage silence.

Awareness of body language

From the moment they step into the treatment room and lie on the mat, clients display body language that can provide glimpses into their physical, psychological, and emotional states. An accomplished Thai therapist observes this body language, tries to interpret it, and proceeds with the treatment while remaining sensitive to the client's needs. When a client lies down on the mat, are her palms turned up or down? Are her legs and feet close together or apart? Are her hands resting on top of her stomach, her chest, or near her genitals? Is one foot pointing more upward than the other? What could each of these things be saying? Very often, our interpretations and explorations of these observations can determine a correct course of treatment for each client we see. See "Considering Body Language" in this book.

The element of time

A complete Thai massage simply cannot be done in one hour. In many cases, even ninety minutes is barely enough time to adequately address the entire body. In Thailand, it is customary to administer sessions of two to three hours in length, but in the West, with the busy daily schedules of therapists and clients, this is sometimes not possible. Nevertheless, it's best to allow between ninety minutes and two hours for each session, and even more when necessary.

Spiritual healing

Thai massage, at its essence, is a spiritual healing art, not simply a physical therapy. In Thailand, massage belongs to one of the branches of Thai medicine, and it incorporates Buddhist healing principles. Never underestimate the power of meditation and stillness while at work, both for the giver and the receiver. Stay grounded; be silent and encourage silence; focus your energies on your hands and on the other parts of your body that come into contact with the person you are touching; send metta to the receiver as you work; observe breath, both yours and the client's; try to keep your mind empty of thought, as in *vipassana* meditation; try to sense blockages in the sen lines as you work, then try to dissipate them before you move to the next area of the body.

Providing comfort and maintaining safe boundaries

It's best to keep the practice room at a comfortable temperature. A person who is lying motionless on the floor can become cold, not only because of room temperature but also because of internal energy movement. Take extra care to keep the client's hands and feet warm, and consider covering portions of the body that are not being touched or moved for extended periods. Respect boundaries, both physical and psychological. When you apply acupressure and assisted yoga stretches, don't push beyond the client's level of comfort. Maintain regular contact with your client's face, look for signs that display discomfort or pain, be patient and humble in your approach, and always work within the natural limitations of each individual.

At the beginning of a session, and periodically during the treatment, check the person's body language to see if you can read anything about their potential protection zones. As you approach those private or "guarded" areas, take extra care to not directly invade them. If sexual thoughts or energies ever arise, whether they are initiated by the giver or receiver, momentarily stop the session. If they continue, terminate the session.

Balancing energy

One of the main goals of a nuad boran session is to free blocked energy *(lom)* in the sen, and to encourage free flow of that energy throughout the body. Displaced lom, however, can remain trapped in a client after a session if the therapist neglects to balance or forgets to balance the client's energy properly. If a particular line or area of the body seems blocked, you might spend more time there, but also make sure that other points on that line receive your attention. In Thai medicine, lom flows in both directions along the sen, but the most common and respected traditional format is to begin at the feet with the client in supine position, and to end at the head, also in supine position. No matter how many body positions are used during a given treatment, it can be helpful to imagine the client's overall energy as moving from the bottom of the body to the top.

Pre-session preparations and post-session cleansing

Before a session takes place, the room should be neat and clean, and it should be free of lingering energies from any previous activities. Take time to meditate or pray, focus on your altar, loosen your body through yoga, breathe slowly and deeply, and clear your mind. After the session is finished, and especially if it was an intense or emotionally charged treatment, make sure to cleanse the room properly, and also take time to rid yourself of any outside energies that you may have taken on during the treatment. The essay in this book called "Self-Protection Techniques for the Thai Therapist" suggests pre- and post-session techniques that may be of interest.

Dignifying Thai healing arts

One of the most wonderful things about Thai massage is that it is not static, and that it will continue to evolve and expand as a healing art well into the future. Despite this wonderful capacity to expand and grow, however, it is important to study and practice Thai massage within the contexts of Thai healing traditions, Thai Buddhist spirituality, and Thai culture.

In recent years, some Westerners have combined Thai massage concepts with other practices and therapies, and even some teachers and schools in Thailand promote treatments and courses of study by using the word "Thai," when these curricula are not true to Thai healing traditions. In my opinion, there's nothing wrong with combining techniques and concepts from different sources, as long as the result is promoted as a hybrid form or a new creation, and not as a traditional healing art.

Traditional Thai massage is a unique and powerful vehicle of healing, and it deserves to be practiced, taught, and promoted within the context of traditional Thai medicine, not Indian Ayurvedic medicine, Chinese medicine, Western medicine, or any other body of knowledge. Some people speak of Thai sen lines in relation to Chinese meridians, but traditional Chinese medicine has never had any direct influence on the evolution of the traditional Thai medicine system. Many Thai massage lovers are also avid yoga practitioners, and since they are familiar with yoga philosophy or Ayurveda, they blend them and present the result within the framework of traditional Thai massage. Fortunately, these days, there is a growing interest in learning more about traditional Thai medicine, and qualified teachers are becoming more accessible to serious Thai massage therapists in the West and in Thailand. I hope this trend will continue into the future.

I encourage all students, practitioners, and teachers of Thai massage to be diligent in their approach to study; to evolve slowly, patiently, creatively, and respectfully as practitioners of this noble healing art; and to dignify and elevate traditional Thai massage by practicing it within the framework of the traditional medicine, culture and spiritual values of Thailand.

Traditional Thai Massage: An Overview

KIRA BALASKAS

Traditional Thai massage is a unique and powerful healing art that combines acupressure, stretching, and assisted yoga. As Thai massage has grown in popularity around the world and in Thailand, it has taken on many names. The terms *nuad boran*, Thai yoga massage, traditional Thai massage, Thai yoga therapy, and Thai yoga bodywork are used interchangeably, since they all refer to the same healing art that has been practiced in Thailand for many years.

Nuad boran is not massage as it is known in the West, and the term "Thai massage" is somewhat of a misnomer, since the human energy system, not only the physical body, is affected during treatment. Elements of nuad boran have been incorporated into modern forms of massage, bodywork, physical therapy, and yoga, but there is no real substitute for the mind/body healing process that unfolds during and after an effective Thai session.

History and origins

Thai massage traces its lineage to Jivaka Kumarabhaccha, a legendary doctor from early Buddhist scriptures. Thai people refer to him as Shivagakomarapaj or Gomalapat, and throughout Thailand he is honored as the father of Thai medicine. Statues and images of a bearded Indian man in flowing robes, sitting in cross-legged position, may be found throughout the country. Protection amulets bearing his image are worn by healers and also by those who seek healing. Thai massage teachers and practitioners say prayers each day to honor Jivaka as an ancestral teacher, and as an intercessor for healing.

Epigraphs at Wat Po showing energy lines and pressure points

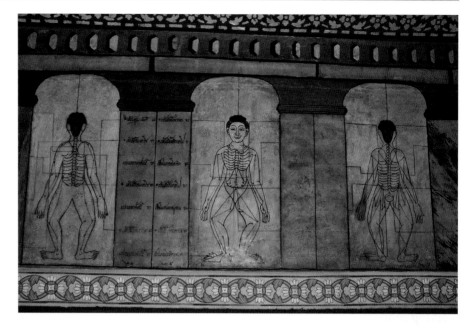

It's not clear exactly how and when nuad boran developed in Thailand, but its origins almost certainly may be traced back to Indian Ayurvedic principles and early Buddhist traditions. The exact origins have remained obscure, and this is partly due to the fact that for centuries Thai medical knowledge was passed down orally from teacher to pupil. In addition, early Thai medical documents that were kept on palm-leaf manuscripts were destroyed during a war with Burma in the eighteenth century.

Thai massage today

A general revival of Thai massage took place in Thailand during the last two decades of the twentieth century. Prior to this, the popularity of Western medicines, combined with government efforts to modernize Thai society, had greatly diminished the roles of traditional healing arts, including massage and herbal medicine. In rural areas, however, traditional teachings were kept alive by healers who followed the traditions of their ancestors. Westerners, seeking knowledge of alternative forms of healing and spirituality, began to arrive in Thailand in the 1980s, and treatment centers such as Wat Po in Bangkok and the Old Medicine Hospital in Chiang Mai played major roles in keeping these healing traditions alive. The influx of foreign students seeking knowledge of Thai healing arts also encouraged a resurgence of Thai massage among Thai people in Thailand. Since then, traditional Thai massage has continued to increase in popularity, both in Thailand and all around the world.

Those people familiar with traditional Thai massage recognize that it is highly effective in the treatment of many ailments. It can benefit stroke victims by returning mobility and sensitivity to their limbs, and it is effective in treating frozen shoulder, asthma, back pain, and many other conditions. Today, a variety of teachers and schools throughout Thailand offer courses in nuad boran, and storefronts offer massage treatments on the streets of major cities. Because of the lack of regulated standards of study and practice, however, the quality of treatments varies greatly. All around the world, it's difficult to know if you'll get an experienced and sensitive therapist, or someone who has had little training. It's often best to choose by personal recommendation, to receive a session from a teacher at a Thai massage school, or to seek out a traditional healer.

In many Western countries, licensed table massage therapists may legally practice Thai massage if they have studied only at the most elementary level, and even sometimes if they have never studied Thai massage at all. Knowledge of table massage doesn't automatically qualify someone to give an effective Thai treatment. As with any discipline, one must be adequately trained before offering professional services. Local and national governing boards, seeking control and revenue, may one day attempt to regulate traditional Thai massage under the aegis of another modality, such as table massage. This is a matter of great concern for Thai massage professionals and also for the general public.

Nevertheless, there are many dedicated and experienced Thai therapists and teachers around the world today who aspire to high standards. The Sunshine Network, established under guidance of the late Asokananda, is a loosely woven network of teachers trained under shared guidelines. Thai Healing Alliance International (THAI) is an international nonpartisan network of students, therapists, teachers, and schools that adhere to and promote basic standards of study and practice of traditional Thai massage around the world.

Styles and variations

It is often said that there are two general styles of Thai massage: Northern and Southern. The principal school to promote southern-style nuad boran is based at Wat Po in Bangkok. What is known as the northern style was largely developed at the Foundation of Shivagakomarpaj (Old Medicine Hospital) in Chiang Mai. Today however, a wide variety of schools and teachers promote northern, southern, or a combination of these two styles.

Whether studying the northern or southern approach to nuad boran, you will encounter great diversity in techniques, and many therapists and teachers currently incorporate a mixture of styles and techniques into their work. As you travel from place to place in Thailand, you will rarely receive the same form of treatment twice. Some practitioners concentrate on energy lines, working in a slow and methodical manner; some incorporate extensive stretching techniques; while others pluck the tendons with thumbs and fingers, a style sometimes known as *jap sen*. Length of the sessions varies, and some therapists and schools use hot herbal compresses for every session.

Rather than making distinctions between northern and southern styles, some argue that there are only two legitimate forms of Thai massage: Royal (*ratchasamnak*) and Folk (*chaloeysak.*) As the name implies, royal style was developed long ago in order to treat Thai kings, queens, and other members of the royal family. There are strict rules covering protocol for working in a respectful manner, and only hands may be used. In addition, the practitioner must take care to maintain extra distance from the receiver, and prone position (face down) is never used during the course of a treatment. Royal style is still used in some places to treat the general public, and because it utilizes strong thumb acupressure, it can bring about good results in a short period of time. The more common folk style disregards the etiquette reserved for royalty, and instead utilizes hands, feet, elbows, knees, and other parts of the body to execute postures and techniques. The overwhelming majority of practitioners around the world and in Thailand practice in the folk style.

Thai massage theory

Thai yoga massage is based on a belief in a life force that circulates through energy pathways in the body. Indian yoga philosophy calls this life force *prana*, the Chinese refer to it as *chi* or *qi,* and in Thai medicine it is called *lom*. It is said to be absorbed into the body from the food we eat, from the air we breathe, and from the living energy all around us. In Thai massage, these pathways comprise an energy system of pathways or lines (*sen*). A blockage in any line may impede or prevent the free flow of lom, and therefore may lead to aches, pain, and disease on physical, emotional, and spiritual levels. Thai yoga massage focuses on ten major lines, called *sip sen* (ten sen), and a thorough Thai treatment usually affects these ten sen lines.

The Indian origins of Thai yoga massage are clear from its basic theory. The link becomes even more obvious if we compare the names of three of the main Thai sen lines with their Indian equivalents, known as *prana nadis*. The Thai energy line called *sumana sen* is known to Indian yogis as *sushumna nadi*. Similarly, the two *sen* known in Thai as *ittha and pingkhala* are derived from the Indian nadis called *ida* and *pingala*.

Some people claim that Thai sen lines are the same as the meridians in Chinese medicine and, by extension, other modalities such as Japanese shiatsu. This is definitely not the case. The sen lines and Chinese meridians do intersect at important acupressure points along the body, but they follow different pathways. Also, lom in Thai medicine is believed to flow in both directions within individual sen, whereas chi in Chinese medicine is believed to flow from one point to another in only one direction. What-ever the differences in form, technique, and theory, how-ever, Thai, Chinese, Indian, and other ancient Eastern healing systems are all concerned with locating and dimin-ishing blockages so that the free flow of energy may be restored, balanced, and fortified.

Spiritual elements

It's important to understand the spiritual nature of Thai massage, and to work in a spiritually focused manner. Tra-ditionally, nuad boran was offered on the grounds of Bud-dhist temples and was an extension of spiritual practice, particularly meditation. Accomplished therapists strive for a sense of awareness of each moment as they work on the receiver's body. The effects of Thai massage are greatly enhanced through a practice known as *metta,* or loving-kindness meditation. When we send metta to our clients as we work, we offer them unbridled compassion through our healing touch.

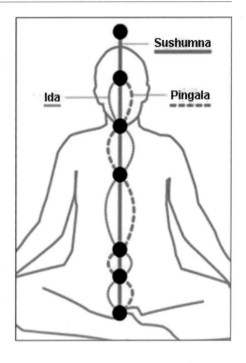

The Indian nadis sushumna, ida, and pingala lend their names to three important Thai sen lines

An important aspect of Thai massage is the intention with which we carry out a treatment. A session given with awareness, metta, sensitivity, and care will feel totally different from one given in a mechanical or technical way. Per-forming the work in a meditative way also engages the relaxed parasympa-thetic state in the nervous system of the receiver, allowing the heart rate to slow down, intestinal and glandular activity to increase, and the muscles to relax. Practicing in a calm, meditative way allows both parties to feel balanced and peaceful, and it helps the therapist to develop intuitive abilities and to sense blockages in the sen lines.

East and West

Without an understanding of the Eastern thought process, Thai massage can become stuck in a Western field of perception, one that is more limited in scope. Systematic and analytical Western viewpoints can make it difficult to understand and experience the intuitive and spiritual healing that takes place in nuad boran.

In the West, we often seek out one absolute truth, one solution, and one answer to each issue. Eastern thought, however, allows for many ways to deal with matters, and personal intuition, inclination, and spiritual direction are very important. The Eastern mind searches less for final answers, and works with what is available at each moment in order to fulfill an immediate purpose. Since there is not a single, standard solution to every problem, one must be intuitive and creative during a Thai massage treatment. If what we do doesn't work, we might try something else. In the Western medical approach, most patients who see a doctor for symptoms that point, for example, to a stomach ulcer, will be given the same treatment or prescribed the same type of medicine in almost every case. In Eastern medicine, if several people go to a traditional doctor, each one might receive slightly different treatments. By extension, the same holds true for Thai massage. We cannot use the same sequence or routine for every person we treat.

Another difference between the two approaches is that unlike Western massage, nuad boran has little relationship to anatomy and physiology. In ancient Thai society, human dissections were probably not performed, and healers did not systematically study the basic structure of the body under the skin. Instead, they studied the workings of the human energy system, and how massage, point pressure, and manipulation bring about healing by releasing blockages in the body's energy channels.

These days, many students wish to apply their knowledge of anatomy and physiology to Thai massage, but anatomical knowledge doesn't necessarily improve the effectiveness and quality of Thai treatments. It is important that the Western analytical approach not interfere with our innate abilities to sense blockages and to feel energy. Learning to be still and aware enough to feel energy is crucial to practicing Thai massage in an intuitive, creative, and effective way. At an advanced level of practice, intuition, mindfulness, and spiritual focus are the most important elements of our work.

Effects and benefits

Many benefits may be gained from a Thai massage session. Properly balancing the energy systems of the human body can have a profound effect on the receiver. One often feels an immediate sense of grounding and openness, and perceptions such as taste, touch, smell, and vision may be dramatically enhanced. It can sometimes take several days for the energy rebalancing to take full effect, and clients often continue to feel positive effects for many weeks after the session.

Two common responses to a Thai massage session are tiredness, or a dramatic spike of energy. Whatever the initial reaction, energy is in the process of being rebalanced, and even if we feel tired immediately afterward, once the lethargy passes we will usually feel much more energetic, alive, and aware. Other benefits of Thai massage include greater flexibility in the joints, enhanced blood circulation, improved body alignment, straighter posture, deeper breathing, and stimulation of internal organs, which helps them to function at an optimal level.

General conditions for practice

Before and during a Thai massage session, it's important to take into consideration a number of factors related to health conditions, environment, body positioning, breath, flow, and pressure.

Know your client's health history

Before you begin a session, make sure to ask the receiver about their current health and their health history. It's important to know about any condition that could make your work unsafe or cause harm in any way. If you practice Thai yoga massage professionally it's essential to keep a health history for each client, so that you have a permanent record of their information. You can find samples of professional intake forms on the Internet, you may create your own, or you may download the client intake form from the Thai Healing Alliance website.

Maintain good posture

The most common postural mistakes in Thai massage are bent arms, a hunched back, tense shoulders, and using muscle strength to apply pressure. Working in this way is bound to leave you feeling achy, tired, and drained after giving a massage. You may also be more likely to absorb the receiver's tension and be more sensitive to negative energies released during the session. Always keep your back and arms straight, and apply pressure and stretches using your body weight. If you remember to do these two things, you should feel energized, relaxed, and pain-free after giving a treatment.

Due to relative body size, there may be a few exercises where it may be difficult to keep your arms straight or to use your body weight effectively. If you're attempting to do a stretch that requires muscle power, or if you anticipate straining of any type, simply eliminate that exercise or technique. While performing Thai massage, stay aware of your posture, and especially notice if your shoulders begin to creep upward. If they do, take a breath, relax, and let your shoulders release downward.

Breath awareness

Once you become aware of your own breath, you can tune into the rhythm of the receiver's breath. Breath awareness helps you to stay calm, concentrated, and relaxed in your own body. Being aware of the receiver's breath helps you to relate more deeply to him during the treatment. This, in turn, allows you to tune into his energy body, and to be aware of his needs in a more intuitive way.

During the massage, try to bring your attention to your breath as often as possible. If you're feeling tense or frustrated, bring your focus back to your breath and you should immediately feel calmer and more connected to the receiver.

Applying pressure

Thai yoga massage is a strong and vigorous bodywork treatment. The pressure you use shouldn't be painful, but generally it should be right on the threshold of pain – just before it becomes painful. The amount of pressure needed to reach this level varies from person to person, and it is vital that you apply the correct amount of pressure for each individual. This is not only important for the well-being of the receiver but also for the effectiveness of the treatment itself. If you work too gently, your pressure may not reach the energy body. If you work too strongly, you may cause the receiver to feel tense and be closed to the work.

Discovering the right amount of pressure for each person is an art in itself, and it takes practice and experience. At first, you may need to ask your clients for feedback. As you practice, don't hesitate to occasionally ask about the level of your pressure. If you don't ask, many people will not say anything at all, even if the pressure is too strong for them. It is even more common for people to remain quiet if the pressure is too gentle.

There are particular points or areas on the body that are usually more painful than others. These are mostly therapeutic pressure point areas, where it is normal to feel a certain degree of pain. This is sometimes referred to as "good pain." Good pain is generally beneficial, as long as it is bearable, and as long as the receiver can breathe into the pain and stay relaxed and open. Good pain usually disappears as soon as the pressure is released. "Bad pain," on the other hand, lasts after the pressure has been released. This usually indicates that pressure was applied in the wrong place or in the wrong way. Don't press too hard until you are confident that you're in the right place and that you aren't pressing on bone. Your confidence and sensitivity will increase with practice and time.

Maintaining a connection with your client

Establishing and keeping a constant connection to the receiver is vital for a good, healing massage. Even without speaking at all during the treatment, you can still develop a silent form of communication that gives the receiver a sense of trust and a feeling of being nurtured. This helps clients to relax more deeply and to surrender on physical and emotional levels. Watch the receiver's face, and look for signs that may indicate if your pressure is too strong, if an area is painful, or if the client isn't comfortable with something you're doing. Listen to the receiver's breathing and to your own breathing, and try to harmonize them with each other as the treatment progresses.

Rhythm, flow, and balancing energy

An important meditative aspect of Thai yoga massage is gentle rocking. Constant rhythm is very relaxing and nurturing for both the giver and the receiver. Ideally, your pace should be established at the beginning of the massage and continue all the way through to the end. It takes practice to hone your ability to develop a vision for the entire session. This means being totally present in each moment while at the same time holding a vision or intention of the next step. Continued practice is what helps the massage to flow as smoothly as possible. Think of Thai massage as a painting. As you gain more experience and knowledge, you understand better how to use shape and color. Sometimes, when you look at a blank canvas, you immediately have an idea of how your painting will take shape; other times, you simply start painting and see what develops. When you first touch the receiver, you may or may not have a long-term idea for your treatment, but it's important to stay present, and to maintain a good flow and a steady pace that will carry you through the entire session.

A good system to follow throughout the treatment is to begin work on the dominant side of your client. A woman's dominant side is the left, and a man's is the right. Try to always work the dominant side first. If you work on a woman with strong male energy, you may start on the right side, and if you work on a man with strong female energy, you may start on the left. The idea is to begin on the same side first during the entire treatment. When you work with one foot at a time, for example, work on the dominant foot first. When you work on one arm at a time, go first to the dominant arm.

Intimacy and body space

Although the receiver is fully clothed, Thai massage is an extremely intimate form of bodywork – a close dance between two bodies and energy systems. Awareness of body space is essential to allow the receiver to fully relax and let go. Many people have experienced some type of invasion or physical or emotional abuse in their lives. This makes it important to be extremely careful to not overstep physical boundaries. Watch the receiver's face when you are near sensitive areas, and don't go any further if you detect any signs of discomfort. Working in this way provides the receiver with an experience of a wonderfully nourishing, safe, and intimate form of nonsexual touch.

A lifelong pursuit

Only so much can be said about Thai massage in an introduction such as this. After all is said and done, we are shaped by our own personal experiences, by individual learning experiences with our teachers, by feedback from our colleagues and clients, and by a sincere and humble dedication to the work. The practice of Thai massage is a lifelong pursuit. Only after many years of practice and ongoing study can the sensitivity and skills required to give effective healing treatments begin to develop.

Common Myths Associated with Thai Massage

C. PIERCE SALGUERO

In the late 1990s I spent several years in Chiang Mai and Isan, Thailand, where I studied with traditional healers and Buddhist teachers. During this time I became fascinated by how traditional medicine and Buddhism interact so much with each other. When I returned to the United States to study this topic in graduate school, however, I was stunned by how much of what I had learned was, in fact, mythological. As Thai massage has become increasingly popular in recent years, these same myths have continued to be spread by teachers, practitioners, and students all around the world. I hope that this article helps to dispel some of these popular misconceptions, so that the true facts become better known to the international Thai massage community.

Myth: Thai massage is an ancient tradition

It's quite common for people to claim that Thai massage is 2,500 years old, and that it is an ancient tradition that has its origin during the Buddha's lifetime. Such statements can be effective marketing pitches, but they don't accurately reflect facts. It is true that Thai massage incorporates ideas that can be traced back to India during the time of the Buddha, and possibly even earlier. The concept that the body contains a type of energy – one that is usually associated with wind and/or light, and which can be manipulated by breath and through mental and physical exercises – dates at least to the Upanishads, which were written in India in the first millennium BC. These ideas were further developed in subsequent centuries, and they came to characterize several Indian religious and healing systems (such as hatha yoga, for example) that reached their full development between AD 1000 and 1500. What is known today as Thai massage or Thai yoga massage is related to this larger context, but there were no routines, steps, or protocols that were assembled or developed in ancient India and then transmitted to Thailand as a coherent system of healing.

The history of medicine in Thailand has a long and complicated timeline. Since the Silk Road and the Indian Ocean maritime routes were developed around 2,000 years ago, multiple waves of influence have washed up on the shores of Southeast Asia, including various forms of Buddhist, Ayurvedic, Chinese, and Western medicine. The Thai people themselves have only lived in the territory of modern-day Thailand for the last thousand years or so, and when they arrived, they almost certainly brought with them indigenous traditions of spirit-based healing. In this vibrant and dynamic historical context, it is virtually impossible for any one aspect of human culture, let alone something as complex as Thai massage, to remain static and unchanged for millennia.

Traditional Thai massage is the remarkable result of the combination of many historical and cultural influences, and it's a uniquely Thai creation. Although it is often promoted as an ancient healing art, most popular Thai massage routines that are learned and taught by Westerners today were prepared by the Wat Po school and the Old Medicine Hospital school in the last quarter of the twentieth century, with the specific goal of developing formalized protocols to teach tourists.

Myth: Thai massage was invented and spread by Jivaka

Both Thai people and *farang* (foreigners) like to tell stories about Jivaka (also known as Shivago, Chivok, "The Father Doctor," and by other names), and these are a wonderful part of traditional Thai medical culture. Jivaka Kumara-bhacca is a Buddhist hero who is recognized in many traditions throughout Asia as a wonderfully effective healer. In some versions of these tales, he performs procedures that may be characterized as truly medical, such as craniotomies and abdominal surgeries. Other details are more mythological, such as when a magical gemstone or the branch of a magical tree grants him x-ray vision in order to see into his patients' bodies. In the sacred writings of Theravada Buddhism practiced in Thailand and in other parts of Southeast Asia, Jivaka performs several surgeries, uses *ghee* (clarified butter), applies ointments, and even heals the Buddha with a purgative. These were all standard procedures among Indian doctors of the time. What is conspicuously missing from this story, and from accounts of Jivaka's life in any canonical Buddhist text, is the mention of massage.

It is impossible to say to what extent the legends of Jivaka that are retold today are based on a historical doctor who lived during Buddha's life, or on an imaginary, idealized, and archetypical doctor of the day. If Jivaka lived and practiced in India twenty-five centuries ago, there is no chance that he traveled to Thailand to teach Thai massage. Most probably, he is credited as the founder of traditional Thai medicine and worshipped as the patron saint of Thai healing arts because he is the only important figure associated with medicine in the Pali Buddhist texts.

Myth: Thai massage is closely connected to Chinese medicine

On the surface, Thai healing arts appear to share some features with traditional Chinese medicine, and this leads many people to imagine that there is a strong connection between them. Some Thai *sen* line maps feature pathways in the arms, legs, and torso that appear similar to portions of Chinese meridians, and some hand techniques used in Thai massage are similar to those used in Chinese massage styles such as *tuina* and *anmo*. Thailand has a long history of association and economic exchange with China, but the ideas behind Thai massage have far less of a connection with Chinese medicine than they do with Indian traditions.

There is one exception to this generalization, which has led to confusion. In the mid-1990s, a Chinese style of foot massage that uses a carved wooden stick to apply pressure to Chinese reflexology points was introduced from Taiwan to several of the major tourist schools. This became a commercial success, and massage schools all over Thailand soon began adding this technique and other forms of massage to their curricula in order to attract an increasing number of Western tourists. By the early 2000s, many types of Eastern and Western massage techniques in Thailand became available in schools. Today, they are sometimes still promoted as coming from the Thai massage tradition, regardless of their actual points of origin.

In contrast to the wooden stick foot massage, the full-body routines that most people consider as Thai massage share little or no theoretical ground with Chinese medicine. The theories guiding Thai therapy are not those of reflexology, of yin-yang, or of the Chinese Five Elements. To anyone familiar with the theoretical basis of traditional Asian medical systems, it is clear that Thai massage has much more in common with the Indian model of traditional Ayurvedic medicine.

Myth: Thai massage is interchangeable with Ayurveda and yoga

Much of traditional Thai medicine is derived from Buddhist healing and Indian Ayurvedic medicine, while the basis of Thai massage is more closely aligned with yoga. Although Thai massage is largely derived from Indian ideas, there are some important differences. The apparent similarity between Thai massage and yoga often leads practitioners, teachers, and clients to conclude that Thai massage is a form of interactive yoga that can be modified to fit into modern yoga training curricula and other lifestyle industries. Thai massage and yoga do exhibit many similarities because they both belong to a larger family of Tantric traditions of mental, physical, and spiritual cultivation. This family also includes practices such as Tibetan yoga and Thai *reusi dat ton.*

What is most interesting about Thai massage, however, is not what it shares with these other traditions, but rather how it differs. Because Thai massage is a unique variant among healing practices worldwide, these differences are worth exploring. Thai massage deserves to be studied and promoted as a unique cultural heritage, rather than being modified to fit into more familiar and marketable consumer trends.

Myth: There are authentic Thai massage routines and sequences

There is, in fact, no single authentic, traditional, or correct Thai massage routine. Until recently, there were no standardized training curricula and government regulations of Thai massage. Even after the Thai Ministries of Health and Education got involved, free-form improvisation has remained the norm. It is difficult to receive the same massage twice in Thailand unless it's by a teacher or school that uses a specific sequence that is promoted in their place of business. Otherwise, an accomplished Thai massage therapist creatively mixes together many different techniques, following his or her intuition, in response to an individual client's needs.

Before the advent of commercial schools, instruction in Thai massage involved a long-term apprenticeship with an acknowledged master (*ajahn*), who in turn had apprenticed under an acknowledged master. This teacher-student lineage was generally traced back through many generations. Each practitioner, therefore, was part of a lineage, and had to formally commit to carry forward the teachings of their particular line of teachers as a condition of their training.

This teacher-student transmission was never done in a static or robotic way. Practitioners were free to add stylistic twists and techniques, guided by their own expertise and intuition. When practitioners studied with multiple teachers, they often mixed techniques and practices learned from each of their teachers. Before textbooks and national standardizations arrived on the scene, Thai massage represented a living tradition. It was a body of knowledge that was constantly changing, developing, and evolving. For serious and accomplished modern-day practitioners, the same holds true today, as Thai massage continues to evolve into the future.

A problem for historians, however, is that throughout history, lineages have almost always been based on oral transmission instead of on written texts. Because of this, we have very few texts, artifacts, or other windows into the history of these early practices. There are a few references to massage in texts from the Ayutthaya kingdom (AD 1350–1767), but these are not guidebooks and they do not describe specific techniques in detail. There are also examples of sen line and point charts from the Bangkok period (AD 1782–present), the most famous of which are the epigraphs housed at Wat Po. However, all these artifacts present only snapshots of moments in time during a constantly evolving tradition. They do not provide evidence of one true or original style of Thai massage.

Myth: The Wat Po epigraphs represent a pure and ancient transmission of Thai massage

The medical artifacts at Wat Po include not only the above-mentioned charts, but also herbal medicine tablets, statues depicting *reusi dat ton* postures, and other materials. These were produced during the reigns of the first three Thai kings (AD 1782–1851) in their attempts to reconsolidate the kingdom and showcase achievements in the arts and sciences. A number of medical experts from across the country were brought together to produce these collections, and they no doubt had diverse backgrounds and medical skills. Further standardization of this material took place during the reign of the fifth king (AD 1868–1910), before the Thai medicine texts that are used today were published. Analysis of some texts by the scholar Jean Mulholland has shown that they represent a diverse and mutually contradictory collection of ideas. This is most likely because the project brought together a wide range of opinions from different parts of Thailand rather than accurately representing any one particular tradition. By extension, we cannot consider the Wat Po epigraphs as a pure transmission from the ancient past.

Myth: Massage was an important part of healthcare in ancient Thailand

Though massage always played a role in folk medicine in Thailand, it has only recently emerged as an influential part of the healthcare system. Massage is mentioned in texts from Ayutthaya, but based on records from the kings' courts, it appears that Chinese, Indian, and even Western medicine concepts were more valued and accepted than local healing traditions. Despite the activity at Wat Po, interest in traditional Thai healing arts was sporadic during the Bangkok period. From the mid-1800s through the 1970s, the country as a whole focused on modernizing the healthcare and public health sectors by emulating Western models and by developing an infrastructure for scientific medicine. Of course, traditional healers continued to treat patients, but they operated in legally marginal settings, and they were often the targets of suppression.

This situation changed in the late 1970s, when the World Health Organization and other global agencies began to take an interest in promoting traditional medicine in developing countries around the world. Since that time, there has been a resurrection of interest in traditional healing arts in Thailand that parallels the revivals of traditional Chinese medicine, Indian Ayurveda, and other medical traditions.

In Thailand, more than anywhere else, massage has played a major role in this process. Massage was specifically promoted by the government's Thai Massage Revival Project, beginning in 1985. However, the most dramatic surge in popularity of Thai massage came from Western tourists. Curricula were specifically targeted to this market first at Bangkok's Wat Po, and later at Chiang Mai's Old Medicine Hospital. From there, it rapidly spread outward. As a result of the increased interest in massage, the Thai government soon got involved in regulating and taxing the industry, and eventually in the 2000s, national licensing and training standards were established. Today, the Thai government and business sectors aggressively promote the country as a haven for traditional medicine, alternative healthcare, and the spa industry. In recent years, thousands of massage schools and clinics have emerged. All of this has allowed massage to play a more important role in the Thai economy, and to have a larger presence in Thai cities than ever before.

Myth, history, and authenticity

Much of the above information can be summarized by stating that no teacher or school in Thailand has a historically verifiable claim to a system of Thai massage in use before the 1800s. In fact, the routines that most Westerners study today date only from the past few decades, and all claims of "ancient" and "traditional" are simply not accurate. Yet these historical myths persist, perhaps because they are excellent marketing tools, and also perhaps because practitioners seek validation of their own training as something that has been handed down by sages over thousands of years.

I encourage all students, practitioners, and teachers to consider authenticity as something that comes from within oneself rather than from a particular style or technique. In my own view, to be authentic is to be clear about one's own goals and intentions, and to study deeply with knowledgeable people. Authenticity has little to do with the history of the technique being learned.

I realize that the deconstruction of the above myths may be difficult for some practitioners to accept. My intention is not to offend anyone or to challenge the validity of Thai massage as a whole. I simply wish to identify what I see as the misuse or even abuse of history by the Thai massage industry in the West and in Thailand, and to encourage Thai massage professionals to engage in constructive conversations about where true authenticity lies. If Thai massage continues to be marketed based on myths, then factually incorrect information will continue to mislead clients, students, and therapists. Understanding the true history of Thai massage gives all of us the opportunity to deepen our knowledge, and to fully appreciate the healing art that we love so much.

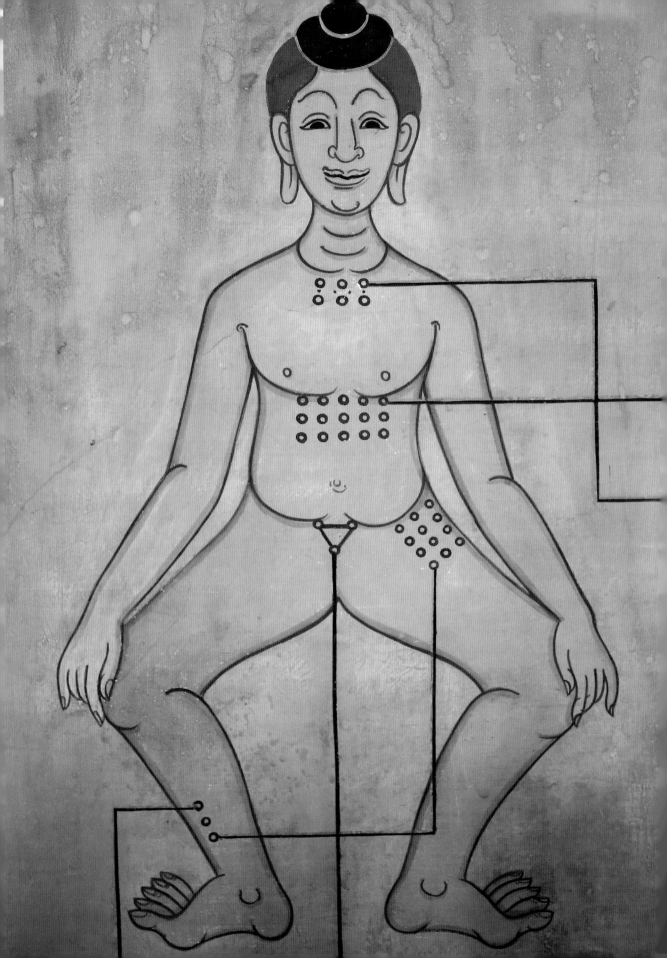

Section 2

Mastery of Practice

The Care and Feeding of Your Thai Massage Practice

BOB HADDAD

When we first begin to study Thai massage, we are often most concerned about memorizing the basic sequences that we learn from our teachers. As we become familiar with techniques and sequences, we settle into patterns that seem comfortable for us. Here is where problems can begin. Without continued guidance, ongoing study, and feedback from our colleagues and clients, we are prone to get stuck in the patterns we develop for ourselves, whether or not they are effective for our clients or healthy for us in the long term.

This essay presents ideas that may be helpful to deepen your work as you progress in your learning and practice. These include practical considerations such as maintaining your room and altar, using props, marketing and advertising ideas, and client maintenance tips such as record keeping, maintaining boundaries, and offering self-care recommendations. Finally, I offer suggestions about developing your work through ongoing study and refinement of techniques. Maintaining flow, moving gracefully, working slowly, supporting and locking clients in place, using sensing and intuition during a session – these are all signs of an advanced Thai massage practitioner. I hope the information offered here is interesting and helpful.

Tools for effective practice

Your practice room

Your Thai therapy room is a sanctuary – a sacred healing space for your clients and for yourself – and it should be equipped and maintained for that purpose.

It is best to use the room only for treatments, yoga, meditation, and similar activities, but if this isn't possible due to space limitations, try to carry out your Thai work in one area and allow for other activities to take place in a different part of the room. In large rooms such as yoga studios or in multipurpose spaces, a private area can be demarcated using a folding screen or a large piece of fabric hung from the ceiling. Privacy is important, so keep your space protected, secure, and comfortable.

Keep the room clean, always remove shoes before entering, and clear the energy from one session to the next by opening windows to allow air circulation, spraying a natural fragrance (see later in this section), and changing sheets and pillow cases regularly. An unscented candle can also help to burn away lingering odors.

The mat

A wide variety of mats may be used for traditional Thai massage. In many cases, your choices will be limited to space restrictions and the accessibility of materials. Naturally, you should choose a mat that is comfortable to work on and practical for your surroundings.

An important factor to consider is whether you, as the therapist, wish to work mostly on the mat or off the mat. The size and height of the mat determines your ability to position yourself in relationship to your client, and it also affects your balance. My preference is to work at the same level as the client, whenever possible, and I suggest that you try to work "on" the mat as much as possible.

I find that when I am sitting or kneeling even one inch lower than my client, I have to constantly adjust my balance and body posture in order to compensate for the difference in height. If the mat is too small, a therapist may have to keep one foot on the mat and the other foot off the mat. This can contribute to instability. In my opinion, most of the commercial Thai massage mats on the market today are too small for effective Thai therapy. Some of them are also quite expensive. If you have enough space and you generally don't travel to give your sessions, consider using a very large mat.

High-density foam rubber is a practical and economical mat substance. Depending on the density, 1–2 inches in height will be sufficient. High-density foam is often dark in color, and is used in furniture and automobile upholstery. An even harder variety is used to pad surfaces such as gymnasiums and recreational areas. It can be bought through foam distributors, upholsterers, or exercise companies. The surface should be comfortable but quite firm. If your room is large enough, use the widest mat possible, either queen size or king size (193 x 203 centimeters / 76 x 80 inches). The foam can be placed on top of a large rug or in a room with wall-to-wall carpeting and then covered by a large cotton sheet with the ends tucked underneath. If you are working on a hard surface such as cement or ceramic tile, consider using gymnasium padding as a base; place a rug or a large piece of carpeting directly underneath, to keep the area as clean and warm as possible. On a medium-hard surface such as a wooden floor, a rug may also be used underneath, one that is bigger than the mat itself. If you are working in a room where there is plush wall-to-wall carpeting, you may be able to use a large "mattress topper" as your mat. "Memory foam" is now widely available, and it is reasonably priced. This type of foam adapts to the relative shape and weight

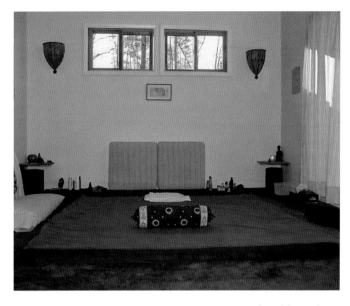

A comfortable and well-equipped practice room

of each individual, and it is extremely comfortable to lie on, but only when the surface underneath is fairly soft. If it is placed on top of a thick rug or on a sheet of high-density foam, it can work very well as a Thai therapy mat. If you travel to give sessions, a variety of fold-up and roll-up mats are available, and most of these are made of foam or cotton.

Pillows

For supine position

Pillows of several sizes are important for your practice. Consider using small, thin pillows for the head, such as those that are supplied by airline companies for long flights. Generally speaking, it is best to not use a thick pillow for your client's head in supine position. A thick pillow can raise the neck to an unnatural position and can minimize free flow of oxygen. It also gets in the way and crimps the neck when you perform techniques such as plow, or do leg compressions toward the upper torso. If your client doesn't need or want a pillow for their head, don't use one.

For side position

For working in side position, however, an extra large and very thick pillow for the head is important. The large width allows you to turn the client on her side, and still give her plenty of pillow support. The extra height provides natural ergonomic support when the client is in side-lying position, and it keeps the neck and spine straight. Many people need extra support in side position, so keep another large pillow in the room to wedge against the client's stomach and to keep him from slipping toward the floor. Tubular pillow rolls, such as those used underneath the knees in table massage, are also helpful to wedge into the stomach and to place between the client's extended arms while in side-lying position. Large oversized pillows and foam bolsters are important when you work with pregnant women.

For prone position

Most people can tolerate short periods with their necks twisted to one side in prone position, but a small pillow placed under the collarbone can lift the upper torso slightly, and allow the person to rest his chin or forehead on the mat without having to twist his neck to one side. For longer periods in prone position you might try using a "doughnut" pillow or a sloping foam pillow, which is specially designed with side air vents for the purpose of lying on the stomach. These are available at bedding stores and on the Internet.

For leg and knee support

After finishing leg and lower torso work in supine position, Thai therapists usually proceed to the abdomen, chest, and other parts of the upper anterior body. Before you begin working on the stomach, consider placing a pillow roll under your client's knees. This elevates the upper legs and the sacrum a bit, and it provides a more comfortable position for the client to receive work on the upper body. Tubular or half-moon–shaped pillows work well. Massage supply stores carry several varieties, but I find that the plastic-covered ones are sometimes too cold and rigid. I use cloth-covered tubular pillows that I stuff with cotton or fiber fill to the desired firmness. If you can't find a suitable tubular pillow where you live, roll up an extra-large bath towel and place it under the knees.

Keep several small pillows nearby to support your clients' knees when compressing and butterfly-pressing in "tree" position. Foam rubber bolsters covered with cotton work well. I also keep a few small round cushions, which work perfectly under the knees when extra support is needed.

Blankets and covers

I almost always use lightweight covers during my work. As we work in nuad boran, we help to move energy from one part of our client's body to another, and this energy movement often results in extremities such as the hands and feet becoming cold. Because of this, and especially in colder climates and during the winter, it's important to keep our clients warm as we work. Light, natural fabrics such as rayon, silk, or light cotton, usually work best as coverings.

I keep a variety of rayon sarongs nearby, which I use to cover parts of the body that are not being touched. Since we begin Thai massage at the feet and legs, it's often helpful to cover the upper torso until we start working there. Light sarongs provide a layer of warmth, and allow the client to keep their arms and hands under the cover, while feeling pampered and secure. When you finish working on the legs, and you move to the abdomen and upper torso in supine position, you can slide the cover down over your client's feet and legs. You may not be touching them there for many minutes, and they could easily become cold. In cold weather, or in drafty or damp locations, a heavier blanket may be more appropriate, but avoid wool or other materials that might cause itching or allergic reactions.

Tissues, towels, and clock

It's a good idea to keep a box of tissues in your treatment room for hygienic needs and for occasional emotional responses. Keep a small towel nearby to dry hands if they become sweaty. If possible, keep an electric clock in your room, or one that doesn't make a ticking noise, which could be distracting to you and your clients.

Accessory tray or bowl

Keep a small tray on the floor near the head of the mat, where your client can put jewelry, watches, and accessories. Keep a few elastic hair ties in the tray so you can tie back long hair, especially when you work with your client in sitting position.

Water and tea

Pour a fresh glass of water for each client and one for yourself before each session. Keep them nearby, but out of the way of the work area. Plastic, rather than glass, is best for the practice room.

I remember that I felt pampered when I was first served herbal tea immediately after a Thai session. If you have hot water handy, or if you prepare a thermos of herbal tea each day, your clients will probably appreciate a cup before they leave. Don't pre-sweeten the tea, but put a small sugar cube on the tray if you wish.

Balm, talc, and *nam ob Thai*

Massage oils are not generally used in nuad boran, but several types of balms and creams may be used on the feet, and at the end of the session while working on the shoulders, neck, and face. Thai analgesic balms, made of eucalyptus, peppermint, and camphor are excellent for applying to sore muscles, problem areas, and even to the feet, but remember to wash and dry your hands immediately after applying them to your client's body and before you continue the session. Keep some water and a hand towel nearby, or use a commercial sanitizing gel from a pump bottle.

Unscented talcum powder can be helpful for sweaty hands, feet, and bodies. I sometimes find it helpful to sprinkle a little talc on my hands if I do an abdominal massage directly on the skin. If you have sweaty hands or feet, apply unscented talc to them before working.

A lightly scented herbal balm, made from a base of beeswax, is excellent for finishing touches on the neck, face, and forehead, when the client is in final supine position. Just a small dab on the third eye area of the forehead can help you work the entire face. Unscented or lightly scented cream or lotion may also be used.

After I finish working the face and giving a head massage, I like to anoint my client's face and head with a bit of *nam ob Thai*, a lightly scented perfume water. Sprinkle a few drops in your hands, and gently refresh your client's face and hair in a soft, stroking fashion before you offer your final *wai* and leave the room. If you can't find nam ob Thai, you may consider rose water, orange water, or iris water, which are available from food and baking distributors or ethnic grocery stores.

Your altar

An altar is an essential feature of your practice room, and it should hold items of guidance and spiritual focus. Thai massage altars in Thailand usually contain statues or images of the Buddha and Jivaka, candles, incense, flowers, and other spiritual items. Whatever you use as a stand, platform, or small table, place it at the head of the room or in a corner, away from the working area. The altar should be at eye level as you work on the floor (about 1–1.25 meters / 3–4 feet high), so you can gaze at it as necessary during a session.

It's important to have a statue or image of Jivaka on the altar. In Thailand, it is common to offer food and water to deities. If you wish, you may place a small amount of water or food (even just a few grains of rice) on your altar. Remember to freshen up the offerings on a regular basis. According to Thai custom, if you place a Buddha on the same altar where you have a Jivaka image, the Buddha should be in a higher position. Photos of teachers and your parents (especially if deceased) as well as other meaningful items may also be placed on the altar. In Thailand, many people also keep an image of a *reusi* (practitioner of esoteric sciences) on their altars.

It is good practice to light a candle for each client you see. A tea light placed inside a clear votive cup works well, because each candle lasts about three hours, and extinguishes itself neatly in its aluminum sleeve.

Take a few moments to focus on the altar before beginning your work, and bring your attention there for guidance during a session whenever necessary. After your client leaves the room and you are cleaning up and clearing energy, you might take another moment to connect with your altar.

Air and energy cleaners

Clients' energies can linger in your room long after they have left. Whenever you or your client have experienced a difficult session, or one in which there were energetic or emotional releases, it's a good idea to cleanse the room after the client leaves. Open a window to allow fresh air to circulate freely, and change the sheet and the pillow cases. Rather than incense, which can be unpleasant for many people, consider spraying a lightly scented neutralizing substance into the air. A few drops of essential oil mixed with water and a bit of clear alcohol works well. Avoid using strong scents, heavy incense, synthetic chemicals, or commercial deodorizers.

Donation bowl

If collecting money from your clients sometimes feels a bit awkward, you might leave a donation bowl in your treatment room, along with a pen for clients who pay by check. A donation bowl can be less intimidating, and sometimes clients leave little gifts and offerings there, too.

Clothing and hamper for clients

It's a good idea to keep an assortment of lightweight clothing for your client's use. Lightweight, baggy cotton or rayon pants such as Thai fisherman pants work extremely well. Keep a few shirts in different sizes for men and women. T-shirts and collared shirts restrict access to the neck and shoulders, but tank tops and V-necks work well. Keep a small hamper or basket nearby for used clothing.

Socks

Many people get cold feet during a Thai massage session. For this purpose, and especially when you work in colder climates, it can be helpful to keep clean socks handy. The half socks that are used for airline travel cover the soles and tops of the feet, without constricting the ankles. Consider wearing socks yourself when you have cold feet, so you don't transfer the cold temperature to your clients as you place your feet against their bodies. Also consider using socks if your feet or your client's feet are excessively sweaty.

Accessories for your practice room

Music

In the West, we often associate massage therapy and bodywork with candles, incense, and relaxing music. But in Thailand, music is hardly ever used to accompany a traditional nuad boran treatment. One problem with music is that it can attract the listener to a particular melody or rhythm, when one of the most basic ideas of giving and receiving this work is to be present and "empty" as much as possible. If the listener is drawn to a melody being played, his mind may become more focused on the song than on the session or on his breath. Music can also distract the therapist, and minimize his ability to hear the client's breath, which is an all-important barometer for proper execution of techniques. Sometimes, silence is golden. This is not to say that music can't be used during your practice. Before each session you might ask your clients if they want music or if they prefer silence. Some people who usually like music occasionally request silence. If you don't ask, you won't know what they want.

If you do use music, keep the volume very low – low enough that you can hear your client's breathing or converse in a very soft voice when necessary. Rhythmic music is generally more intrusive than music with spaces of silence in it – soft acoustic instrumental music with an open and airy feel usually works best.

Foot washing bowl and supplies

In Thailand, before you receive a treatment, you are often handed a bowl and a towel and asked to wash your feet. Occasionally, your feet may be washed by the therapist. I remember the first time my feet were washed before a session – I felt so humbled and grateful. Immediately afterward, I decided to incorporate foot washing into my practice. In addition to the practical aspect of washing your client's feet, it is also affords a great opportunity to take a few moments to ask your client how they are feeling before you begin your work. Ultimately, it helps to create a mood of gentleness, trust, and peace.

Fill a small plastic bowl with hot water, and mix in a few drops of natural oil or essence. Peppermint essential oil works very well. Place a small towel under your client's foot. Soak a washcloth in the solution, wring it out, and clean your client's feet gently yet thoroughly. (Make the water as hot as possible without burning your client or your hands). Dry the foot thoroughly with the towel, and repeat on the other foot.

In cases where you have no access to hot water, you can spray your client's feet with a solution of water and a natural essence.

Electric blanket for colder climates

For people living in colder climates, it can sometimes be helpful to place an electric blanket on your mat, under the sheet. This helps the client to remain warm and also keeps your own feet and legs warm as you work. If you use an electric blanket, make sure to ask your client if it is acceptable. Some people have objections.

Herbal compress steamer

Luk pra kob are steamed compresses filled with medicinal herbs and rhizomes. Compresses are applied before, during, or after a nuad boran session, and they are extremely relaxing. If you work with herbs, you will need to have a steamer handy.

Record keeping

In all major forms of medical treatment, physical therapy, and bodywork, keeping accurate client records and health histories is not optional; it is required. I am concerned when I hear of Thai massage practitioners who don't keep detailed notes of their sessions or maintain health histories of their clients. It's clear that more teachers and schools should stress the importance of record keeping for a professional practice in traditional Thai healing arts. Today's holistic health practitioner must take more responsibility for his clients' welfare and for his own professional development. Session notes and client intake forms are valuable tools that can take your practice to a new level of growth and professionalism.

Client intake form

The first time you see a new client, allow a few minutes to discuss their health history, and make sure they fill out a client intake form beforehand. The intake form should include your client's name and contact information, their health history, emergency contact information, specific medical conditions, medications, and other relevant information. Many therapists also take this opportunity to have the client sign a waiver of some sort, to address personal liability claims or declarations that Thai massage sessions are strictly nonsexual. A client intake form can help a therapist to work more effectively and address each client's needs more appropriately. If you don't already have a health history form, samples may be found on the Internet. Thai Healing Alliance has a form that may be downloaded by the general public and modified according to each therapist's specific needs. A sample client intake form appears on the next pages.

Confidential Client Information Form

name: _____ date: _____

home tel: _____ cell: _____ e-mail: _____

address: _____

date of birth: _____ profession: _____ referred by: _____

emergency contact info: _____

are you currently taking medication? _____

describe any special medical conditions: _____

_____

indicate if any conditions apply:

surgeries ☐   spinal/disc problems ☐   heart problems ☐   high blood pressure ☐   osteoporosis ☐   hernia ☐

diabetes ☐   arthritis ☐   wear contact lenses ☐   pregnancy ☐   back pain ☐   neck pain ☐

broken bones/fractures ☐   constipation ☐   diarrhea ☐   other ☐

describe in more detail any of the above conditions:

_____

_____

On the diagrams to the right,
circle any problem areas,
and indicate as follows:
tension "**T**"
pain "**P**"
surgeries "**S**"

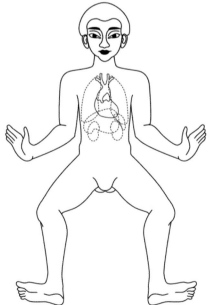
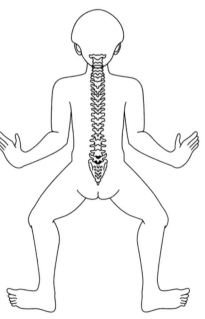

Do you have any restrictions in movement? _____

Are there any movements or stretches you think may be harmful? _____

Do you generally like to hear music during a session? _____

Is it OK to use lightly scented lotion or balm on your face? _____

Do you have any other comments or requests? _____

Client consent and agreement — Please read and sign below

- It is agreed and understood that Thai massage therapy is intended for relaxation, and that it is not meant to diagnose, treat or remedy any illness, disease, injury, physical condition or mental disorder.

- Except in cases of emergency, I agree to pay for all sessions that are not cancelled at least 24 hours in advance.

- Traditional Thai bodywork is strictly non-sexual. Under extenuating circumstances, either party reserves the right to immediately terminate the session.

- I understand that the practice of all forms of body therapy is subject to local laws and ordinances.

signature   date
_____

date (d-m-y)   **total session time**

Session notes

date (d-m-y)   **total session time**

Session notes

Session notes

A practice log is a written record that describes a progression of treatment sessions. You may devise your own form, or staple a blank page to each client's intake form in order to record your notes after each session. Written records of each session provide invaluable information about the client's condition and about the therapist's work. They allow the therapist to track changes, and to note client preferences and responses to certain techniques and therapy routines. By keeping accurate session logs, the Thai therapist may quickly and efficiently review previous sessions, and therefore be better prepared to work with his clients from one session to the next. Written records can also be helpful if an insurance claim is ever made against the therapist, or if a client's treatment history must be shared with another healthcare professional.

Always keep a written record whenever you conduct a Thai session. As soon as your client leaves the premises, and while the session is still fresh in your mind, write your thoughts on paper. Don't just write short, simple descriptions. Describe things such as the client's physical and emotional states, which positions you used during the session (supine, prone, side, sitting), and how your client responded to what you did that day. Describe any special conditions that may have had an effect on the session today, whether positive or negative, and mention the techniques you used that you thought were beneficial. Take note of anything you could have done differently, and give yourself suggestions for the future. The next time you work with this person, review your notes from previous sessions so you can see the "big picture" of your ongoing therapeutic interaction with this particular client.

Samples of session notes, each of which was written by a different practicing Thai therapist about one of their own clients, are included on the next page for your reference.

Marketing and promotion

Mail and e-mail

We often don't like to do it, but most of us need to engage in marketing and promotional efforts to maintain the clients we have and to bring in new clients on a regular basis. Sometimes just following up with your regular clients is enough to sustain them, but an occasional e-mail or post card to advertise your services to regular and prospective clients can be a good idea. Printed materials such as brochures, flyers, postcards, coupons, and special offers may be sent by mail, but e-mail announcements are cheaper, faster, and easier.

You may choose to use one of the many html-based services to create your own e-newsletter, with announcements, photographs, and hyperlinks. The professional contact services that are available on the web for this purpose

Sample Client Session Notes

date (d-m-y)		special conditions		total session time	1:45

session notes

Good session, very flowing. Worked in supine, prone and seated position. I sensed that her mid-section was blocked, so I worked there as much as possible. Did compressions, spinal twists, cobras, and line work. Worked the hips with pulls and suspensions in side position, and also worked the back lines. Gave a fairly deep stomach massage to try to open her mid section; did blood stops. The rest of the session was based on a normal sequence. Next time, check the mid section, and continue to work there in different ways if needed.

date (d-m-y)		special conditions	smoking support	total session time	2:00

session notes

Supine and seated position. He returned after two years because he recently stopped smoking and he wants some reinforcement to remain smoke-free. Used a compress especially on the chest, stomach and throat, and applied balm to the chest area and on the back in prone position. I had him breathe in the vapors and he coughed phlegm several times into a tissue. Lateral leg lines were blocked, worked them with feet. Shoulder and neck work in seated position, and face and head in final supine position. In the future, continue to use hot herbal compresses to help clear the lungs !

date (d-m-y)		special conditions		total session time	1:50

session notes

Three months pregnant, so I worked mostly in side position, with extra pillows. Avoided pressure points in feet, ankles and head. No blood stops! Her lateral legs were blocked, especially the right side, but she opened up with compressions on her calves and thighs, and she said she liked the work very much (do it again in the future). Did light circular stomach massage only, very little pressure. Worked sen kalathari and sumana down the center of the back of legs. Did some gentle back openings in side position. Worked her head and face and neck with large pillows to support her in semi-seated position. A good session.

date (d-m-y)		special conditions	recent injury	total session time	1:30

session notes

Knee problem, right ACL injury. I avoided excessive bending and rotating but I did work the pressure points around the knee and worked the lines with thumbing on both legs. Complained of low energy due to menopause, so I worked at a steady pace to try to energize her. Used all 4 positions, focused on low and middle back in prone position, and shoulders and neck in sitting. She said she felt lighter and more open. Afterward, I showed her some yoga poses that she can do to help strengthen her back.

date (d-m-y)		special conditions	shoulder pain	total session time	1:50

session notes

Mysterious pain in the shoulder, left side. Osteo-arthritis in right hip, severe pain so I was gentle with direct contact and compressions. Worked in all 4 positions, spent time on her feet (one at a time) and worked her leg lines with palming and then thumbing. All techniques on the hip required a slow, careful approach, and I used pillows to prop her up in seated position. I tried to be sensitive to her right side in general. She said she felt significant pain relief in her hip. It was good to see how the work helped her. Next session, take more time to examine and prevent occurrence of pain in right side, especially near hip.

have a variety of templates to choose from, and prices vary according to the number of people on your list and the number of e-mails sent per month or per year. For the purposes of a professional Thai massage practice, a quarterly newsletter (four times a year) is usually enough.

Print advertisements

Advertising in local newspapers and health digests may also be an effective way to attract new clients. With print advertising, it's almost always better if you run a small advertisement over a long period of time rather than a large ad only once or twice. Research shows that it is the frequency of exposure that helps to "brand" a product or service of any type. For the most part, classified text advertisements work well, and sometimes you can add a graphic or a logo for a bit more money. If you decide to advertise in local publications, think of your total investment as occurring over a period of time, say for six months, and make a commitment to pre-pay for your advertisement for the entire trial period. After several months of exposure, you'll know if your investment is a good one, and then you can decide to continue advertising in that publication, to try a different publication, or to discontinue the advertising altogether.

Local exposure and word-of-mouth

Grass-roots types of marketing are always helpful, and they are often free, or cost very little. You can print flyers to post on bulletin boards at community centers, yoga studios, and other places that are visited by health-minded people. You might offer to give a free demonstration or a discussion on Thai massage to community centers, libraries, yoga studios, or other public gathering places. Personalized color postcards from online printing services are inexpensive, and brochures and business cards can often be left at local businesses.

The best way to get new clients is by personal recommendation. Your clients will recommend you to others if they are happy with your work.

Client maintenance

It's a good idea to ask first-time clients to contact you a few days after their first session, and to tell you how they are feeling, and if they've noticed any changes in themselves as a result of the treatment. If they forget to do so, you can send them an e-mail or leave a phone message inquiring about their health. This shows that you care, and may also encourage the client to contact you for another session. If the client reports a strong response, whether favorable or unfavorable, add it to their session notes for future reference. If you let your clients know that you are there for them, they will often volunteer information to you that can be helpful for future sessions. If you don't ask for feed-back, many people will not offer it.

Inquire about their state

Before you begin a session, take a few minutes to ask your client how she is feeling today. You might do this while you're washing her feet. Inquire about her physical condition, if she has any tension, pain, or soreness, and if so, how it came about. You may ask to view, touch, or even gently manipulate and explore the affected area, so you can better understand your client's physical condition on that particular day, and so you can adjust your work accordingly.

If your client has previously confided in you about a difficult situation she is going through, whether emotional, psychological, or otherwise, you might ask about it to show that you care. Be careful not to pry, however, or to invade your clients' privacy, or tell them what you think they should do. You are not a counselor; you are a Thai therapist trying to serve your clients in a more holis-tic way. Be there for your clients, with all your compassion, with all your *metta*.

It's important to develop a professional rapport with clients, and to help sustain them from session to session, but it's usually best to not become close friends with your clients or to socialize with them frequently outside the con-text of your services. When that happens, the professional relationship and boundaries between client and therapist can easily become altered, and this may have adverse effects on the therapy itself.

Client self-care

An important element of holistic healing arts is the underlying concept of self-care. You may occasionally recommend certain activities or exercises to cli-ents, for example. For clients who consistently exhibit "holding" in certain areas, you may suggest yoga exercises to do at home that you feel could help the client to release those pockets of tension. For people with lower back prob-lems, you might suggest a series of plows, cobras, or spinal twists, or exercises to strengthen their core. Clients who have shallow breathing might benefit from a *pranayama* (yogic breathing) exercise. If you are knowledgeable about diet and herbs, you may suggest that they modify their eating habits in a way that might benefit them. Be careful to only recommend or suggest things that lie within your scope of practice, however. You may also refer clients to acu-puncturists, specialized bodyworkers, or Chinese and Ayurvedic doctors, if you feel they could be of help. Ultimately, it is our responsibility as therapists to encourage and help our clients to maintain optimal health.

Keeping your client comfortable during the session

It's important to keep your client comfortable at all times during the session. Nuad boran is most effective when the client is fully relaxed, with open energies and deep breath, and when a strong sense of trust and confidence has been established with the practitioner. Physical, emotional, psychological, and spiritual issues come into play during a typical Thai massage session. Try to be aware of the following:

Work at an appropriate level of pressure

As we work with our clients, it is extremely important to maintain even, steady pressure, whether through point work, palming, thumbing, compressions, or yoga stretches. As you work, look at the person's face on a regular basis. It may seem difficult to do, but actually it is quite easy, and it serves as an excellent exercise in metta, or focused compassion. Pour your metta into your clients as you work with them, and while you do, watch for any signs of physical discomfort such as wincing, raised eyebrows, or other facial expressions or body movements.

You don't want to give an overly soft session, but you never want to make your client uncomfortable with your pressure or movements. It's best to always work at a level just below the client's threshold of discomfort. Usually, you will get a good sense for the right amount of pressure within the first 5–10 minutes of a session. This is a good time to check in with your client, ask how they feel, and inquire about the depth of your pressure.

Once you establish the correct depth, continue uniformly in this fashion, keeping in mind that various parts of the body can withstand more pressure than others. Watch your client's face and body throughout the session, and ask whenever you are in doubt. This way, you'll have a good indication of how your pressure is being received.

Don't cross boundaries

This means all boundaries – physical, emotional, sensual, and psychological. Watch your client's face and body language in response to your techniques and body contact. If a client tenses up unexpectedly, it could be a manifestation of physical discomfort, emotional uneasiness, or both. If you sense at any time that what you are doing is violating that person's private space, you should immediately stop, or at the very least, you should ask the client if you can proceed. Sometimes, just gently asking "Are you okay?" or "Is everything alright?" will allow your client to tell you something that you may not have suspected. If they say all is fine, then you may proceed with caution.

Watch your own boundaries, too. Sensual triggers work both ways. Don't allow your mind to be drawn into lustful thinking when you are working. If you catch yourself being sexually attracted to a person you are working on, immediately calm yourself, gaze at your altar, and refocus your energies. You might silently recite in your mind the Thai massage *wai khru* or any other mantra or prayer. If you ever encounter a case of sexual stimulation, whether initiated by the client or by yourself, it is best to immediately cease physical contact with your client. Simply remove your hands from that person's body. If the stimulation came from you, you might excuse yourself and leave the room for a moment in order to compose yourself. If you sense that the stimulation was directed at you by the client, move to another technique or body position, or stop your work and discuss the issue before you continue any further. In severe cases, you should simply terminate the session without accepting compensation.

Encourage silence

I have witnessed Thai massage sessions by Western therapists who talk to their clients quite a bit, comment on their condition, and coach them about when to breathe and what to do during a session. This is not recommended, and it is not in keeping with the traditions of Thailand or with the spiritual nature of the work. Try to be as silent as possible when giving a treatment. This work is, after all, a form of meditation for both parties. There are ways to flip a person from one body position to another without saying a single word. Learn and practice those moves, and learn how to be as silent as possible when you work with your clients.

Sometimes clients can be chatty at the beginning of a session. Try to avoid engaging them in conversation, and simply allow the nervous tension that is manifesting in speech to subside. If it becomes necessary to calm someone down a bit, ask them to take a few long and deep breaths. You can even ask them to take three deep breaths simultaneously with you. This will often stop the talking.

Allow for a bathroom break when necessary

Some people are shy about having to use the toilet. After you finish working on the lower torso, and when you're ready to begin on the abdomen and upper torso, you might gently ask if they need to use the restroom. If you need to use the restroom, simply excuse yourself, and do so.

Cultivate good flow in your practice

Flow might be described as the fluidity with which you move from one posture to another as you work with your client. True mastery of flow is when we support our clients' bodies as we work, and when we integrate breath, good body mechanics, rocking movements, and effortless transitions from one posture to another.

Move gracefully, and integrate rocking and alternating movements

In your work as a Thai massage therapist, you will find that moving gracefully helps to maintain focus during a session. It can also help conserve your energy and keep the session moving along at a comfortable pace. Each one of your graceful movements transfers directly to your clients. It feels good to have one's body moved gracefully, and feeling good encourages relaxation and well-being.

Try to integrate more rocking and alternating movements as you work. In many ways, nuad boran is a healing dance that we perform together with our clients. Stay loose, but stay focused as you work. Allow your inner self to move and sway and make gentle rocking movements as you apply pressure. Pivot and rotate from your *hara,* and lull yourself (and your client) into a peaceful dance of healing movement and pressure. Many palming and thumbing techniques can be executed with slight alternating or rocking movements. If you keep your body too rigid as you apply pressure, the muscles in your shoulders, arms, wrists, and hands will probably work harder than they need to. If you allow your weight to sink into the body of your client, and you engage with that person in gentle rocking movements whenever possible, it will feel better to the client and will require less effort on your part.

Develop easy transitions

The way in which a Thai therapist transitions from one posture or technique to another can have a profound effect on the outcome of the session, for both the therapist and the receiver. Try to maintain physical contact with your client as you move from one posture to another, and whenever possible, don't abandon one part of the client's body until you make contact with another area. Be creative, and structure your sequence based on easy transitions. Use your own body – whether your hands, arms, chest, legs, or feet – to move your client into the next position in a flowing and graceful fashion.

Lock your clients in place

One of the most valuable lessons you can learn in your Thai massage practice is to understand the importance of gently locking your client in place against your body before you execute certain maneuvers. Try to stay aware of ways to keep your client's appendages and body gently interlaced with your own body before you begin to execute a specific technique.

Support your client as you move

Try to support your client's body as you move from one position to another. Making contact with an extra hand or a foot can help the client to relax and to stay open to movements and energy flow. When you release a client's arm or leg to the mat, support the elbow or ankle with your other hand as you let it down softly. Client support is important in all four body positions: supine, side-lying, seated, and prone.

Work slowly and allow for moments of rest

One way to remain composed and deeply focused in nuad boran is to work slowly. Take your time as you work with your partner, and proceed from one part of the body to another at a relaxed pace. When you apply pressure, always begin lightly at first and then deepen your touch progressively until you reach the person's first point of resistance. You might choose to move on from there, or to remain at that depth. If you remain there, hold your pressure firmly but gently until she yields more space to you. Then, on her exhale, move in a little deeper. As she inhales, release your pressure just a little, so she knows you are aware and listening to her body. Proceed in this manner throughout the session.

Work slowly

In many cases, it's better to work slowly and to target key areas rather than to move quickly through a full-body sequence. Try to never begin a Thai massage session with a pre-determined course of action or outcome. That kind of pre-planning may color your mind and diminish your sensing and intuitive abilities. It's not necessary to work with your client in three or all four body positions in order to achieve good results; an excellent session can be carried out in only one or two positions. With women in advanced stages of pregnancy, for example, an entire treatment should be given only in side-lying position.

Work slowly. Work slowly as you apply acupressure, and move slowly as you stretch your client into assisted yoga poses. Whenever it is appropriate, gradually increase and decrease pressure in repeating cycles of three or five, and always try to coordinate your pressure with your client's breathing. For the client, the rewards of slow, progressive work are deep relaxation and a heightened sense of self. Working slowly also helps the therapist to remain focused, and it reminds us that traditional nuad boran, in essence, is meditation in movement.

Resting poses

I believe it's very important to allow yourself and the client to experience moments of stillness during a Thai session. Silence and stillness are sometimes necessary for a client to fully assimilate the work and for a therapist to remain calm and focused. Imagine the power of a deep *savasana* (corpse pose) at the end of a yoga workout. There you are, lying motionless on your back, yet you can feel energy surging through you. Your relationship to time and space in that motionless pose allows you to relax, to unwind, to assimilate positive energy, and to become renewed. I am not suggesting that we should allow our clients to rest motionless for long periods during a Thai massage session. But short breaks of up to 90 seconds, especially after strenuous movements or emotional releases, can be very beneficial to the client. We, as therapists, also need to take some moments to relax during our work. There are many concepts and techniques you can use to calm things down during a session. Here are a few of my favorites:

Sacral squat in child's pose

At some point during the course of a Thai session, we usually get our clients into a version of the traditional yoga "child's pose." Child's pose is especially important after you have been stretching the back in the opposite direction, with assisted cobras, bridges, locusts, and reverse leg pulls, for example. By the time you have reached this point in the session, you have probably been working at a steady pace. Rather than the traditional palm-pressure techniques for child's pose that are taught in most Thai massage courses, here's a way to take a few moments to relax while your client benefits from a wonderful compression to the sacrum and back. After helping your client into child's pose (remind her to inhale as she gets up from the floor), turn around with your back facing her head, and gently sit on her sacrum. Support about 50 percent of your own bodyweight with your feet, and sink your weight down gradually to the first point of resistance. Keep your back straight, and breathe in and out as you feel your client's body expand and contract.

A variation to remaining still is to slowly shift your weight slightly downward at a 30-degree angle toward the mat. Slide toward the mat by releasing some of the pressure in your supporting legs and shifting your body weight forward. Then gently release the downward pressure as you re-engage your legs and pivot back up to the starting position. The movement of your client's body should be minimal, perhaps only a few inches. Repeat this slow rocking movement several times.

When you are ready, release your weight gradually as you come to a standing position, preferably on your client's inhale, and while you are also inhaling (30–60 seconds for this technique).

Shoulder compression using feet in supine position

For many people, few things are more relaxing and therapeutic than deep shoulder and neck work. If during the course of your session, you haven't spent much time with your client in sitting position, or if you haven't addressed the shoulders and neck on a deep level, you can try this technique. It's best to use toward the end of a session, in final supine position, right before you begin to work on the face and the head. By this time, your work is coming to a close, and it's a perfect time to slow things down. Make sure your client's arms and hands are close to the sides of his body. Sit behind your client and place the middle of your soles on the fleshy part of his shoulders, in between the shoulder bone and the base of the neck. Your feet should be straight, with toes pointing upward. Don't fully extend your legs; keep your knees upward. Allow sufficient space so that your legs are comfortable, and so that you can press forward and maintain steady pressure.

When you're ready, press forward simultaneously until the first point of resistance, and hold with even pressure. Try to press each foot slightly in the direction of the client's opposite hip, toward the center of his body. Wait for your client to relax in the position, and when he exhales, move in just a little deeper. Continue in this fashion, and always release a little bit of pressure as your client inhales. In addition to working simultaneously with both feet, you may also alternate the pressure with your feet. First push on the right side, then, as you release, press forward on the left side. You may move closer to the neck area

Shoulder compression using feet in supine position

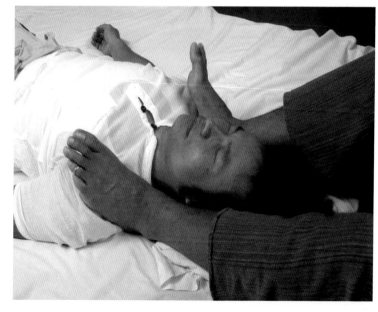

too, but be careful to only use the fleshy center of your feet, and take care to not touch the sides of the client's head with your calves or ankles. Avoid rubbing the skin at all costs. Move slowly, and always work with the client's breath, pressing as he exhales and releasing as he inhales. End with simultaneous pressure to both shoulders and then release slowly with the client's inhale (60–90 seconds for the entire technique).

Sen sumana in supine position

An effective way to calm things down during a session is to lightly work *sen sumana* while the client is in supine position. This can be done after working on the abdomen and chest, and before finishing in supine position. The therapist exerts practically no effort at all, and the client lies motionless; however, the effect of this technique can be extremely powerful.

Sit alongside your client with your dominant hand near the client's upper torso. Lightly touch the hara with two fingers of your hand, locate sen sumana, and try to sense the energy within. With your index finger and third finger, press down and maintain light to medium pressure against her body for a few seconds. Release gently and slide your fingers upward to the next spot. Continue in this way upward along the line, passing the upper abdomen. Work slowly and send metta to your client through your fingers. Take note of her breathing patterns, and time your pressure and your releases accordingly. When you reach the rib cage, you can begin to make slight and slow circular movements with your fingers, as you maintain the pressure. Don't remove your fingers from the body as you circle; maintain contact as you transmit subtle rotating energy to your fingers. Then release and move to the next spot. Continue slowly upward, to work the entire center of the rib cage and the sternum. When you reach the neck, use your thumb on one side and your second and third fingers on the other. Continue pressing very lightly against the throat as you ascend toward the chin, working slowly and gently. When you reach the chin, gently grab hold of it with your thumb and two fingers, and slowly rotate or move it up and down to make sure the jaw is relaxed. You may work downward and upward with light finger pressure once again, if you feel it's necessary, but try to always finish upward, at the chin. Work slowly and meditatively (60–90 seconds for this technique).

Open the wind gate in side position

In elementary Thai massage training, students are taught to use their palms to execute "blood stops." In Thai, this technique is called *bpert lom* ("open the wind"). Opening the wind gate may be done more than once during a treatment when necessary.

Wind gate openings may be carried out using palms, fingers, knees, feet, forearms, elbows, and also by sitting. When we use arms and legs to balance our body weight, we risk transmitting shaking or trembling feelings from the therapist to the client. A sitting blood stop, however, applies solid and steady pressure, and it is also a convenient resting pose for the practitioner.

Make sure your client is resting comfortably in side position, with her head on a pillow and with her spine straight. Turn around, so that your back is facing the client's head, and squat down in position. With several outstretched fingers of your hand, locate the pulse area in your client's upper thigh, below the buttocks. Then lower yourself into position with the focused weight of your sit bones right over the pulse. Don't let your entire weight fall into place, but instead, use your arms and hands to lean on the floor as you settle into position. Allow your thigh to rest directly on your client's thigh. Your other foot should be half standing and slightly outward for good balance. Your inside hand should rest on your outstretched anterior thigh, and your outside forearm should rest and dangle over your opposite knee. Make sure your back is straight, and sink as much weight as is necessary into your client. Make sure you can feel your client's pulse beneath you. Hold the pose for 60–90 seconds and then slowly release your weight as you inhale and move out of position. I find it's best to slide off gently by rolling your body toward one side of the mat.

These are just a few of the many resting poses that may be integrated into a Thai massage session. Don't deviate too much from Thai tradition, but when you feel a need to slow down, or if you feel your client is being stressed, treat yourself and your client to one or more brief periods of rest during a session.

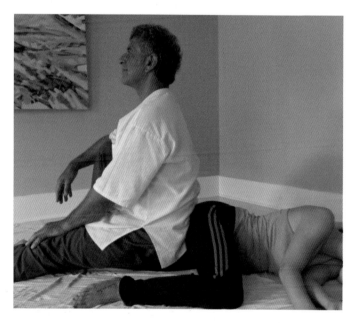

Opening the wind gate with client in side position

Sensing and the intuitive nature of nuad boran

As Thai massage therapists, we utilize specific postures, techniques, and acupressure as we go through routines with our clients. These sequences can become quite mechanical and commonplace if we allow ourselves to get stuck within them. Since every client is different, and since each person has specific needs, we need to maintain awareness of our clients' bodies and energies, so we can constantly adapt and modify our work according to each person we touch. As we become more experienced practitioners, we learn to change the ways in which we work with our clients. We shake ourselves free from the all-purpose fixed routines that we learned as beginning students, and even from the routines that we ourselves may have developed. Two important vehicles for this important and necessary change are sensing and intuition.

Sensing

One of my most influential teachers, Ajahn Pichest Boonthumme, has been known to say: "*Farang* (Westerners) always do, do, do. But *how* to do?" In other words, how do we treat each person in accordance with his needs? We're all human beings, but each of us is different, so Thai massage therapists cannot treat each individual in the same way. We need to utilize sensing. We do this by listening to and staying aware of our clients' bodies and energies as we work. We work "with" them, instead of "on" them. Rather than working mechanically, we pay attention to subtle differences in each individual and allow those differences to guide us effectively through each session.

From the very moment you touch your clients – for example with your hands on their feet in supine position – try to utilize sensing to detect any tensions or blockages. As you progress through the entire session, take note of what you feel (or what you *think* you feel) as you focus on the sen lines and on the energy flow within them. Try to calm your mind and be free of thoughts, and send metta to your client. Here are just a few hypothetical scenarios in which our innate abilities for sensing might guide us as we work:

- When you put their feet in your hands and open their legs to start palming techniques, what do you feel? Is one leg heavier than the other? Is there an energy restriction or blockage of some sort, or is what you're feeling on the physical level? Are you drawn to a particular place? If so, should you go there now to investigate, or should you come back to it later, when you're working in a different body position? If you do feel an inconsistency, is it coming from the ankle, the calf, the thigh, or the hip? Could it be symptomatic of something farther up, say at the upper lateral leg, or at the lower back? How might these sensations help to guide you through the session?
- As you press their feet laterally to the ground, does one foot sink farther or more easily to the floor than the other? Is one foot more erect than the other? If so, what could that mean? To where might you trace the problem?
- As you palm or thumb the leg lines, do you sense a slight shaking or vibration at one point along the line, but not at other points? Do you think that vibration is the epicenter of a blockage, or could it be a radiating point? Are you sensing that you should stay there for a while and try to dissipate it?

Or would it be better to work up and down that sen line a few times to see if you can detect a corresponding point that needs your attention?

- As you lift a client's legs to do leg presses, leg pulls, rotations, or plows, can you feel any resistance? If so, where is the resistance: in the hips, in the legs, the lower back, the abdomen? Can you do anything to soften it? How can your perception of what you feel help to guide you through the rest of the session?
- Is your client unconsciously "holding" a particular part of her body? Can you identify that part of the body and direct your work in ways that might help to release the holding?
- Is your client trying to "help" you, rather than remaining fully relaxed? If so, are you okay with his reactions, or has he begun to annoy you? Should you work in that area for a few minutes to try to dissipate the tension and help him relax more deeply? Should you stop doing the technique that is causing that particular reaction? How are all of these feelings influencing the direction and the quality of your work today?

Sensing should be going on throughout the entire treatment session. Simply put, the more attuned we are to our clients and to ourselves, the more effective our work will be, and the more rewarding the experience will be for all concerned.

Intuition

I once asked my teacher Asokananda if intuitive abilities could be taught. Here's what he said:

Only to a certain extent. You can teach people how to develop their sensitivity, but intuition has to come by playing with the energy lines and feeling the energy. Ultimately it comes from within, and most people have the ability to tap into it.

So what is intuition, and how do we use it? How do we know when to linger and when to move on? What does energy feel like? How do we know where to work, and which techniques to use? This intuitive sensitivity comes from within, and flows out of each person, and naturally, it becomes stronger the more we practice and study. However, there are some basic guidelines which can help to encourage the development of strong intuitive abilities.

Try to stay present at every moment during the session

This is easier said than done, and it is a life-long lesson. But as we go deeper in the practice of Thai healing arts, we must learn to detach from outside stimulation and distractions and be more present and in the moment. That means we must always be listening to and sensing our bodies and the bodies of our clients. Just as in meditation, it's important to bring ourselves back to inner stillness whenever we become distracted.

Don't get stuck in the usual sequences and routines

As mentioned earlier, each person is different, and not all techniques work the same way for all people. A tall practitioner working on a short client may need to modify his approach to a particular technique, and not simply do it the way it was taught in a classroom. Try to not follow the same basic routine for each client. Be as aware as possible about what your client needs at each moment, and don't be afraid to deviate from a routine that you were taught in order to serve your client in the best way possible.

Trust your judgment

Rely on your senses and your instincts. If, when you pick up your client's legs, you feel that she is holding in the upper lateral thigh, consider going there to see what you find and make a quick assessment before you continue your work. It's important to work consecutively from the bottom of the body to the top, and to follow the running of the sen lines as you work, but you don't need to spend a lot of time working in an area that you sense is already "open." If you sense that one area is more blocked than another, you might decide to spend more time there, rather than moving on to another position or technique. If necessary, check in with your client to get their feedback, direction, or approval, if you sense a blocked area. If you allow yourself to follow your instincts, your sense of intuition will naturally become sharper and deeper.

Seek guidance and study with a variety of teachers

Nuad boran is a living art form, and it has never been stagnant. From the earliest influences based in Indian and Buddhist healing principles, through its development in Thailand, traditional Thai massage has continued to evolve to the present day. One teacher does it one way, and another prefers to do it differently. How will you know which way works best for you? I've known students who have studied almost exclusively with one teacher or at one school, and even after years of practice, their view of nuad boran can be a bit narrow, and their range of techniques and applications may be somewhat limited. It certainly is important to have an anchor, a mentor, a home base; but it's equally important to study with a wide range of teachers who integrate and utilize different styles, techniques, and concepts.

Summary

A professional practice in traditional Thai massage involves much more than helping people relax by performing assisted yoga stretches. Traditional Thai massage is a complex blend of physical, energetic, and spiritual healing, and dedicated Thai therapists should practice ethically, professionally, and in accordance with Thai healing traditions.

Maintain a clean and well-equipped practice room, and keep records of your clients and notes of each session you perform. Try to not get stuck in usual sequences, be as empty of thought as possible, cultivate graceful transitions from one movement to the next, and always listen to the body to help guide you through each session.

A true master never refers to himself as such. He knows that there is always something more to learn, and that humility is one of the most important virtues of true mastery. As you continue in your study and practice of traditional Thai massage, always seek guidance from teachers, colleagues, and clients, and remember that the study of this marvelous healing art is an enriching, enlightening, and lifelong pursuit.

Thai Acupressure and the Wat Po Treatment Protocols

NOAM TYROLER

When I began studying Thai massage, I was mostly interested in the pleasure, fun, and magic of giving and receiving *nuad boran*. Only later, when I started to learn about treatments for specific ailments, was I drawn to the medical uses of this ancient healing art. Some of my clients were suffering from chronic pains, and over time I began to acquire tools in order to help them. In 1997, I traveled to Thailand in search of medical knowledge and found the Wat Po collection of treatment protocols. By the end of the following year, I'd compiled my own personal notes from my studies, and I began to share what I had learned with my students. Much later, I published a book called *Thai Acupressure*, which covers in detail the major treatment protocols from the Wat Po collection.

There are 55 points (plus six special points) in the treatment protocols of royal-style Thai massage (*ratchasamnak*), and more than 200 points in the Wat Po protocols of folk-style Thai massage (*chaloeysak*). In royal style, the practitioner presses the lines of the legs, abdomen, arms, back, and neck using only the thumbs, and there is a general lack of stretches. Royal massage is comprised entirely of line and point work. In folk style – the type of Thai massage that is best known – the exact same lines are treated, but the practitioner is not limited to thumb pressure and also uses palms, elbows, knees, and feet to work the body. In folk style Thai massage, practitioners also use a wide variety of stretches to open the lines and to work the joints. Regardless of the style of Thai massage, working the *sen* lines is the most important component of a treatment session.

Most people understand the word acupressure to mean the skillful application of applying pressure to therapy lines and points on the body in order to bring about healing. Treating pain and chronic conditions calls for accurate and skilled acupressure, but even Thai massage routines aimed at relaxation should incorporate a considerable amount of acupressure in addition to assisted stretches.

These days, Western students and practitioners tend to neglect line and point work and are often more attracted to the beautiful stretches and assisted yoga postures found in Thai massage. Some teachers don't even include line work in their courses. Although a treatment comprised solely of stretches can be fun and relaxing, it is not true to Thai tradition. In my opinion, a Thai massage treatment is not complete without extensive line and point work. In this article, I hope to familiarize the reader with the Wat Po method of acupressure, which has become an important part of my practice and teaching.

Thai acupressure

As we work the sen lines in a Thai massage treatment, we pay close attention to the pressure that we apply with our thumbs, hands, elbows, knees, and feet. We sense how deeply we should press, how long we should stay there, and how fast or slow we should work. We work some lines only once, but others seem to need two or more repetitions. As we work these lines, we are drawn to specific points, some large and some small, where we sense our pressure is needed. Whenever we use pressure in a Thai massage session by accurately working a line or a point, we are practicing Thai acupressure.

Thai people appreciate and eagerly seek out treatments offered by practitioners who know the body well. Many of these practitioners have never formally studied massage, but they have a keen sensitivity, a passion to help others, and thousands of hours of experience behind them. Good therapists, whether trained or untrained, rely on their ability to work pressure points accurately. They locate particular points and lines that need stimulation, and they concentrate on them. They don't waste much time on parts of the body that are not in need, and they give special attention to lines and points that need their work.

Fixed-point treatment protocols

One field of knowledge in Thai massage is the use of ready-made treatment protocols based on a fixed set of therapy lines and point combinations. Fixed sets of lines and point combinations are widely used in different acupuncture and acupressure traditions. Traditional medical massage in Thailand relies heavily on the use of fixed protocols aimed at treating specific conditions.

Some focus on the sen lines and view the points as secondary, while others place more emphasis on point pressure.

An advantage of fixed-point treatments is that they can be very effective, even when carried out by practitioners with only basic training in manual therapy. In addition, fixed-point combinations allow for development of intuitive awareness, and eventually lead to a deeper understanding of the body and its conditions. Experienced practitioners are creative in their treatment of pain and use different techniques and different approaches with each client. They don't feel obliged to follow the exact steps of the treatment protocols they have studied. The correct protocol is the basis of their work, but they add relevant points that they find along the way, and use different techniques to effectively treat the painful areas of each client.

After I first learned the protocols of Wat Po, I went to meet a practitioner near Chiang Mai who had an excellent reputation as a healer. I asked him to treat my lower back pain, and I received an extremely effective treatment. He didn't follow the protocol I had learned for my specific type of lower back pain. Instead, he used different techniques, and he interpreted the work in his own unique way while working the same lines and points I had learned. I later watched him treat my wife for acute hip pain in lateral rotation. Again, he worked in his own beautiful and unique way, while at the same time concentrating on the correct lines and points for that ailment.

I asked him if he had studied the Wat Po treatment protocols, and he replied that he had never done so. I asked him how he knew how to treat my lower back pain. He told me that shortly after completing his studies at the Old Medicine Hospital, a person from his village came to him with very intense lower back pain. He treated the man based on what he had studied, but the treatment was not effective, and as a result he became frustrated. Afterward, he had a long talk with Dr. Shivago, telling him he could not let that man suffer any longer and that he needed help to relieve that poor man's pain. That night, Shivago came to him in a dream and showed him the specific lines and points to use, and how to effectively treat his patient. He summoned the man the next day and gave him a treatment following the specific instructions he had received in his dream, and this time the treatment completely relieved the man of his pain. That practitioner was the now famous healer Pichest Boonthumme.

Another well-known healer from Chiang Mai, the late Chaiyuth Priyasith, once explained to me that he is not the one who gives the healing. "It's him," he said, as he pointed to a painting of Doctor Shivago. He told me that Shivaga Gomalapaj can also be channeled by *farang* (Westerners) if they truly believe in him.

Whether or not you are able to access divine intervention from the Father Doctor as you work with your clients, a solid external knowledge of treatment protocols will be very helpful in your practice.

The point combinations of Wat Po

This essay focuses on a well-known collection of treatment protocols, which I have been practicing for many years. They are made up of 52 traditional Thai routines that were collected and organized in 1955, during a series of seminars with a group of teachers arranged by Ajahn Preeda Tangtrongchitr, the founder of Wat Po Massage School in Bangkok. In these seminars, knowledge was shared and exchanged in order to arrive at a standardized general massage routine aimed at relaxation, and also to standardize traditional point combinations that treat simple orthopedic disorders. These two bodies of knowledge have been taught since then at Wat Po. The basic Wat Po sequence (and its Chiang Mai variation) are widely practiced today in Thailand and around the world, but the treatment protocols for individual ailments are much less known.

Simple orthopedic disorders

The routines of the Wat Po collection address the most common orthopedic pathologies treatable through manual therapy. These include soft-tissue ailments such as muscular hypertonicity and myofascial trigger points; muscular weakness; disorders such as tendinosis, tendonitis, and tenosynovitis; muscle and ligament sprains; osteoarthritis; neurovascular entrapments; and neural tensions. The routines do not treat serious pathologies such as fractures, joint dislocations, or orthopedic ailments created by viral, bacterial, internal, or systemic diseases. The collection does not include other routines that are practiced throughout Thailand to treat other pathologies and conditions. You may study varying point-based treatment routines with different practitioners in Thailand, but it's best to first determine their effectiveness, and not to automatically assume their validity.

Point-based treatment routines are inviting to use because they go directly to the painful points and immediately provide

Routine for radiated leg pain, also used for hip pain in outer rotation

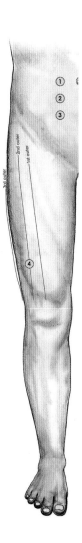
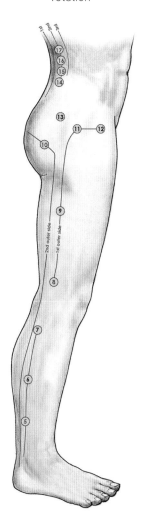

relief – the client gets a feeling of "Ah! This is exactly what I need." In order to treat orthopedic pain, you must know how to search for, and locate, sensitive areas, lines, and points. Your client needs you to locate his "special" points. He may often try to reach those points on his own, and may even be capable of directing you to some of them. Sensitive and experienced practitioners can locate many of the relevant and needed points for an effective treatment. I recall observing treatments in Thailand by practitioners who had never studied fixed-point combinations, and I was amazed at how they could find a complete set of points. Such a high level of work may be attained only after many years of study and practice, and after thousands of hours of treatments.

Orthopedic conditions bring about sensitivity in certain lines and points, which must be worked in order to bring about healing. Predetermined point combinations can guide practitioners in their search for those points that are in a state of excess or deficiency. Not many practitioners have the experience or ability to find all the relevant points of a given condition through self-exploration; therefore, most practitioners greatly appreciate a body of knowledge of proven point combinations. Following a brief diagnosis of our clients, using simple guidelines, we can determine which specific combination of points to use. We will know where to find the points in need, and we'll be attracted to those points that invite our touch.

Acupressure treatments are best carried out on a floor mat, but they can also be done on a massage table, on a bed, or on a chair when treating upper-body ailments. The client remains fully dressed. In Thailand, men are sometimes treated with their shirts removed.

Treatment routines versus general massage

From a Thai medicine perspective, general treatments work best as a preventive measure. Unlike a general treatment for the entire body, a point combination treatment routine is aimed at treating an existing disorder, and focuses only on a few areas, lines, and points. Sometimes stretches are integrated. The lines and points of a specific routine are the core of the treatment, while other parts of the body are not touched, or they are treated only if time allows. When a specific problem exists, treating irrelevant body parts can waste time. Your client wants to feel that their pain is being treated directly, and it can frustrate them if this is not done.

Acute pain is usually treated first, then, if time allows, the rest of the body is treated. In chronic conditions, you can begin with a general massage, but make sure to save enough time to use a protocol that fits the specific ailment you are treating. Two hours or more is the ideal time needed to bring about good results.

Short treatments of 20–30 minutes, using point work only

When time is limited, only the points are addressed and point pressure comprises the entire session. The first point of the routine is worked, then the second, and then the rest of the points follow. After completing one round of pressure points a second round begins, then possibly even a third round of points, until the end of the session. Each point is pressed for as long as the therapist feels is right. The pressure is usually applied for 10–15 seconds, though at times it can last longer, and is usually deep and, ideally, the strongest pressure the client can receive without making him wince in pain or pull away from your touch.

Full treatment sessions of 90 minutes–3 hours

Ideal treatment sessions last for as long as the client is in need of the application of pressure on the selected points. Some disorders can be thoroughly treated within 30 minutes, while others may require a full treatment session of up to three hours. Lower back pain, for instance, needs longer sessions to bring about lasting relief, but it can be treated effectively in short sessions as well. Ideally, the treatment should continue as long as the condition improves, and as long as the client wants additional therapy. The treatment is stopped when the points become "tired," that is, when they become overly sensitive to the touch. An experienced therapist should be able to sense when the points no longer need pressure.

Acute and chronic conditions

In acute conditions, only the sen lines and acupressure points that correspond to the particular condition should be used. These same points and lines are treated over and over again until the energy seems restored in those areas. Lines, points, or body parts that are not relevant to the treatment are avoided. Non-relevant stretches, such as those that are found in a general massage treatment, may sometimes aggravate a particular condition being treated. When treating a chronic condition such as lower back pain, where the main discomfort is stiffness rather than sharp pain, it may prove effective to cautiously apply general massage stretches to your client's legs and back. As the client's condition improves, you can integrate more elements of general massage.

After focusing on the specific painful area with line and point work for the first few treatments, you can continue using a whole-body general massage in future sessions, while paying extra attention to the relevant lines of the client's particular condition. General massage is used in the beginning and at the end of the long-term protocol. At the beginning, it is used as a preventive treatment, and at the end it is used as a rehabilitative treatment. Weekly or bimonthly general massage helps prevent the majority of disorders that are treated by acupressure routines.

Thai acupressure treatment steps

Warm-up

When time allows, a treatment should begin with general palm pressure along the sen lines of the legs, arms, or back, or with a general massage to the upper back or the abdomen, if those are the areas that will be treated in more detail.

Energy lines

Following the warm-up, we continue with deeper application of thumb pressure on the specific energy lines of the routine. The lines on which the points of a specific routine are located should be worked prior to the treatment of the points themselves. Working the relevant lines before working the points will make the treatment much more effective. Treatment of the relevant lines alone can be effective, but not as much as when the acupressure points are integrated.

Point combinations

Now you are ready to work the acupressure points themselves. The point combination is executed for several rounds, as needed, up to a maximum of ten rounds. When session time is limited consider working only the points, after a short treatment of the lines themselves.

Optional complementary procedures

After completing the therapy point treatment, and if time allows, additional supportive work may be done. When treating a chronic neck condition, for instance, you might work lines along the back and hip, and execute stretches that correspond to that specific neck routine. When treating chronic conditions, using complementary procedures will prove very effective.

General treatment procedures

When time allows, and after completing all of the treatment steps, you may apply general massage to different parts of the body. You should make sure, however, to not apply pressure or to otherwise create pain in sensitive body parts that have just been treated with point pressure.

Diagnosis: Choosing the right point combination

Specific Thai acupressure routines are chosen according to the location of pain, the pattern of the pain, or the movement that brings about or aggravates the pain. The therapist selects the routine that is most appropriate, based on the condition of his client. Diagnosis by an experienced therapist takes only a few minutes. "Radiated pain to the leg" for example, is a Thai acupressure lower back routine that is used whenever there is a radiated pain to the leg. "Lower back pain while bowing face down" is another lower back routine that is used when the pain is aggravated during lower back flexion. "Lower back pain while standing and bowing backward" is used when the pain is felt when bending backward, rather than forward. If, for example, either of these two conditions is accompanied by a radiated pain to the leg, the therapist can use two routines to treat the problem more thoroughly.

Locating the pain

Ask the client to point out where he feels the pain. Then ask the client to demonstrate the movements and postures that create or increase the pain. When the pain is created or increased, ask him to point again to the location of pain. Locating the pain in this way is usually more accurate. Once you have the exact location, investigate further for yourself the movements that create or aggravate the pain.

Choosing an appropriate routine

A routine is chosen according to symptoms that are relevant to the Thai diagnosis, regardless of the Western medical definition of the condition. Whenever the symptoms of the client match the symptoms described by one of the routines, the practitioner should try it and observe the client's reaction. If the pressure is welcomed, the treatment may give good results. If an improvement is noticed, the therapist should stay with the same routine until there are more complete healing results.

Some conditions are based on two related disorders occurring simultaneously. These cases may be treated by using two separate routines, but using two routines when only one is actually needed is usually a waste of treatment time.

When using a point-based treatment routine, first verify that you've chosen the right routine. Begin the treatment, and check whether or not the lines and

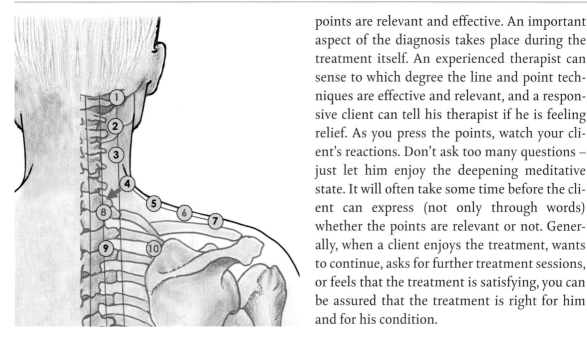

Treatment routine for one-sided neck pain

points are relevant and effective. An important aspect of the diagnosis takes place during the treatment itself. An experienced therapist can sense to which degree the line and point techniques are effective and relevant, and a responsive client can tell his therapist if he is feeling relief. As you press the points, watch your client's reactions. Don't ask too many questions – just let him enjoy the deepening meditative state. It will often take some time before the client can express (not only through words) whether the points are relevant or not. Generally, when a client enjoys the treatment, wants to continue, asks for further treatment sessions, or feels that the treatment is satisfying, you can be assured that the treatment is right for him and for his condition.

Relevant and effective points

Some clients can help you locate the exact spot of an important point, and the proper amount and duration of pressure that is needed. Others may not be so precise with direction, but will respond positively once you locate and press a relevant point. Some clients will not be able to help their therapist much at all. In these cases, therapists must rely on their sensing and intuition and must work through a routine that they feel is most applicable for the condition.

The first indicator of a point in need is that it will feel stiff and very "full." These types of points respond well to repetitive work. The client may feel these points as painful and sensitive but also as pleasant or in need of pressure. Other points are not as easy to find but are equally important in treatment. They feel stiff but "flat." They are not "full," and they don't rise above the surface of the skin. They feel closed, empty, and lifeless. The intuitive therapist will have an urge to press such a point deeply and for a long period of time in order to get a response. The client will feel such a point as numb and without much sensitivity. Other types of points feel very deep to the touch, and draw the therapist's thumb deeper and deeper into the body. For these "hungry" points, it's best to gradually increase continual pressure for 30–60 seconds, or even for a few minutes. Release when you feel that your thumb is being naturally pushed away from the body. The client may feel sleepy upon release of your pressure.

Concentration

Thai acupressure, like other manual healing methods, works through the power of concentration. Our role is to let our clients develop deeper meditative states and to disturb them as little as possible. Talking more than needed, or allowing for other types of disruptions, will hinder the body's ability to heal through concentration. A meditative mood doesn't always require complete silence; the objective is simply to avoid unnecessary disruptions. Maintaining a continuous rhythm in our work and using the right amount of pressure are factors that contribute to a meditative mood. Pressure that is too light doesn't catch the attention of our clients, and pressure that is too deep or painful doesn't encourage them to relax. Deep and focused pressure will usually result in a calm and meditative state.

Feeling what we do

The effectiveness of a treatment varies, depending on the quality of our technique. Even with a correct diagnosis, the right routine, and proper location of all the points, the effectiveness of a treatment depends on how well we press the lines and points. It is typical for beginners to work technically, moving through the lines and points of a routine without feeling much of what they do. When learning acupressure we must first locate the points, but once we learn the point locations and treatment procedures, we naturally become more playful and insightful with our movements and postures, and we start to feel and sense on a deeper level.

As you work, try to focus your bodyweight into the point you are pressing. Make sure your posture is comfortable enough to apply prolonged pressure for at least 10–15 seconds. Once you can press deeply while still feeling comfortable, your treatment will become more effective. Feeling our thumbs, sensing the points, and viewing our client through the points are what make our treatments so effective.

Before making contact, ask yourself: How should I approach this point? How is this point going to feel?

While working, ask yourself: Is my touch wanted here? In which direction does my thumb want to press? How deeply does this point want me to go? Where is the deepest spot in the point? Is the pressure strong enough? Is the pressure too strong? Should I release my pressure a bit? Should I stay longer? Has this point had enough?

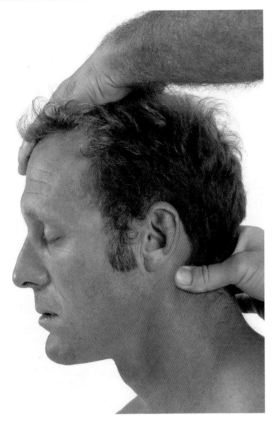

Apply pressure incrementally, and in a supported fashion

Disorders without matching point combinations

Sometimes we have to treat a condition we are not familiar with, or for which there are no ready-made point combinations. In such cases, try to locate relevant therapy lines and points that you feel may be beneficial. Start with a general massage at the area of pain, beginning with palm pressure and followed by thumb pressure on the sen lines. As you treat your client, you may sense that certain lines and points are relevant for treatment. They may seem stiff and full, or closed and lifeless. These lines and points are in need of pressure, yet at the same time they may be very sensitive. If your client is responsive and sensitive, he may lead you to the lines and points that are in need of your touch.

Treatments for different types of conditions

A traumatic injury may result from a car accident, a sports injury, a fall, or a blow from an external source. Thai point combinations are effective in treating some trauma injuries, but it is unwise to treat any serious trauma, especially in an acute phase, before an evaluation of the condition by a specialist. Inflammations and spasms sometimes hide pathologies such as fractures; joint dislocations; tears to ligaments, tendons, or muscles; and damage to nerves, blood vessels, or internal organs. Treatment of a trauma in the chronic phase is safer and may bring about good results, but you should nevertheless exercise caution.

An injury due to overuse usually manifests in soft tissues, bones, and fascia, and often has its roots in poor postural awareness, stress, lack of physical activity, and aggressive physical activities. Thai line and point protocols are appropriate, safe, and effective in the treatment of overuse injuries, but acute cases should be treated with care and/or referred to a physician.

Thai acupressure routines do not treat orthopedic pains and disorders that are caused by internal or systemic disorders. Bacterial infections, viruses, tumors, autoimmune diseases such as gout or rheumatoid arthritis, nutritional deficits, and genetic disorders all fall into this general category. If clients with these conditions seek our help, we should recommend they visit a doctor. Treatment of orthopedic disorders in clients who have an unrelated internal disease (diabetes, for instance) is perfectly fine. General Thai massage treatment may help ease chronic conditions in between the flare-up phases of rheumatoid arthritis or gout, but the acupressure routines of Wat Po are not meant to treat such diseases.

Integrating Thai acupressure into a general Thai massage treatment

In our quest to learn more about Thai medicine, we may study the diagrams of points and lines at the Wat Po medicine pavilion, or research other charts of Thai lines and points. Finding them is a good start, but then you need to learn from someone who has been using them for years, someone who has the knowledge in his hands. We can't rely on maps alone. Individual instruction and guidance is needed.

Practitioners of medical massage in Thailand tend to view general massage for relaxation as separate from point and line protocols that are meant to treat specific conditions. They administer general massage when there is no complaint of pain, or they will use a specific protocol to address a specific complaint. Sometimes, treatment plans are determined by time limitations. Even when time limitations allow treatment of only one specific body part, it is absolutely essential that the client's entire body has entered into a state of relaxation before beginning a specific protocol.

Incorporating a specific protocol into a whole body treatment is often the most effective plan. Take, for instance, a neck pain condition. If the pain is acute, it will be painful to move the neck or even to lie down. In most acute conditions it is, therefore, better to begin with the lines and points of the protocol first. Acute neck pain creates tension throughout the entire body, and so, in a way, it is a pain of the entire body. Once the specific pain is addressed, and the neck's lines and points are recharged and satisfied with our pressure, then we can move on to treat the entire body with a general Thai massage.

If the client is able to lie down comfortably and find a resting posture without any neck pain, then we might begin with a general massage. We could begin with the feet, then work the legs, abdomen, hips, and back, and all of this can be relevant for the neck condition. Our client will be able to experience how working on other parts of the body can help to relieve his localized pain. Nevertheless, since we started with a general massage, we must still allow sufficient time to insert the specific neck protocol. So to summarize, for non-acute conditions, treat the client with a general massage first, while focusing as much as possible on the lines and points of a specific protocol for a localized condition. Working in this way is most effective when there is no time restriction, since 2–3 hours will be required for a complete treatment.

Even when we treat clients with no specific complaints, we should still try to find hidden conditions that may come to the surface in the future, or just use sensing to work on body parts that we feel are in need. Needy areas may feel stiff, weak, and lifeless, or they may display restricted range of motion. Just focus on the lines and points in need, and utilize your knowledge of acupressure to the best of your ability. It's always a good idea to look for these areas early in the session, so you can dedicate enough time to work on them. Basic Thai massage routines treat the whole body, but they also give us the opportunity to find the "hungry" areas, lines, and points that need extra attention. Listening to the body with our hands, and giving these lines and points what they need, is the best way to administer acupressure. Receiving a treatment from someone who doesn't take the time to sense and to work on lines and points can be a frustrating experience, and will bring about only limited results. A treatment by a sensitive practitioner that is responsive to the lines and points that need attention is an entirely different experience.

The importance of acupressure

Many students of Thai massage, especially Western practitioners, become fascinated with the beautiful stretches in traditional Thai massage, but they sometimes neglect the core of nuad boran: working on the sen lines and pressure points. This problem is compounded because some Thai massage teachers don't even include line and point work in their courses and workshops.

A Thai session made up entirely of stretches is not necessarily bad; it's just not a complete Thai massage. Working the lines, whether with palms, feet, elbows, or thumbs, is an inseparable part of the practice of Thai massage. For a practitioner, it is extremely important to sense blocked areas and points along the sen. I don't mean only a few lines that may have been taught in a basic Thai massage workshop, but rather every line that is relevant to your client's condition. As sensitive practitioners, we must work these lines, seek out the "hungry" places that need our pressure, and give them all the time that they need during a treatment session to unfold and surrender to our touch. Thai stretches may be used after a good line workout, or interspersed with point work during a session. Stretches can complement the line work, encourage flow of *lom* along the lines, and can be effective in rehabilitating chronic conditions.

Whether treating an existing condition, or working the lines and points in a session that is aimed at relaxation, accurate pressure is a key component to the healing that results from traditional Thai massage. Seek out continued guidance and instruction in Thai acupressure, and never underestimate the important role that acupressure plays in the overall healing process of nuad boran.

Introduction to Thai Element Theory

NEPHYR JACOBSEN

All around the world, traditional medicine systems hold one thing in common: element theory. In ancient civilizations based in the Americas, Europe, Asia, and elsewhere, element theory is based on the idea that all things are made of earth, water, fire, wind, and space. Each culture has its own unique way of assessing and addressing these elements, but when we look beyond the structure of each system, the basic concept is the same: elements are the component parts of all things.

When we speak of elements as components, we mean everything from dirt, metal, and bones to dreams, thoughts, and desires. Not only are flesh and blood made of elements but also human character, tendencies, and disposition toward certain diseases. It is the balance and imbalance of the elements within us and around us that affects our emotional and physical well-being.

In Thailand, element theory is a unifying factor for the five branches of traditional Thai medicine. These branches are internal medicine (*paetayasaht*: treatment of the internal body); external medicine (*kayapahpbambat*: bone setting, external application of herbs, Thai massage); spirit medicine (*saiyasaht*: shamanistic healing with spirits, incantations, magical tattooing, amulets); divinatory sciences (*horasaht:* numerology, astrology, and palmistry used to determine elemental and disease predisposition); and Buddhism (*putthayasaht*), which may be viewed as the mental health branch of Thai medicine. All five of these branches incorporate two primary components: Buddhist principles and element theory. These two intrinsic ingredients bind the branches of Thai medicine. Traditional Thai doctors may specialize

Branches of Traditional Thai Medicine		
Internal Medicine	*Paetayasaht*	Herbs, diet, treatment of internal body
External Medicine	*Kayapahpbambat*	Massage, bone setting, eternal application of herbs etc.
Spirit Medicine	*Saiyasaht*	Healing with spirits, incantations, mantras, objects, shamanistic
Divinatory Medicine	*Horasaht*	Using systems such as astrology, numerology, palmistry etc. to determine medical predisposition and remedial measures
Buddhism	*Putthayasaht*	Bringing about cessation of suffering through study and practice of the Buddhist dharma

in one branch, but they will also have a strong background in the other components.

The elements are easiest to understand as they exist in nature, outside of ourselves. A boulder is primarily earth element, a pond is primarily water element, a forest fire is primarily fire element, and the movement of wind through the tall grass is primarily wind element. In our bodies, earth and water make up our flesh and blood (anatomy), and fire and wind are the animating forces that bring us to life (physiology). Earth is the container, water is the fluidity, fire is the heat, and wind is all movement. All things contain all elements in varying amounts. To better understand the elements as they manifest in our individual bodies, let's take a closer look at each element.

Earth *(din)*

Earth element (*din*) has the qualities of being hard, stable, and heavy. It provides resistance and support and an experience of solidity. These attributes are important to understand when we deal with element theory.

One role of din is to be a container or vessel for water, fire, and wind. Imagine a slowly moving, warm jungle river. The riverbed and riverbanks form the container, and they are made primarily of earth element. The river itself is primarily made of water element. The warmth of the river comes from fire element, and the movement of the river is wind.

Earth element dominates physical structures, such as buildings, tree trunks, coconut shells, and mountains. It provides a structure within which other elements may interact. In our bodies it is the structure (but not the movement) of bones, skin, nails, teeth, and organs. Earth supports us, grounds us, and protects us, and it provides defined shape. On a cellular level, our bodies have the same elemental interplay as a river. The cell walls are earth, the fluid within the cells is water, the temperature of the cells is fire, and the movement within is wind. This interplay of elements is constant, and it is everywhere. Because earth element is the heaviest element, it is the slowest one to change, and it is often the last one to be affected.

Water (*naam*)

The primary qualities of water element (*naam*) are that it is moist, fluid, and soft. It provides cohesion and fluidity. Water element dominates all fluids, from tree sap to motor oil, from dew to oceans, from tears to blood. Water provides lubrication and malleability, and it is the glue that holds all things together. Water is a sticky binding agent. If you put two drops of water together, they join to form one drop. Even a boulder, which by its nature is primarily earth element, contains water that holds it together. Without the water, the boulder would be dust.

When considering the element of water, it is helpful to think of still water such as puddles, baths, and ponds, since rivers and oceans also contain a large amount of wind element. Water is the second heaviest element, and therefore, like earth, it is also slow to change.

Fire *(fai)*

The primary qualities of fire element (*fai*) are that it is bright, reactive, and sharp. It has the function of providing transformation and ripening, and the experience of heat. Fire heats our bodies, breaks down our food, encourages transformation, and is the impetus for change. Fire's primary role in the body is the digestion of food. Just as the flames in an active fireplace burn paper and wood, the element of fire in our digestive system breaks down and transforms food into absorbable nutrients. Fire is much lighter than earth or water, and it changes easily.

Wind *(lom)*

The primary qualities of wind element (*lom*) are lightness, mobility, and dryness. The function of wind is to provide growth and vibration, and it has the experience of movement. I am intentionally not using the word "air." Air can be static, but wind is inherently representative of motion. The secondary qualities of wind are cool, light, rough, non-unctuous, subtle, and non-slimy.

Like fire, lom is more of a metabolic force than a physical structure such as earth or water. Wind is movement. From the slow upward growth of a tree to the rapid movement of a ball being kicked; from the flowing of blood in our circulatory system to the rotation of the earth on its axis; from the transfer of electricity between a wall socket and a lamp to the energy of thoughts swirling in our minds. In Thai element theory, all of these motions are considered to be wind element. Though fire is the impetus for movement, wind is the very movement itself. As one of the lightest elements, wind is often the first element to be affected by most circumstances. It changes easily and often.

Space *(aagaasathaat)* and consciousness *(winyaanathaat)*

If earth is the container in which water, fire, and wind interact, then space is the canvas upon which they all exist. Space has the qualities of being expansive and subtle. Its function is to provide nonresistance, and a field of activity in which the other elements can exist. The experience of space is openness. In recent times quantum physics has shown us what the ancients knew: that there is more space than there is matter. It is the lightest and most pervasive of all the elements.

In traditional medicine systems, space is often linked to consciousness, and in Thai medicine, knowledge of the element of space includes study of the Buddha's teachings of the Five Skhandas: form, sensation, perception, mental formation, and consciousness. We will not discuss the skhandas here, but when studying Buddhism in relation to Thai healing arts, they are important to understand. For a Thai massage therapist, working with space involves the experience of sinking into the receiver's body – allowing thumbs, fingers, palms, and elbows to pass by fascia and muscle, while maintaining awareness of the space between all matter.

Counting the elements

Some traditional medicine practitioners separate consciousness from space, thereby counting six elements. Since space is much more esoteric, some healers base their work on the four most tangible elements: earth, water, fire, and wind. Further, since it is difficult to affect change on earth element, three-element theory is sometimes used, in which only water, fire, and wind are primarily considered. Regardless of the number of elements with which a practitioner works, all the elements exist. Three-element theory, for example, does not negate the existence of earth and space.

Elemental constitution *(thaat jao reuan)* and imbalance

In the first five or six years of human life, our *thaat jao reuan*, or core elemental constitution, is established. During this process, individuals are weighted more toward one specific element. If, for example, you have a predominance of water element, your thaat jao reuan is water. As a water element person, you will have certain physical and mental characteristics, as well as certain disease predispositions. Some people have more than one element in nearly equal amounts, in which case their thaat jao reuan is a mixture of two, or rarely, of three elements. Earth element is seldom part of a person's core elemental constitution.

Factors that affect thaat jao reuan include the season of conception, genetics, geography, diet, and karma. Once a person's thaat jao reuan is fully developed, it remains that way for the rest of that person's life. This is not to say that the balance of elements is not prone to shifting, In fact, the elemental balance within a person is constantly shifting, but this is seen as a motion in and out of elemental balance, not a change in thaat jao reuan. Thai medicine views thaat jao reuan as a baseline for understanding each individual, but it seeks out specific imbalances in order to determine a course of action or healing.

Earth thaat jao reuan

Earth element is not often found as part of a core elemental constitution. When it is found, it is often paired with another of the elements.

Physique: A preponderance of earth in a person's makeup will be reflected in a very large skeleton and bone structure. They will also likely have large eyes, a squared figure, a deep resonate voice, and thick hair and nails.

Characteristics: Earth element in a person's core makeup often results in several of the following characteristics: loyalty, being grounded, slowness to change, and a compassionate and balanced nature.

Water thaat jao reuan

Physique: When water is the dominating element, it results in physical characteristics such as a large frame, thick hair and eyelashes, large "sweet" eyes, a fleshy body, well-hydrated skin, and a soft melodious voice.

Characteristics: People with a lot of water element tend to be intuitive, compassionate, emotional, malleable (they easily follow other people's lead), and slow to change. They are frequently the glue that holds a relationship or a family together (water is cohesive), and they tend to enjoy sleep, sweets, and less active lifestyles. They learn at a slower pace, but they learn thoroughly, and with long-lasting retention. They can tend toward depression and fear-based anxiety.

Fire thaat jao reuan

Physique: People with a strong fire component tend to have medium-sized frames, strong athletic bodies, and reddish coloring (red hair almost always indicates fire element). They often have soft hair that grays early, oily skin, and sharp clear eyes. Oftentimes, their eyes are one of the first things you notice about them.

Characteristics: Fire people are generally intellectual, and they learn quickly. They stay focused in communication, and they often become teachers, politicians, or they assume other roles that require public speaking. Fire people are motivated and follow through on their goals. They tend to be passionate and accomplished. Fire also manifests in a disposition that can easily be brought to anger, and fiery people can sometimes overpower those around them, with or without the intention to do so, as they accomplish their goals.

Wind thaat jao reuan

Physique: People with a strong wind element can have either tall or short bodies, but will often have a thin skeletal frame. They often have dark coloring, small eyes, and dry skin.

Characteristics: Like fiery people, windy people have a sharp intelligence. They tend to be creative, and often excel at mathematics and at work that requires calculation. Wind-dominant people often have a lot of ideas, but since the nature of wind implies movement, they often begin projects without finishing them. They are inclined to speak circuitously, and can stray from their subject of focus.

Imbalance

Elements exist in six states: balanced, excited, weakened, deranged (disturbed), broken, and gone (lost). When an element is deranged, it fluctuates between excited and weakened. A broken element implies a serious condition, with life in danger, and when an element is gone, the person is dying or already dead. There are other pathologies related to states of imbalance than those mentioned in this brief overview, but since Thai massage therapists work mostly to restore balance, we will only discuss the states of excited and weakened.

Earth excited: Earth element doesn't go out of balance very easily. As the most dense and most heavy element, it is the last to change in disease progression. When earth is out of balance, it usually results in a serious disorder such as cancer, fibrosis, or organ damage. An earth imbalance can also cause a person to be stubborn and rigid.

Earth weakened: A weakened earth element may result in weak tissues and bones, a lack of focus, and a sense of being ungrounded.

Water excited: Water element in an excited state can result in excessive emotions, depression, obesity, reproductive issues, and diseases of agitated water such as colds, mucous, respiratory conditions, and water retention. The more watery we are, the more we tend to retain toxins in our body.

Water weakened: Water in a weakened state can cause dry skin, constipation, rigidity, reproductive issues, problems with lymph glands and blood, dehydration, and other symptoms. Weakened water may also contribute to excess fire and wind conditions.

Fire excited: Excited fire may lead to heat stroke, rash, acne, and other symptoms of redness. It may also contribute to liver damage, temper and anger issues, fever, and overdigestion of food.

Fire weakened: Low-functioning fire element can lead to poor digestion, lowered body temperature, lack of will and strength, and it may fuel symptoms of excited water or wind.

Wind excited: Wind in an excited state can cause anxiety, pain, headaches, arthritis, insomnia, diarrhea or constipation, and obsessive-compulsive and other mental health disorders. It may bring about dry skin, result in the inability to concentrate or to stay warm, and it may fuel symptoms of weakened water element.

Wind weakened: A low-functioning wind element can cause lethargy, poor circulation, headaches, constipation, poor digestion, and neurological conditions that inhibit movement.

Thai bodywork for balancing the elements

For the most part, elemental imbalances are corrected through dietary change, lifestyle modifications, and internal herbal medicine; however, bodywork can and should be used to complement and support these changes. Thai medicine is a holistic system, and external therapies support internal healing, and vice

Thai Massage for Elements	
Water	Stretching • Twisting • Cupping • Dry heat therapies • Warming balms and liniments • Faster rhythm • Work towards the core • Use care with pressure
Fire	Moderate rhythm • Deep sen work • Plucking • Compression • Cooling balms and liniments • Cupping and scraping • Work away from the core
Wind	Calm rhythm • Balanced work • Sequence work • Traction • Use warming oils •

versa. When using bodywork to treat elemental imbalances, Thai therapists should only attempt therapies in which they have been adequately trained. Elemental balance is encouraged by specific techniques, adjusted speed and rhythm, and sometimes by using tools such as balms and liniments.

Thai bodywork for excited water

People with excited water benefit from invigorating bodywork that is done at a faster pace. Stretching and twisting are recommended, and also Thai fire cupping therapy. Dry heat therapies, such as dry hot herbal compresses, dry saunas, and warming balms and liniments can also be beneficial. Be careful not to work too deeply, especially with point work and *sen* line work, since those with excited water can bruise easily. Work toward the body's core, where water and stored toxins can be processed by the body.

Thai bodywork for excited fire

Those with agitated fire should be treated at a moderate pace, to encourage states of relaxation and calm, but don't work so slowly that it makes the receiver frustrated. Deep sen line work, stretches, plucking, and compression are indicated, as are cooling balms and liniments. Thai cupping and body scraping can help to release excess heat. Work away from the core of the body to disperse excess heat.

Thai bodywork for excited wind

People with overly active wind require very balanced, slow bodywork. Work in a smooth, flowing way, move your client as little as possible, and focus on calm grounding movements and techniques. Standard Thai massage sequences are fine, as long as they are not based entirely on stretches. Traction to the joints is beneficial, but deep, extended stretches are not. Focus more on compression and sen line work, and don't move your client around more than necessary. Rubbing warming oils into the sen lines, or even performing an oil massage is often beneficial for excess wind. If a client has excited mental wind (anxiety, can't stop thinking, worrying), try working from the top of the body down to the feet.

I have not suggested ideas for bodywork with regard to earth element because imbalanced earth brings about conditions such as cancers and tumors that cannot be adequately addressed with Thai massage. Of course, people suffering from these types of afflictions can benefit from bodywork, but the work can't be a course of treatment for the disease. Earth element is always important, however, because it's what the therapist primarily touches; it is the dominant element in the structure of skin, muscle, fascia, tendons, and ligaments. In fact, earth and wind are the main elements that all bodyworkers address when they work with clients. By freeing blockages, we encourage movement (wind, lom).

A doorway into traditional Thai medicine

When I first began learning Thai massage, I believed that what made it "Thai" was the lack of a massage table, the client being clothed, assisted stretches, the concept of sen lines, and the lack of oil. I understand now that traditional Thai massage is not complete without the use of Thai medicine theory. If Thai element theory, sen line theory, acupressure theory, and other Thai therapies guide your bodywork choices, then you are working within the Thai tradition. Sometimes this doesn't seem like the type of Thai massage that is taught to most Westerners. It is entirely possible, for example, to apply Thai medicine theory to rub a person's body with sesame oil, or to not perform stretches, or to work on some areas of the body and not on others.

This essay is meant to be a doorway into the elemental theory of traditional Thai medicine. Understanding Thai element theory can be transformational in a Thai massage practice. It launches the work from systemic maintenance to knowledge-based therapy which can be used to address imbalances, injuries, and chronic troubles. Unfortunately, most people who learn Thai massage are not taught theory. When I first became interested in Thai medicine theory, some people told me that all the Thai theory was lost when Ayutthaya was destroyed. Others said that Thai medicine was entirely taken from Indian Ayurveda. It's difficult for Westerners to find teachers and schools that can properly explain Thai medicine theory, but excellent teachers do certainly exist. I encourage all who are interested to seek out this training.

The Sen Sip: Understanding Thai Sen Lines

FELICITY JOY

The word *sen* in Thai language means line, string, or pathway. It is the movement of energy along these channels that maintains health. The *sen sip* are the ten most important energy channels in the human body. Often, when we press a particular point on a sen line, the effect can be felt somewhere else along that line.

For me, working the sen lines is the most important part of Thai massage. They transcend the assisted yoga and stretching portions of Thai massage, and allow for deep healing sessions. This is not to say that a session consisting mostly of stretches is not a wonderful thing. Stretching, however, is only one part of traditional Thai massage. Without working the sen lines, Thai massage is not complete.

There are disagreements among teachers, schools, and practitioners as to exactly where the lines are and how they run in the human body. As more Westerners come to study in Thailand, anatomical terms have begun to be used to aid in understanding. Western empirical beliefs, however, are difficult to apply to Eastern understanding. The body is a vehicle to access the human energy system, so relying entirely on anatomy to find the lines can create confusion. Where there is injury, illness, or damage to the body, the sen can change their qualities. Maps and line charts cannot show you exactly where the individual sen lie; this is something that you must feel and sense and learn when you touch your client's body. My experience with sen lines is based largely on my teacher Asokananda's investigations, and on the work he completed just before he died. I also learned much from Chiayuth, whose ability to stimulate the movement of energy was on a level I could never have imagined.

Long ago, ancient healers learned about and studied referred pain. They knew that finding a painful area of the body didn't always mean there was a problem in that exact area. They found that treating the referred pain reduced or healed the symptom. So it is with sen line work. As we follow the lines up and down the body, we find places that are painful to the touch, but that, when properly addressed, relieve the symptom. One doesn't need to know anatomy or physiology to be a good Thai massage practitioner, but one certainly must understand the ways in which the body moves within natural law. Knowledge of the body's processes helps to deepen our understanding of maintaining the body's balance.

The Thai word used to describe life energy is *lom*, which translates as wind or air. It is known in other medicine systems as *qi, chi,* and *prana.* This force is believed to come about by the absorption of the elements. It enters the body and runs through the sen in order to maintain optimal health. It is what provides movement to an otherwise motionless form. By compressing and releasing the body in different ways, the sen are stimulated to encourage the free flow of this energy. Incorrect diet, unhealthy lifestyle, negative thought processes, and injury may create blockages along the energy lines.

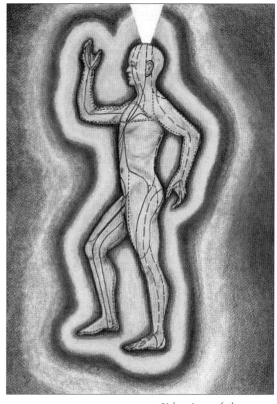

Side view of the sen sip in traditional Thai massage

Sumana

Sen *sumana (su-MAHN-a)* is the central line of the body and is nearly identical to *sushumna nadi* of Indian Ayurveda. It is also similar to the Chinese meridian *ren mai,* and is known as the functional line in other healing traditions. In the Indian tradition, it passes through seven major spiritual and energy centers known as *chakras.* In this way it touches all that one is, and all that one has the potential to be. Sen sumana may be worked to treat respiratory problems, asthma, bronchitis, throat issues, colds, coughs, chest pain, and physical and emotional heart problems. Digestive disorders are also addressed through sen sumana, as are nausea, abdominal pain, and back pain.

Ittha and pingkhala

Sen *ittha (EE-ta)* runs from the feet along the entire left side of the body and embodies female energy. Sen *pingkhala (PING-ka-la)* is a mirror image of ittha, running on the right side of the body, and it represents male energy. Ittha and pingkhala meet at the third eye in the middle of the forehead. Ittha stimulates pingkhala out of its dormant male state into a fiery energy that can be used therapeutically. These vital energies may be employed therapeutically for ailments such as multiple sclerosis, broken bones, Parkinson's disease, nerve function issues, and old, recurrent injuries. Sen ittha is a soothing energy, which helps ailments that require a more subtle approach in order to address long-term underlying issues. Ittha influences intuition and the creative process, and pingkhala is said to strengthen logic and analytical processes. Both lines are used to treat headache, colds, coughs, sore throat, chills, fevers, nasal problems, and dizziness. Pain and stiffness in the back, shoulder, and neck may also be positively affected, as well as internal organs and intestinal and urinary tract issues.

Kalathari

Sen *kalathari (ka-la-ta-REE)* is an important energy line with a very strong quality. On the arms and legs it manifests as the second of three main lines. It is known as the emotional and psychic line, as it affects the subconscious, hidden memories, and many emotions. Working on kalathari can facilitate emotional release, so it must be approached with respect and sensitivity. It can sometimes be painful for a client to receive work on this line, as it contains many major acupressure points. Kalathari can be helpful in treating emotional, mental and psychic disorders, schizophrenia, depression, hysteria, attention deficit disorder, bipolar conditions, autism, epilepsy, shock, posttraumatic stress disorder, and addictions. It may also ease constipation, indigestion, stomach ache, hernia, paralysis of arms and legs, joint pain, arrhythmia, and autoimmune disorders.

Sahatsarangsi and thawari

These are known as the detoxification lines of the body, and because of their ability to release toxicity, they serve to strengthen the four previously mentioned lines. They often bring about an itchy sensation or a feeling of "good pain" when they are stimulated. *Sahatsarangsi (sa-hat-sa-RAHNG-see)* and *thawari (TA-wa-ree)* may have low energetic signatures or may feel weak to the touch. The lines traverse areas and contain points that are helpful in treating issues such as lower back pain, shoulder and neck immobility, and knee problems. They therapeutically treat disorders of the face, eyes, teeth, and throat, and may also be used for sinusitis, skin disorders, and bad breath. Gastrointestinal diseases, jaundice, appendicitis, pancreatitis, and arthritis are also positively affected by working these two lines thoroughly.

Lawusang and ulangka

Sen *lawusang (LAH-wu-sahng)* runs on the left side of the body and sen *ulangka (u-LANGH-ka)* runs on the right, and they are shorter in length than the previous six lines. From the solar plexus, they cross the nipples and move to the throat, where they join part of sahatsarangsi and thawari to the ears, and then move up to the head, where they enter the brain. Applied pressure generally brings about a localized effect, rather than a radiated one. The lines are good for treating balance problems and inner ear issues, including hearing loss. Chest and solar plexus disorders, throat pain, cough, asthma, and other restrictive breathing problems may also be positively affected. They may also benefit facial paralysis, sneezing, coughing, hiccups, heartburn, and indigestion.

Nanthakrawat and khitchana

Sen *nanthakrawat (nan-ta-KRAH-wat)* and sen *khitchana (kit-CHAH-na)* are separate lines, but may also be viewed as aspects of sen sumana. Sen nanthakrawat runs from the naval to the anus and deals mostly with issues of excretion. It treats bloating, gas, hernia, diarrhea, cramps, and abdominal pain. Sen khitchana runs from the navel to the urethral opening, and it deals with sexual and conception issues. It treats menstruation issues, infertility, and endometriosis. In men it treats impotence, premature ejaculation, priapism, and prostate issues.

Summary

I am aware of the debates and disagreements about the sen lines, about where they may exist, and about how to work with them. I also know, however, that disease and chronic disorders can often be relieved in several sessions by engaging in extensive line work. We feel the lines, we sense where there are blockages along the lines, and then we work them using a variety of Thai techniques, be they traditional palming and thumbing, stretching, herbal compresses, *tok sen, yam khang,* traditional oils, or topical herbal poultices.

The main goal in treating our clients is to help them become healthier and happier. The more healthy and happy we all are, the more we can contribute to healing and peace throughout the world.

Using Your Feet in Thai Yoga Massage

RALF MARZEN

In Thailand it is extremely rude to expose the soles of the feet to another person. You would never see anyone sitting with their legs outstretched if their feet were pointed in the direction of others. Once, while asleep on a boat journey between two beautiful islands in the Gulf of Siam, I was awakened by an apologetic woman who, although embarrassed to interrupt my sleep, wanted to be sure she wouldn't step over my body in order to get to her seat on the boat.

One of the many delightful contradictions in Thai culture is that the feet, long considered the most impure part of the body, are used extensively in traditional bodywork. If you have explored the art of traditional Thai massage for any length of time in Thailand, you've probably had the experience of being flattened like a pancake by a little old lady walking on your back, smiling, with surprising ease and confidence, and with the perceived weight of an elephant. At other times, you may have felt the therapist's feet close to your neck and shoulders, working from different angles and positions, in the most natural of ways. In these moments, one forgets the difference in connotation and sensation between hands (the traditional bodywork tool) and feet, especially if the therapist uses their feet in a skilled way.

In Thailand, most practitioners of Thai yoga massage use their feet to some extent in their practice in order to apply pressure to various parts of the client's body. There are even a few classic Thai massage moves that use the feet in a "paddle boat" type of movement.

Of the many *nuad* practitioners I have encountered over the years, a few have made the use of their feet a central element of their work, almost a trademark. Those who have been practicing Thai massage for many years may remember the late master Chaiyuth Priyasith of Chiang Mai, whose work with his feet was so powerful that more than once after a treatment with him I may not have remembered my name if you'd asked me! A younger woman named Khun Su who practices in Nathon/Ko Samui is also well known for being skilled and innovative with her feet. I learned from her a number of techniques that I now use in my practice and teaching.

Most experienced Thai massage therapists enjoy using their whole body during treatments. Rather than relying on our hands, we incorporate our knees, elbows, forearms, and feet into our work. Aside from the many energetic benefits for both therapist and client, which will be discussed later, the creative variety of the whole-body dance between giver and receiver is precisely what makes Thai yoga massage such a unique and amazing form of bodywork.

Grounding

The single most important reason for the extensive use of feet in Thai massage is the physical and energetic grounding it provides – not only for the therapist but also for the client. In the early years of my practice, while I was almost exclusively working with my hands, I would often feel somewhat displaced and ungrounded after giving a treatment. Through lots of experimenting, I realized that the more I used my feet, the less I had this problem. When I used my feet, I could walk away from most treatments feeling centered and grounded. This newfound awareness made the entire experience of giving Thai massage treatments so much more enjoyable. My clients felt great after a treatment, and so did I.

Energetically speaking, grounding is where everything starts. If we're not grounded, it is not possible for our energetic and physical bodies to come to a complete state of rest and relaxation. Grounding can be defined as a sense of stability and solidity, of being connected to the earth. When we're grounded, we have a solid sense of personal identity, while at the same time we're able to welcome the world and other people into our energetic field.

When we're not grounded, our energy moves toward the upper parts of the body, especially the head. With an accumulation of energy in our head, we can lose touch with reality and fall victim to a thought-created world. This energetic movement can manifest as stress. It starts with some type of agitation in the nervous system, based on either internal or external stimuli. If the agitation isn't met with clear awareness, it turns into stress energy that rises in the body and eventually creates an imbalance and loss of grounding. We become disembodied, and we reside and experience most things in our heads. Once in this state, thoughts and noise and confusion expand in the head, and we can experience the world outside of ourselves as stressful. The more we experience the world and life as stressful, the more agitation gets created on an energetic level. This is the stress loop.

So, what's the antidote? In other words, how can we live and act from a place of relaxation and grounding rather than stress? As bodyworkers, we are familiar with a number of techniques and practices that can help our bodies and minds to relax – yoga, meditation, t'ai chi, exercise, a pleasant walk in nature. Consciously connecting with the earth on physical and energetic levels usually has an overwhelmingly positive effect on our nervous systems. Generally speaking, the key to relaxation is to become fully aware of the agitation that arises in the nervous system from time to time. Most often, agitation runs on a subconscious level, and because of this, it has a lot of power over us.

The very moment we choose to fully experience our feelings instead of closing down to them, we give the stress an opportunity to release itself. When we pay attention to the body and its energy movements with a soft and relaxed focus, our nervous system can more easily maintain a state of rest and balance. The stress energy dissipates, and we experience ourselves as grounded and embodied once again, rather than stressed and stuck in our heads. All aspects of life in general, including Thai yoga massage, are much more enjoyable when we're grounded.

Subtle energies

Years ago, when I was living and working in a small Lahu hill-tribe village in northern Thailand, where my late teacher Asokananda founded his Thai massage school, a course in *chavutti thirumal* was being held at the same time as the Thai massage workshop I was taking. In this fascinating form of Ayurvedic oil massage from Kerala in Southern India, the practitioner uses his feet exclusively for the entire treatment. This is done by holding on to a rope that hangs from the ceiling and by applying long and firm strokes with the soles of the feet to the client's body.

Luckily for me, one of my friends was taking the course, and I later received a session from him. The feeling of grounding that I had after that treatment was amazing. My body felt solid, relaxed, and heavy in a pleasant way as a result of the deep pressure I had received from his feet. That experience strongly influenced my decision to use my feet more often in my own Thai massage practice. In chavutti thirumal, the practitioner learns to receive the energy from above through the crown *chakra*, to draw it in and store it in the *hara* (the energy center in the lower abdomen), and then to transfer it to the client's body through the legs and feet. As Thai therapists, we can also apply these principles during the course of a Thai massage. When we work with our clients from a standing position, it is helpful to imagine our energetic channels as being open from above and below, so that we can act as energy transmitters in our work. As you practice Thai massage techniques in a standing position, try to draw in energy from above through the crown of your head, and then let it pour down through your body and out through the soles of your feet.

Especially in Western cultures, where people generally don't have a strong sense of grounding, it is wise to maintain awareness of solidity and grounding. This applies to the practice of Thai yoga massage, for both the therapist and client. As previously mentioned, it's relatively easy for a practitioner to maintain a sense of grounding, and to feel the downward flow of energy while standing and/or working with the feet. When we practice in this way, the energy that gets transmitted onto and into the client's body is more solid and balanced. When this happens, the energetic quality of our work usually improves.

Working the abdomen with the sole of the foot. Remember to visualize downward movement of energy from the crown to the feet

For clients who tend to be agitated, stressed, and ungrounded in nature, a Thai yoga treatment done at a reasonably slow pace, incorporating a lot of work with the feet, will have a very beneficial effect.

The importance of energetic grounding is fairly clear when you consider a traditional sequence of Thai massage. The therapist starts at the feet and usually spends a lot of time working on the legs and the leg lines before moving to the upper parts of the body. The main reason for this is that without grounding and balancing the lower part of the body, intensive work on the back and shoulders will not have a long-lasting effect. Ajahn Pichest of Hang Dong stresses this point over and over again in his teachings, and he constantly reminds his students to do more "warming up" on the lower part of the body before they start working on the back and shoulders. Sometimes newcomers to Thai massage, whether students or clients, are surprised at the extensive amount of legwork found in a traditional sequence. But it doesn't take too long until they become equally surprised when their upper body tension melts away as a result of all the extensive, deep work on feet, legs, and hips.

Grounding the energy always frees up the upper body. In Eastern martial arts, especially t'ai chi, this principle plays an extremely important role. Practitioners learn to focus on, and move from, the body's center of gravity in the

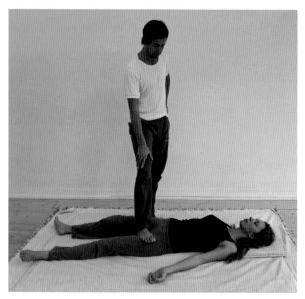

Opening the wind gate in standing position

lower abdomen. This place is called *dan tien* in Chinese and hara in the Japanese tradition. The goal is to root the lower body, to create lightness in the upper body, and to cultivate awareness in the dan tien. By dropping or "sinking" the energy into the lower body, our movements become easier and more efficient, and our minds become clearer and more alert.

As an experiment, while sitting or standing, let your attention drop into your hara. Bring awareness to that core part of your body and your consciousness, and see how that feels. More than likely you will notice a calming of the mind, a greater feeling of ease, and a stronger sense of grounding.

Technical aspects

As you first start incorporating more use of your feet into your Thai practice, it may feel a little unfamiliar at first. After all, we were taught to mostly use our palms and thumbs to work the legs, arms, back, and shoulders. At first, you may not feel comfortable about executing techniques in standing position, or about touching someone else's body with your feet. Your feet may also lack the sensitivity to detect blockages and areas of holding that you may have already developed in your hands. In my personal experience, both in my own practice and also by observing students, these initial difficulties usually subside as you practice using your feet more often, and as you develop more confidence with foot techniques. As always, the key is to practice, practice, practice!

It is also very useful to have some type of physical practice that allows you to energize the lower part of your body. Many of us don't bring a lot of awareness and energy to our hips, legs, and feet. If your energy doesn't easily flow down to the lower extremities, you won't have much sensitivity in your feet, either. And if your feet aren't alive with energy, your sensitivity there will be greatly reduced when you use them in your practice. Yoga postures that incorporate legwork, balancing, and standing are often helpful to increase energy flow to the feet. Martial arts as well as athletic practices can also be very helpful.

As you introduce more footwork into your practice, you may also want to experiment with the different qualities and effects that can be achieved when different parts of the feet are applied to someone's body. Working with the toes can be compared to using your fingers. For example, there is a similarity between using the big toe of your foot and the thumb of your hand while working pressure points. The arch of the foot can simulate traditional Thai palm pressure, and the pressure can be broader and more consistent over a larger surface of the body.

The ball of the foot has a more pointed and stronger quality than the whole arch, similar to using the heel of your hand. And lastly, skillful use of the heel provides a very firm and solid pressure that is well suited for deep work in certain areas of the body. The heel, especially the point at its very center, is energetically connected to the first chakra at the perineum and at the base of the spine. The point in the center of the arch of the foot has a direct connection to the seventh chakra at the crown of the head.

Among the various acupressure and reflexology points on the sole of the foot, one that deserves special mention is found just below the ball of the foot on the central line. This point maintains a strong energetic exchange with the earth, and is also the starting point of the kidney meridian in Chinese medicine, which is extremely important for grounding the body and its entire energy system.

While working with our feet during a Thai yoga session, there are generally three body positions for the practitioner: sitting, half-kneeling/lunge, and standing. Some practitioners like to use tools and props to help them with their posture and balance. If you find it challenging to have good balance while standing and using your feet, consider holding on to the back of a chair with your hand or hands. Some therapists have one or several ropes hanging from the ceiling to help with their balance. I have also seen Thai massage therapists using bamboo walking sticks to maintain their balance during a session. Feel free to improvise with the use of props if it makes you feel more secure. Eventually, after more practice, you may be able to work without them.

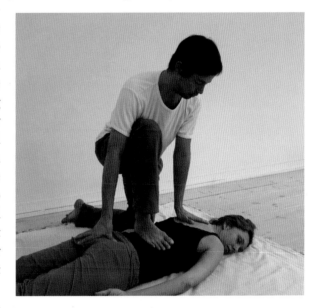

Back compression with the sole of the foot. Notice the hand support on the sacrum and upper back

When using your feet, the guidelines regarding body mechanics are very much the same as with all other Thai massage techniques. First of all, use your bodyweight and not your muscle strength to apply pressure. Lean in, and transfer your weight to your legs and feet. Let your bodyweight sink naturally; don't push it down. The parts of your body that you use on your client's body should be kept soft and still. Your foot acts as the point of contact between you and your client, and it transmits your energy and bodyweight to them.

Explorations with your feet

As you practice integrating more foot work, try to resist the temptation to become tense in your feet and legs. Also, as often as possible, maintain an awareness of energetic connection with the ground as you work. In half-kneeling or standing positions, for example, it's easy to lift up from the ground energetically. Instead, try to sink your weight slowly into the floor as you lean in, and as you change your position to move from one part of your client's body to another. If you work in this way, you won't feel ungrounded or depleted after your sessions, and you'll enhance your personal enjoyment and peace during your Thai sessions.

As you refine your Thai work, practice foot techniques that you already know, work on improving your balance and grounding, and remember to open the flow of energy from your crown chakra downward to your feet as you work. Keep your feet clean, and trim your toenails regularly. Seek out instruction from teachers who use extensive foot work, and as always, practice on your friends and colleagues before you integrate new techniques into your work with clients. The feet are wonderful tools to use in traditional Thai massage. Enjoy your continued explorations with them.

Pregnancy and Thai Massage

BOB HADDAD

Studies have shown that general massage therapy carried out during pregnancy can help to reduce stress, alleviate depression, relieve general aches and pains, improve the potential for successful delivery, and promote good health for the child. It has also been proven that with regular massage treatment, hormones such as norepinephrine and cortisol ("stress hormones") are reduced. In addition, neurotransmitters such as dopamine and serotonin, which are associated with depression when they exist in low levels, are increased. Other beneficial effects of prenatal massage include reduced back pain, improved blood circulation, headache relief, and deeper sleep.

After the first trimester, pregnant women shouldn't lie on their back for extended periods, and for obvious reasons they shouldn't lie on their stomachs, either. Because of this, traditional Thai massage is better suited for pregnancy than Western table massage, since an entire treatment can be carried out with the client in side-lying and seated positions, while resting on a comfortable floor mat.

Pregnancy massage in Thailand

In Thailand, herbal compresses *(luk pra kob)* are used extensively when working with pregnant women. Deep stretches and focused point and line work are generally not performed. Instead, broad pressure is applied to safe areas of the body using the compresses as extensions of the hands. Experienced healers create herbal blends for prepartum work, and herbal teas and decoctions may also be offered to ease pain, aid in relaxation, and help bring about a smooth delivery.

Session time is kept short, usually about one hour, and massage is generally not performed in the first few months of pregnancy. After the baby is delivered, special postpartum herbal compresses may be used to minimize scars, to help the uterus contract, to draw out excess fluids from the mother's body, and to relieve swollen breasts.

Allaying fears and concerns

Although pregnancy treatments in Thailand utilize herbal compresses extensively, many programs of study in the West do not adequately prepare Thai therapists in the art of luk pra kob. This is unfortunate, since herbal compresses are an integral part of traditional Thai healing, and they may be used with great success not only with pregnant clients but with all people. If you're not using compresses, however, your pregnant clients can still derive benefit from Thai massage therapy, as long as you're sensitive, practical, and wise in your approach.

I remember how nervous I was the first time I reluctantly agreed to work on a client who had become pregnant. She was someone I had treated before on several occasions, but when I saw her again, she was already three months pregnant, and I was afraid of doing anything that could cause harm to her or to the baby growing inside her. I consulted the only source that was available at the time for pregnancy in Thai massage: a few guidelines in my teacher Asokananda's advanced book. I corresponded with him by e-mail to make sure I knew which techniques to avoid in my work, and I did research about pregnancy, so I could be as ready as possible for the first session with my client. I had my notes right next to me as I worked. I was so worried and careful during that first session. My pressure and stretching was much lighter than usual, and instead of avoiding only the contraindicated points on feet, ankles, and hands, I don't think I touched her feet or hands during the entire session!

Now, after many years of experience, I am comfortable (and quite excited) when I have the opportunity to work with a pregnant woman in Thai massage. I've worked with some clients throughout their entire pregnancy; from immediately after conception to just a few days before delivery. I consider it a great blessing to be part of two persons' lives at the same time. My sessions with pregnant clients have also proven to be fabulous learning opportunities for me as a therapist, and they have provided me with an enhanced sense of self. When I occasionally have the opportunity to meet a child who was once in her mother's belly on my mat, I feel an immediate connection to that child in a deep, spiritual way.

Precautions, preparations, and tools

Thai massage is absolutely wonderful in pregnancy. An experienced practitioner can resort to many Thai techniques in modified body positions in order to provide a relaxing and balancing full-body treatment for a pregnant woman. Here are some tips and suggestions that may help you to gain the confidence and skills necessary to work with pregnant women:

- Avoid deep point pressure and deep *sen* line work. Instead, work with broad, medium-light pressure, and avoid deep, prolonged stretches. The hormone relaxin exists in highly elevated levels in pregnant women, resulting in pelvic and cervical expansion and a general relaxed state. Because of this, an inexperienced or insensitive therapist can easily overstretch a client, thereby increasing risk to the mother and child.

- Don't practice massage on a pregnant woman until you know the things you shouldn't do. Consider practicing first on non-pregnant friends or colleagues. Do this by running through your normal sequence of Thai massage techniques while eliminating those postures, techniques, pressure points, and stretches that should be avoided for pregnant women. Refine and practice as many side-position techniques as you can, since in mid-to late-term pregnancy, that's the body position you will be using most. In addition to practicing specific techniques on friends, you can also use them in your work with your regular clients, and they won't ever know that you are pretending they are pregnant.

- You will need large pillows and bolsters when you work with pregnant women, so if you don't already have them in your place of practice, buy some. I've found that sofa seat cushions, sofa backrest pillows, and large bolsters work very well. Since you'll be working most of the time with the client in side position, it's best to have a firm and long pillow to use for her head. Normal-sized bed pillows don't work as well. A tubular pillow is also a good tool, since you can use it as a support for your client's top arm when she is in side position.

- Have some large-size loose cotton pants available for clients, and remember to keep your room, your client, and the mat at a comfortable temperature.

- Avoid sensitive pressure points entirely, especially those on hands, wrists, feet, and ankles. Keep reference notes nearby (such as the "Danger Zones" section of this article), so you can remind yourself of specific things you should avoid during a session.

- Always err on the side of caution. Check with your client from time to time to make sure your pressure is not too strong, and that she is comfortable.

How to position the client

As mentioned earlier, Thai massage is especially suited to pregnant women because an entire treatment may be carried out in seated, reclining supine, and side positions. During the first few months of pregnancy, most women can lie comfortably on their backs for short periods of time. Since Thai massage treatments are normally begun by working the feet and legs in supine position, you may continue to do so with pregnant women, at least for the first trimester.

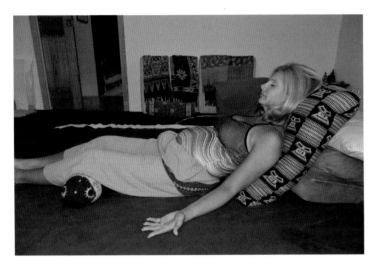

Reclining supine position

But be aware of the clock as you work, and try to not let your client stay in supine position for longer than the first 15 minutes of the session. Remember that you can work the inside and outside legs quite efficiently in side-lying position using compresses, palming, and thumbing, so there is no need to work these areas with the client in supine position. As the pregnancy progresses into the second trimester, avoid keeping the client on her back altogether. Instead, work almost entirely in side position, though, if you wish, you may begin and end the session in reclining supine position.

Reclining supine position

To position a client in reclining supine position, create a firm but pliant back support with large pillows and bolsters such as those used for sofas, daybeds, and other furniture. Make sure there is enough support at the bottom of the stack of pillows, so the foundation doesn't slide. If you are working on a large mat, this will be easier to do. If you are working on a small mat, you may have to place a rug or carpet behind the mat, so the bottom pillows don't slide away when the client leans backward. After you help your client lean back against the pillow support, ask her if she is at a comfortable angle. If she needs to move forward or backward, adjust the pillows until she feels comfortable. You might decide to place an additional pillow behind her head.

When you begin a session in reclining supine position, you won't need a pillow under her knees. But if you end the session in this position, in order to work her face and head, place a tubular pillow or a large rolled towel under her knees for added comfort. If you don't wish to end the session in reclining supine position, you may bring her to a complete seated position, but don't do so in the traditional Thai way of crossing her legs and pulling her up by her arms! That would compress her belly. Instead, gently ask your client to come to a seated position, as you help to push her forward from behind.

Side position

After the initial work in reclining supine position, bring your client into the normal side-lying Thai position. Place one leg over the other, drape one arm over the other, and position her head on a high, firm pillow. I like to use a tubular pillow in front of the chest so the upper arm can drape comfortably. Don't push the tubular pillow too firmly into her stomach, and try to keep her top leg bent at approximately a 90-degree angle.

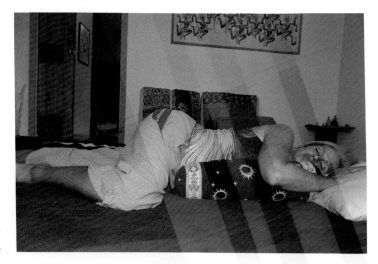

Side position

Now you can begin your leg work. Butterfly-press, palm-press, thumb-walk, and work the points on the female-dominant (left) leg first, and then work on her sub-dominant leg. In the side position photo above, for example, you could first work on the medial (inside) aspect of the left leg, then proceed to the lateral (outer) aspect of her right leg. When she is flipped onto her other side, you would work the opposite sides of each leg, starting first with the dominant leg.

Suggested body positioning sequences

For the first trimester, you and your client may be comfortable starting in regular supine position for the first 15 minutes of the session. Work with compresses, or use traditional Thai techniques, as you work the feet, ankles, calves, and legs. Then bring your client into side position and continue working the top lateral leg and the bottom medial leg. Continue with the hips, sacrum, back, shoulder, and neck. Flip the client to her other side and repeat the sequence. Now, if you wish, you may bring the client into regular seated position and work from behind on her neck, shoulders, face, and head. You can end in seated position, or you can ease her downward to supine position.

After three months of pregnancy, it's best to avoid full supine position, and to use reclining supine position for the beginning of the session. Follow the pattern above in side position, and finish in either seated position or in reclining supine position.

In the last few months of pregnancy, take extra care to not prolong your work in seated or reclining supine position, and work as much as possible, if not entirely, in side position. This is when you can begin to work the entire (top) side of her body from foot to neck, and the medial aspect of the leg and arm that is resting on the mat. Then you may flip her to the other side and repeat the process. Finish in reclining supine or seated position, or just let her remain on the mat in side position, if you prefer.

The importance of working the back

As a baby develops, and as the abdominal wall expands and becomes heavier, a woman's back muscles need to work harder to support anterior weight displacement and to maintain good posture. In the second trimester, back strain may begin, and in the last few months of pregnancy it can become extreme. The added weight can also sometimes have a negative effect on the shoulders and neck.

Fortunately, working in side position allows full access to the sacrum, the lower back, the major sets of back lines, the scapulae, and the shoulders and neck. After you've finished working on the client's legs in side position, you can work the upper hip with gentle leg rotations, gentle backward leg bends (be careful), and light pressure to the boomerang points at the hip. When you return the upper leg to a 90-degree resting position, you can then work on the back.

I spend a lot of time gently working the client's back with my feet. Foot walking provides broad pressure and is a great way to gently open up and relax the entire back. Spend as much time as you like working with your feet on her back. Try to find areas where you can feel the tension, and gently sink your foot in until you feel a slight resistance. Then stay there for 10–20 seconds, at least through one inhale and two exhales. If your client needs more pressure there, you will feel her surrender more space for you to press deeper.

I remember one session with a regular client who was in her last stages of pregnancy. She loved it when I worked with my feet on her back, but one day she asked me to go deeper, and I obliged. Then as she exhaled she asked me to go deeper again. I complied, but I began to worry that I was getting dangerously close to her belly, and therefore close to the baby. I told her I didn't think I should go any deeper. She replied: "You have no idea how much pain I have down there carrying this baby. I can't wait for this baby to be out of me! I need more pressure. Now push harder. I said push harder!"

As a result of that dramatic and comical experience, I learned how important it is to work on the backs of pregnant women. And in my opinion, using foot-presses, rather than palm-presses, is the best way to do this. Spend as much time as you like applying broad and gradually deepening foot pressure. Work only one side of the back for each side-lying position. In other words, if the client is lying on their left side, work the lower (left) side of their back. The posterior portion of your heel will be sliding on the mat, your upper heel and arch will be making most contact with her back, and the upper arch and toes of your foot will surround and cup the spine as you push forward.

Work with your outside foot first (the foot that is closest to her legs), and then gradually introduce your other foot as you begin to pedal against her back with rocking pressure, alternating from one foot to the other. As the back begins to open and relax, it will become more flexible. Then you can do some of the classic Thai techniques, such as gently pulling her leg slightly backward as you anchor your foot against her back. Remember: be gentle, and never strain or overextend your client.

After a while, you can reach over and grab her uppermost arm and bring it backward toward you. Hold each other's wrists, hold her foot in your other hand, and gently begin to pedal first with one foot, then another, in alternating fashion. Make sure to open the arc of her outstretched arm and leg as wide as possible. Don't pull back on the arm and foot. Just hold them aloft as you gently pedal with your feet. Be careful to always work sensitively, and check with your client to make sure she is comfortable and that she is enjoying the work.

Use common sense. Be attentive to your client's signals, work gently and compassionately, and help her to relieve the back stress she is enduring as a result of the extra weight in her belly. Your client will be grateful for all the attention you are giving to her back.

Working the stomach, face, and head

Although you should take care not to press on the stomach at any time, your client may appreciate a soft and gentle belly massage. It's best to ask the client's permission before you touch her stomach. If you have her permission, you can begin in clockwise fashion making a contiguous series of small palm circles. You can also move from one circle to the other by working in a figure eight pattern. If you and your client feel comfortable with gentle compressions, you may do so while following the outside contour of the amniotic sac. If this is the case, cradle the sac with your palms and press it very gently toward her navel, but never press directly downward into the mat.

Working with a luk pra kob compress can be very soothing to a pregnant mother, and it's nice to imagine that the warming effect and medicinal herbs have a positive effect on the baby, too. You can apply extremely gentle pressure with a warm compress on the entire belly, as well as on the chest, shoulders, neck, head, and face.

Working the face and head are not very convenient from side-lying position. Besides, it is nice to work the entire face and head at the same time, as a finishing touch of the massage, Because of this, consider kneeling behind your client and working her face and head while she's in reclining supine or seated position. Modify your kneeling or half-kneeling position so that you have best access to the portions of her face and head that need your attention.

Danger zones: Pressure points, areas, and techniques to avoid

☠   Any type of spinal twist is prohibited for pregnant women. Compression of the belly during pregnancy, whether in side position or in reclining seated position, is forbidden. Avoid "chopping" or any type of percussive technique on the back, chest, or belly.

☠   Avoid all "blood stop" techniques *(bpert lom)*. Never perform extended compressions on femoral or axillary arteries.

☠   Ordinary deep Thai stomach massage is forbidden during pregnancy. Never use palm presses, butterfly presses, elbows, or forearms to work the stomach, and never work stomach pressure points with your fingers. If you wish to make contact with your client's stomach, follow the guidelines previously mentioned in this essay.

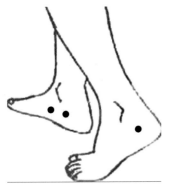

☠   Avoid pressing the point at the outside (lateral) ankle, and the two corresponding anatomical points on the inside (medial) ankle. It is best to avoid giving deep acupressure altogether on the lateral and medial ankles, since stimulation of these areas is believed in some traditions to induce labor. Gentle thumb circles on the top and bottom foot lines, as well as ankle rotations, twists, and pulls are fine.

☠   In addition to dangerous ankle-pressure points, the wrists also contain powerful points that are believed to stimulate pelvic muscles, including the uterus. Because of this, and to be safe, avoid working the pressure points on the wrists. As with the feet, working the finger lines with thumb circles, as well as rotations, pulls, finger bends, and finger cracks, is fine.

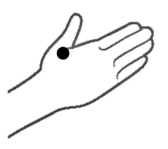

☠   Avoid pressing the point between the web of the thumb and first finger of each hand. This point is called *hegu* in Chinese acupressure. Pressing this point under normal circumstances eliminates or reduces pain, including headache, but this point should be avoided for women in any stage of pregnancy.

Final suggestions

The following suggestions may also be helpful:

- Pregnant women often feel warm, so be careful to not overheat your room.
- Pregnant women can easily become dizzy or feel faint. Having a quick source of sugar nearby, such as juice, may be a good idea.
- If your client has nausea or morning sickness, it is best to minimize rocking motions as you work.

I hope these guidelines and suggestions will be helpful for Thai therapists working with pregnant women. It's natural to be nervous the first few times you work with a pregnant client. Just remember to use common sense, to maintain your focus, to maximize your sensitivity, and to study and research the points, techniques and stretches you should always avoid. Practice safely and compassionately, and your pregnant client (and her baby) will be grateful.

Considering Body Language

BOB HADDAD

It happens quite often. A new or returning client enters your practice space, you chat a bit, and when the client lies down on your mat, she immediately and subconsciously displays body language. Your awareness and interpretation of these displays of physical, emotional, and psychological conditions can help you to carry out a successful treatment. It can also foster good relations with clients, ensuring a comfortable and protected environment within which to work. A client's body language can guide you through your work, and can help you determine what to do (and how and when to do it) during the course of a therapeutic Thai massage treatment.

This essay focuses on interpreting the body language that your clients display during a Thai massage, and working with it in an intuitive and sensitive way. My goal is to raise your awareness of elements of body language in your practice, so that you can more sensitively address your clients' needs.

The science of interpreting a person's inner feelings by observing their body language has mostly been developed by observing people engaged in business meetings, in social situations, while under stress, or in roles of responsibility, dominance, or subordination. Moreover, most studies and books on body language have made their determinations and reached their conclusions as a result of live interactions between two or more people in normal social situations. By contrast, Thai massage clients are generally at rest on a floor mat, with their eyes closed and their nervous systems in a relaxed state. How, therefore, do we apply the determinations and conclusions of body language based largely on external social stimuli to this situation? In this essay,

I propose that the usual standards of body language do not fully apply in the realm of the healing arts. I believe we must reinterpret and reapply our understanding of body language specifically in the context of our work as healers, bodyworkers, and Thai therapists.

Conventional studies and research in body language are often based on what is sometimes known as "cluster theory." In normal social contexts, body language experts look for their subjects to display not just one, but several indicators of their underlying conditions. In a police investigation, for example, when suspects are interrogated, detectives are trained to look for clusters of physical signs that could indicate that a person is lying or misrepresenting the truth. Touching a hand to the mouth or lips; not looking directly into the eyes of the questioner; increased movements in the lower body, legs, and feet; and turning the head to one side are all indications that a person may be lying.

Although cluster theory makes sense and has been proven reliable when it comes to people who actively engage with others during everyday social activities, I don't believe it has much bearing when a client comes to a therapist for Thai bodywork. For one thing, visual stimulation is largely absent from the bodywork dynamic, so this gives the receiver much less to "hide" from. Another factor is that the receiver is being touched, compressed, stretched, and moved continuously. As such, the client has much less idle time, and less reason to react in clusters of several expressions, gestures, or movements at the same time. Finally, there is little or no verbal interaction, so clients cannot show their expressions or sentiments through their voices. I am convinced that a sensitive, aware therapist can decipher meaningful information about a client simply by observing a single action, movement, expression, sound, or physical display.

Indicators of physical conditions

Although conventional body language research is based mostly on social, emotional, and psychological factors, bodywork clients also display indicators that point to specific physical conditions. Accomplished therapists should be aware of both types of body language, and should assess and explore them based on individual determinations that are reached during the course of the client-therapist relationship.

It can be important to look for indicators of physical conditions when working with new clients. Therapists get to know their clients' bodies over a period of time, not just in the first session. In pre-session consultations, we discuss health history, and we learn about prior accidents and surgeries. As we get to know a client's body and energy during the first few sessions, we learn more about underlying physical conditions and restrictions that may result in physical manifestations.

As soon as a client lies down in supine position, for example, if one hand rests comfortably on the mat with the palm facing upward, but the other hand is rotated slightly inward, then this may indicate a physical problem on the inwardly rotated arm. The same could be true if you notice asymmetrical positioning of the feet, legs, shoulders, arms, or other body parts. Though much of the information in this article addresses subconscious psychological indicators, therapists must also take into consideration those bodily manifestations that are caused by underlying physical conditions.

Body language on the mat

Body language is an important determinant of the overall state of a client, and it's important for therapists to watch for signs that may signal possible underlying conditions. Maintaining this awareness as we work allows us to develop into more sensitive therapists, and it helps us to determine what we should and shouldn't do during a Thai massage treatment. If we exist as therapists to serve our clients within their needs, then in addition to knowing their physical bodies, we must be aware of their fears, apprehensions, and concerns, so that we can allay them as best as possible and work with each client within his or her limitations. After all, a successful Thai treatment should not be an imposition of our agenda onto another person. We should always work *with* our clients, not *on* them. Awareness of clients' body language can guide us through even the most difficult sessions, and can allow us to work in accordance with each person's physical, emotional, psychological, and spiritual needs.

Though I've studied conventional types of body language, I haven't found any in-depth information on body language within the context of traditional Thai massage or other forms of bodywork. This is a pity, because if professional therapists were trained to recognize displays of potential stress, fear, discomfort, and pain, they could more adequately and more sensitively attend to their clients' needs. As a result of working with many clients over the years, I've come to some conclusions that have been helpful in my professional practice, and I'd like to share some of them here.

Initial visual assessment

An initial visual assessment based on physical manifestations is important in order to gauge the overall state of the client. Since traditional Thai massage usually begins with the client in supine position, therapists have a chance to view the entire anterior body at one time. Soon after a client lies down, their eyes generally remain closed for a long period of time. This gives the therapist an opportunity to continually and discreetly scan the front of the body for clues and suggestions about the client's overall condition. If you are not currently doing this in your practice, I suggest you start doing so. A few seconds of time spent in this way can sometimes provide valuable information that can guide you and sustain you through the entire session. Here are some things to look for as soon as your client lies down on your mat.

Upward or downward palms

Upward facing palms generally means the client is receptive to the work and open minded and positive about the process and potential outcome of the session. Downward palms can suggest the opposite.

Distance of the arms from the torso

If the client's inner arms are away from his sides, it generally indicates a sense of ease and openness. If they are placed close to the body, it could denote holding, tension, or a protection mechanism of some sort. If the client's forearms are on their sides, with palms facing inward and touching the sides of the body, it could suggest concern, fear, and apprehension.

Distance of the legs from each other

While in a state of relaxation, most people lie on their back with their legs at a comfortable distance from each other. Naturally, the distance depends on the relative size and dimensions of each individual, but if you notice that both legs seem unnaturally close, or are touching each other, it may indicate something on a deeper level.

Breathing patterns

Maintaining awareness of your client's breathing is extremely important, as it can help to determine the course of treatment and types of techniques that may be used during a given session. Someone at ease will generally breathe in a calm, deep manner, with a gentle rising and falling of the abdomen, and a short period of rest in between each exhalation and inhalation. Shallow breathing may indicate a blockage in the stomach and the chest, and if this is the case you may be guided to work more extensively in those areas. Quick, short breaths may indicate nervousness or fear, or they may be physical symptoms of shortness of breath.

Now let's look more closely at individual body parts, and ways in which they may suggest certain physical, emotional, and psychological states.

The face

In Thai massage and most other forms of bodywork, the face reveals considerably less emotion than usual because the eyes remain closed during treatment.

Even with the eyes closed, however, pursing of the lips or tightening of the facial muscles can indicate pain or discomfort, and flaring or slight twitching of the nostrils or lips often suggests that an emotional response is very near. Be cautious, get ready to lessen your pressure, and be supportive and compassionate if you notice any of these displays.

The forehead

Clients can involuntarily wrinkle the brow in response to sensations or emotions such as surprise, fear, pain, or some form of concern. A forehead will often rise straight up toward the scalp if the emotion that surfaces is surprise. Fear, pain, and grief, however, are usually manifested by a wrinkle that engages the muscle between the brows, and pulls it inward toward the nose. The muscles near the temples also move inward toward the nose. People under high stress will often massage the area between the eyes, at the bridge of the nose. They may also rub the third eye in circular fashion with two or three fingers, or press it and then spread their fingers laterally – the thumb to one side and the index and third finger to the other side. This same gesture often indicates a tension headache.

The head

Very few emotions or sensations are displayed with the head when a person is in a static relaxed position. In social body language, many head expressions are also tied to eye movement, and since in massage, the eyes are generally closed, fewer head movements are displayed. Nevertheless, a raised chin, especially if it's accompanied by a forehead wrinkle, could indicate pain or discomfort. Also, when a therapist applies broad pressure to the shoulders, or works the neck or shoulder lines, clients may move their heads from side to side as they attempt to release their own tension in counterbalance to the therapist's pressure.

The hands

Placement of the hands on top of and near various body parts can indicate fear, protection, and other concerns. When hands cover areas of the body, the gesture can indicate a barrier, and a "do not enter" sign to the therapist. In all cases of crossed hands and crossed feet and legs, a therapist should take extreme care to not break through those areas in ways that could startle the client or make him feel uncomfortable. Doing so could jeopardize the cultivation of trust that is necessary in order to facilitate healing.

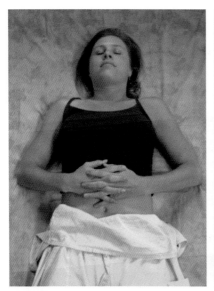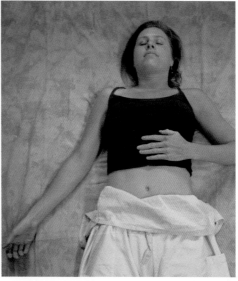

(left) No need to open the hands right away

(right) Be careful as you approach the stomach

Folded and clasped hands

Hands that are folded and placed on top of the stomach can be a signal of protection. When you encounter folded or clasped hands, a good rule to follow is to not unfold them quickly or unexpectedly. If you can work relatively well for a while without uncovering the hands, do so. Folded or clasped hands near the genital area should be taken seriously within the context of bodywork, since this gesture may indicate sexual trauma of some kind. In this case, extreme care must be used when approaching the inner legs with your hands or with any other part of your body.

Regardless of where hands are placed, once a client feels more comfortable, and a level of trust is established, they may unclasp their hands on their own. And if they don't, you always have the option to ask them to do so, or to ask them if you can do so. On the other hand, you may choose to simply take note of their positioning and not touch them there or work in that area at all. In many cases, heeding a "do not enter" sign is the best way to gain your clients' confidence and trust. It's often best to work within the needs and restrictions of the particular person on the mat at that moment in time. Once a safe healing environment is established, fears may diminish and signs of protection may disappear.

Closed hands and clenched fists

Some clients exhibit closed hands – and more rarely, clenched fists – when they are lying on the mat in supine position. One or two closed or clenched hands can indicate different feelings, and the reasons are difficult to determine within the context of a session. For the most part, however, a closed hand or a clenched fist can indicate some sort of resistance, defensiveness, or determination. If you notice a closed hand or fist as you begin working in supine position, take note of it and develop a strategy to slowly move toward that arm somehow, so you can naturally take hold of it, as you would during the process of a regular Thai massage movement.

If, for example, you notice that one hand is more closed than another, you might wait until you begin to work on the upper lateral leg on the same side of the body. As you approach that upper leg, you would have to grab hold of the client's hand in order to open their arm so that you can begin your leg line work. Once you grab their hand to open their arm, this could be a perfect time to explore the hand a bit, to gently massage it, stretch the fingers, rotate the wrist, and press into the palm. Try to release the tension in a flowing, organic way before you bring the arm back to the mat and begin your leg work. Very often, even the slightest touch to an area that is holding tension will bring about an opening.

A slow and natural approach to closed or protected areas of the body is almost always the best strategy. Rather than targeting a particular area by singling it out and working on it aggressively, always try to approach the afflicted area organically and within the context of the whole body. Take time to work the general area around an afflicted spot, instead of jumping right onto the target.

Palms

Palms are very good indicators of a client's openness and disposition. For the most part, palms that are open and turned upward indicate openness and receptiveness to the work. They may also indicate that the client feels comfortable in your presence, and that they don't feel threatened or intimidated in any way. Palms that face inward and upward signal that the arm muscles are not engaged, as they must be when they are positioned downward or outward. From an energy perspective, open and upwardly turned palms allow healing energy to enter the human system more easily, since the very act of turning palms upward results in an internal energy shift. Anyone who works in energy healing knows this.

Try it for yourself. Stand or sit and extend your arms and hands outward with your palms facing downward toward the ground. Now bring all your attention to your hands, and take note of the feelings, sensations, and energies you have there. Now, while focusing your attention on your hands, rotate them outward so that your palms face upward. You should immediately feel different sensations of lightness and openness that you didn't have when your palms were facing downward.

On the Thai massage mat, upward palms can signal openness, receptivity, and non-threatening or submissive energy. Downward-facing palms may indicate defiance, being closed to the work, or they may even suggest a sense of authority or superiority. Submissive, trusting dogs who want to be touched reveal their throats. Humans show their palms. This is not to say, however, that every time you see downward facing palms you should assume the client is closed to your work. Some people's anatomy is such that their arms and wrists are in a relaxed state when their palms are slightly pointed inward, or even if their arms and hands are on their sides, with thumbs facing upward. In addition, women's arms anatomically rotate outward more easily, while men's rotate slightly more inward.

If you have a client with downward-facing palms, take note but begin your work without moving them. You will have plenty of time to investigate the arms and hands when you address them during the course of the session. In many cases, after you work an arm with compressions, palming, and thumbing, the hand will open, palm upward, when you release the arm to the mat.

Self-touching
A client who rubs his fingers together, usually the thumb and index finger, may be engaging in self-comforting. It's the same if he uses one or more fingers to gently rub or caress a part of his body such as a leg, the chest, or the heart area. Take note of these gestures, but don't stop them. Your client may simply be adjusting to your work by comforting himself, and this will allow him to go deeper in the session and to open up more fully to the healing process.

The arms

Body language with arms often involves draping one arm over the body, holding an arm or wrist with the other hand, or gripping one or both elbows with the hands. While these gestures may have different subtle meanings, they almost always indicate some sort of protection or barrier.

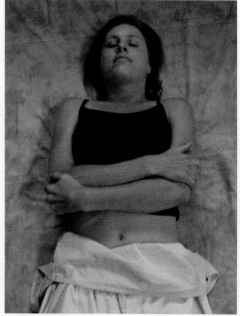

A rare double arm grip. Avoid the mid section, be patient, and work slowly.

Partial arm-cross, self-hugging
In clinical body language, a partial arm-cross, where one arm drapes across the body in order to lightly touch the opposite side of the body or grasp the other arm, is often viewed as a type of self-hugging mechanism. It can indicate that the person is fearful of your work and that she is trying to console herself. This act of self-comforting and self-assurance may further indicate that she is engaging in a process of establishing trust in you as the therapist. Because of this, don't stop or invade that process by quickly unhooking her arms. As always in these types of situations, a slow, organic, compassionate approach is best.

Arm-gripping

When one hand is firmly gripping the other arm, or when both arms are folded together across the chest, a firm barrier is being placed between you and the client. It is a defensive posture, and in addition to being a sign of "no entry" between you and the client's chest, breasts, or heart area, it could also indicate negativity or doubt about the session itself. Though it is rarely seen on the mat, a double arm-grip, where both hands grip the opposite elbows or upper arms, is a very strong statement, and serious thought should be given about how (or if) to approach the client in the area being protected.

The legs

For the most part, clients know that a therapist needs to work on the feet and legs, and that in order to do so, they must be uncrossed and somewhat open. If a client lies down and immediately crosses her legs or places her feet so close together that you need to open them wider in order to work, you've got a situation that needs addressing fairly quickly.

Crossed legs and feet can indicate general protection of the medial legs and the entire inner area of the lower torso. In some cases, it can be a subconscious protective device resulting from sexual abuse. A gentle way to diffuse this type of posture is to let the client know that you will now be holding and moving her legs. Rather than quickly and forcibly opening the legs on the mat, you might try putting both feet in your hands and gently moving both legs together. Double leg movements such as gentle rotations, rocking from side to side, and forward compressions can help to diffuse barriers, warm up the lateral leg lines and hips, and bring about more comfort and ease. In most cases, the legs will release their tension and the feet will relax. When they do, you can open the legs while still holding them aloft and repeat the rocking and rotation movements with one leg at a time. After a few minutes of working like this, when you return the legs to the mat, they will almost certainly be more relaxed and will probably rest comfortably on the mat at a reasonable distance from each other.

The feet

In supine position, clients will sometimes jiggle a foot repeatedly for a few seconds and then stop and start again. When you see this, it is often a sign of nervous energy. Jiggling the feet can also mean that the person subconsciously wants to run away from what is being experienced. Try to imagine how you could work with that person in a way that would help to calm and dissipate that energy. Visualize where the nervous energy that is exiting at the foot may be stored. It may be in the upper lateral leg, for example. If this is the case, gentle, persistent work there could uncover tense muscles, a pocket of stress, or an energy blockage. Foot jiggling can also indicate that a client is bored, and if this is the case, it will stop as you progress through the session with new techniques.

Watch for dorsiflexion of the feet when you work on the feet and ankles. Some people will flex their feet upward when you hold or lift their feet or lower legs. This could be a defensive posture if the client is afraid of feeling pain in this area, or it could mean that they are trying to "help" you. Curling of the toes is often an expression of fear or protection. Be aware that these are usually involuntary reactions, so try to not become frustrated with clients who react this way. Send metta to them, and be patient and compassionate. Work these areas gently but firmly with rotations, compressions, and line work on the anterior and posterior feet. You can bend the toes backward, apply acupressure to the webbing between the toes, and crack their toe knuckles, too.

If a client keeps his feet very close together in supine position at the beginning of a session, consider making physical contact with their lateral legs first, perhaps by doing some palming and thumbing on the outside leg lines. After a while, and once the client feels comfortable with your touch, his feet and legs may open more naturally.

Body language awareness

I hope that these ideas about body language within the context of therapeutic touch will be helpful to the Thai massage community. I believe that awareness of body language in clients is an invaluable tool for all professional bodyworkers. The safest way to address clients' fears and barriers, and the best way to win their confidence and trust, is to work with respect, compassion, and patience.

Remember to take a moment to visually assess your client before you even touch them, and be aware of body language during each session. Observe the body's physical placement and relative symmetry, scan for possible indicators of underlying psychological conditions, and take note of breathing patterns. Your impressions and intuition can serve as tools to guide you through each session, and can allow you to be as sensitive as possible to each client's needs.

When you see a display of body language that suggests "no entry," it's best to not abruptly break your way through that protection zone. Doing so can result in further alienation. First, try to work around those areas, whenever possible, and see if they gradually open up by themselves with your touch. Remember that it's always best for a client to surrender to his own process of self-healing, rather than feel invaded or forced open by a therapist. When and if it becomes absolutely necessary to uncross an arm, or to move a hand from the heart area, or to unclasp two hands from over the stomach, you have several options. You may ask permission to do so; you may softly announce that you will soon be doing so; or you may gradually approach the protection zone by slowly working up to it from a nearby part of the body.

When we work with compassion and patience, we respect the individual before us on the mat, we break away from self-imposed constructs of what we think that person needs, and we encourage the session to unfold with the loving-kindness that is so essential to traditional Thai massage.

Breath and Body Mechanics in Nuad Boran

BOB HADDAD

My intention in writing this essay is to describe elements of body mechanics, ergonomics, and breathwork that I have found to be essential for a professional Thai massage practice. The concepts are presented as guidelines to help Thai therapists in their work with clients, and to serve as a source of inspiration for deeper work in *nuad boran*.

Spiritual and meditative elements of traditional Thai massage

Before we deal with breath and body mechanics, let's stop for a minute and take into consideration the extraphysical aspects of nuad boran. From the Eastern perspective, the human body not only houses muscles, tissues, bones, and fluids but also contains an invisible energy force. In Thai healing arts (and in most non-Western modalities), the body may be used as a vehicle to the inner self. In a deep, focused Thai massage treatment, healing can take place in a way that is not entirely dependent on physical laws or methods. Change can also take place within our energy bodies. With all this in mind, it's helpful to stay aware of the spiritual manifestations of healing that take place during and after a Thai session.

The practice of *metta* (loving-kindness and compassion toward others) is an important spiritual focal point for the Thai therapist while engaged in his work. It's also helpful for the client to feel at peace during the session, and to engage in mindfulness, awareness of breath, and meditation. During the first few minutes of a Thai session (especially with a new client), the therapist may check in with the client to see if his pressure is appropriate and if the client is comfortable. Once a flow is established, however, it is often best if both the practitioner and client "go inward" to their spiritual centers, remaining mostly silent, focusing on breath, and being aware of each moment as the session unfolds. Generally speaking, the more "floppy" the receiver is (in both a physical and a metaphysical sense), the deeper the effect of a traditional Thai healing session will be.

Those who have experienced any form of meditation may think of nuad boran as a type of meditation in movement. As stray thoughts enter your consciousness, note them, but try to not dwell on them. Allow them to drift freely in and out of your mind without significantly affecting your focus on breath and presence. Maintain awareness, do your work, but also surrender to the client's process of self-healing, to which you are merely a witness.

Breathwork

Breathing is an involuntary process, but in order to perform Thai massage to maximum efficiency, especially when using techniques that require body movement, you should maintain breath awareness. Your clients will achieve optimal response from compressions, stretches, and sen line work when they are breathing calmly and deeply. The Thai therapist should also breathe calmly and deeply in accordance with all movements.

Whenever you begin a session, take some time to focus on your client's breathing patterns, and regulate your own breathing so that you are in tune with her body. From time to time during the session, look at the rise and fall of your client's abdomen, so that you know when to apply your movements.

Synchronized breathing is when both you and your client inhale or exhale at the same time. *Oppositional breathing* is when one person inhales and the other person exhales. Both types of breathing may be employed in a typical Thai session. It's important, however, to learn which moves require synchronized breathing and which ones work best with oppositional breathing. This knowledge comes with a lot of practice, and by being fully aware from one moment to the next during a session.

Under no circumstances should you ever hold your breath when exerting pressure, lifting, pulling, or executing any other Thai techniques. In general, your clients should be exhaling as you apply pressure to them or when you dramatically move their bodies from one position to another, and they should inhale when you release the pressure or return them to the starting position. Whether or not you are breathing with, or in opposition to the client depends on a number of factors.

Synchronized breathing

Use synchronized breathing when you work the abdomen, perform palm presses to the legs or back, work *sen* lines on the back, and do compressions on the chest. In general, techniques that are mostly carried out with both parties in close proximity to each other work best with synchronized breathing.

If you and your client have similar breathing rates, they can be synchronized easily. If your client takes quicker breaths than you, you can time your moves to every second breath your client takes. If you get lost, or if you find it hard to establish the breathing rhythm that you need, take a moment to relax, take note of your client's breathing rate, and adjust your breath in a way that will allow both of you to be as comfortable as possible as you proceed through the session.

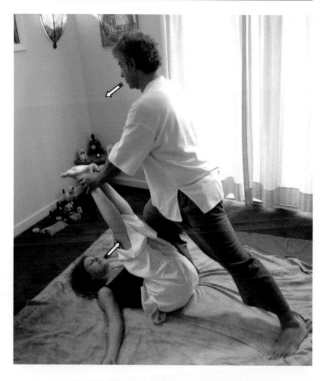

An example of synchronized breathing

Let's apply this information, combined with good body mechanics, in order to execute a plow using synchronized breathing, as illustrated in the photo.

The photo demonstrates a simple assisted plow. But to an experienced Thai therapist, there is much more going on beneath the surface of the technique. To begin, the therapist should inhale as he lifts the client's legs into a straight position of approximately 90 degrees with one graceful movement. (If the extended legs don't reach 90 degrees, stop where you feel they have reached their maximum point of comfort.) Now the therapist places his feet and legs in a position with good body mechanics, with his outside lower leg guiding one side of the client's waist, so the client doesn't wiggle from left to right in the pose. The therapist takes note of the client's breath and establishes synchronized breathing – when the client inhales, so does the therapist. Then on a mutual exhale, the therapist lunges forward slowly, with elbows locked and arms straight, to the first point of resistance.

The client's body energy will tell you where to stop. Be sensitive and try to not go beyond the client's first point of resistance. Stop there, allow for a mutual inhale, and then push forward one or two more times until you reach the maximum depth that is comfortable for your client. With each movement forward, make sure you are both exhaling. With each movement backward, even slight ones, make sure you are both inhaling. Then, when you are ready to end the pose and release into supine or starting position, do so on a mutual inhale.

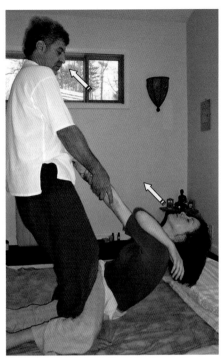

An example of oppositional breathing

Oppositional breathing

Oppositional breathing is when the client and therapist are breathing in opposition to each other. This type of breathing pattern is beneficial for certain movements and techniques that require strength and focus on the part of the therapist, and relaxation (openness) on the part of the client.

For example, when the therapist executes cobras, suspensions, and other lifting postures on another person, the receiver should exhale as she is being brought into position. The therapist, however, should inhale as he lifts her into position, because the increased oxygen to his body will give him more strength as he engages his core muscles and moves his own body.

In addition to assisted cobras, other Thai yoga techniques that can benefit from oppositional breathing are arm lifts in supine and side position, back lifts, cross-leg crunches (the Thai technique that is often used to bring a client into sitting position), and most types of suspensions and inversions.

The concept of oppositional breathing is simple enough to understand, but there is something else to consider. Many techniques that benefit from oppositional breathing while getting into a pose often work best with synchronized breathing as you get out of the pose.

Let's take a simple assisted cobra as an example. As the client is being pulled back into position, the therapist is inhaling and the client is exhaling. But once in position, and after a few breaths, the therapist should synchronize his breathing with the client's breath, so that they are both exhaling when it's time to release the client to the mat. So whether performing a cobra or a suspended spinal twist as in the photo, the client is pulled into position using oppositional breathing (client exhales while therapist inhales), but she is lowered back to the mat using synchronized breathing (both people exhale).

It's not as complicated as it seems, and once you practice this method of breathing, it will make your work easier and more enjoyable. Take some time to consider using oppositional breathing in your practice for certain poses and techniques. And remember to synchronize on a mutual exhale when you release or return to starting position.

Be aware of your client's breath

Occasionally you may wish to remind your client to take a deep breath, and then wait for their exhale to begin or continue the next technique. For the most part, your role as Thai therapist is to coordinate your movements in accordance with your client's breathing patterns. Sometimes this means waiting for your client to inhale or exhale before you begin a new move. Do not repeatedly ask the client to control her breathing, as this will distract her, and take away from her ability to fully relax during the session. Be patient, allow your client to feel comfortable, and remember to direct metta toward your client as you work.

Body mechanics

Proper body mechanics are of utmost importance in a Thai yoga therapy session. The practitioner should maintain awareness of his own body alignment and also that of his client. If a client becomes sprawled in an anatomically incorrect position, take the time to realign the client's body before continuing the session.

Most importantly, be aware of the way in which you apply pressure to your client's body. When you use your bodyweight (and not your muscle strength) to compress, pull, and stretch, you give the client a more relaxing massage, and you save wear and tear on your own body.

Some ergonomic guidelines for your Thai practice

- Always ground yourself from your *hara*, the area slightly below your navel, and let that area be the very center of all your movements.
- Keep your movement confined to what is within your reach, and take care to not hyperextend your body (or your client's body) while executing postures and techniques.
- Always keep your spine straight and your head in straight-ahead alignment. Avoid curving your back forward while lifting. Keep your arms straight when pulling and compressing.
- Remember to inhale when exerting pressure or lifting. Never hold your breath. Always be aware of the receiver's breath patterns, and encourage deep and relaxed breathing when necessary. Try to time your moves in accordance with the receiver's inhalations and exhalations.
- Allow for short moments of rest when appropriate, and allow the client time to transition from one position to the next, especially after deeper postures.

Use your bodyweight whenever possible

Nuad boran is a healing modality that allows therapists to work at an appropriate level for each client. A Thai session can be relatively effortless once the therapist learns to use bodyweight and gravity efficiently.

Let's take a traditional Thai shoulder press as an example. The client is in sitting position, and the therapist lightly supports the client's back with his legs, as he presses downward onto the client's shoulders with his palms. To use body weight effectively in this technique, the therapist's elbows should be locked, his arms and back straight, and the fleshy part of his palms should make contact with the receiver's shoulder muscles. The therapist's energy originates in his hara, runs through his entire body, and exits at his hands as he sinks his weight downward toward the mat.

Whether making contact with your hands, feet, elbows, or knees, use gravity, not muscles. Never rely on muscle power or arm strength. If at any point during a session you find yourself using your muscles, immediately stop and try it a different way. Remember to always keep your shoulders relaxed, and to exhale as you apply pressure.

Work from your center

As you work in nuad boran, try to initiate all body movements from your core, or center. Your center is in your lower abdomen, approximately two finger widths below your navel. To find the center point of your energy and grounding, engage your core muscles, and move your upper torso from left to right and front and back. This balance point is where all your movements should originate.

When you work, keep your arms straight but not rigid, and keep your shoulders relaxed. When you execute movements, allow your hands and feet to become extensions of your hara. Every small movement in your hara should transfer energy to the parts of your body that you are using at that moment. For the most part, whenever you bend your elbows or work from your shoulders downward, you are breaking the connection with your hara. This almost always results in inferior work for you and for your client, and it causes your shoulders and arms to work harder than necessary. Over time, this lack of ergonomic awareness can lead to long-term bodily stress and even injury.

Try to always tune in to your clients' bodies and work in accordance with their breathing patterns. Try to bypass your brain when working with clients. Too much thinking almost always lessens sensitivity and intuition. When you are tuned in to the energy and the body of your client, you can better gauge what type of pressure is best, how to pace your work, and when and where to give more attention.

With straight arms and relaxed shoulders, your arms, hands, legs, feet, and entire body can move as extensions of your hara. Allow yourself to be drawn in to your clients' bodies, to the exact depth that is needed, so you can work *with* them rather than performing Thai massage *on* them.

Maintain rocking or alternating movements whenever possible

To ensure a Thai massage session that is less strenuous for the practitioner and more meditative for both parties, you should rock as you work. By rocking, the practitioner's bodyweight is transferred to the client in a uniform and comforting way. Your rhythm should be repetitive but not mechanical, and there should be periods of stasis (rest), when you are applying pressure. Instead of using your muscles, rocking movements allow your energy to pass from your core and sacral area onto the body of your client, and help to keep you anchored and focused as you work. There are three general ways to rock during the course of a Thai therapy session, and variations of each one of these movements may be explored during the course of a Thai healing session.

Side-to-side movements

With side-to-side rocking, the practitioner is usually kneeling or semi-kneeling. In some cases you can also be in Thai sitting position, with one leg folded inward and the other bent outward.

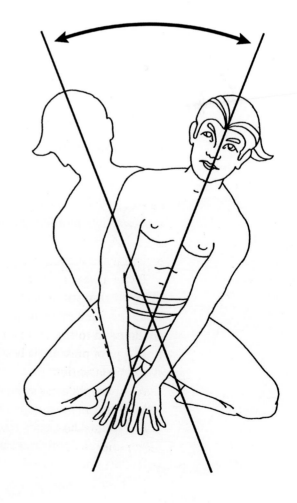

If you are kneeling, you may open your legs and bring your feet together behind you to form a solid base. The tops of your toes should rest against the floor, but you may occasionally bend them backward in tip-toe position. Keep your head and your spine straight. Straighten your arms and move your trunk on its axis from one side to the other, like a stalk of bamboo in the wind.

Examples of Thai techniques that lend themselves to side-to-side rocking include:

Supine position: alternating foot palming, alternating lower leg palming, working inner thighs with your feet, working the shoulders with your feet;

Sitting position: shoulder rolls with forearm, side-to-side mobilization of the head;

Prone position: forearm rolls on the back, with client's leg above your lap; and

Side position: working leg lines, thumbing and palming back lines, thumbing hip pressure points.

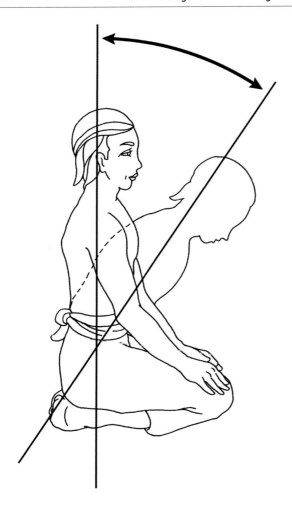

Front-to-back movements

With front-to-back rocking, the practitioner is usually kneeling, although some techniques may be applied with this type of rocking in semi-kneeling and standing position. When kneeling, your knees may be together or apart, but keep the tops of your feet against the floor to get a wide range of motion. If you are half-kneeling, make a steady lunging movement forward and backward. If you are standing, place one leg ahead of the other and lunge forward in a *t'ai chi* type of movement. Keep your back straight and your sacrum relaxed but strong. Oscillate the torso from front to back, like a rocking chair.

Examples of Thai techniques that lend themselves to front-to-back rocking are:

Supine position: Foot and leg compressions and pulls, foot and leg palming, butterfly presses and palming on thighs, most types of plows;

Sitting position: Shoulder stretches, backward arm pulls;

Prone position: cross leg presses, palming, butterfly pressing and thumbing back lines, cobras;

Side position: working back lines with your feet; and

Child's pose position: sacral compressions, working back lines.

Circular or spiral movements

With circular rocking, the practitioner is usually kneeling or semi-kneeling. Keep the same ergonomic posture as in the above examples, and allow yourself to slowly gyrate in a spiral movement. Circular movement doesn't have to be exaggerated in order to be effective. Sometimes, even the slightest circular movement can transfer a sense of peace and comfort to your client. The direction can be clockwise or counter-clockwise, and the range of your movement can be tight or wide, depending on the Thai technique you are using and the size of your client's body relative to your own body. Try to not get stuck rotating in one direction, and vary the rotations from clockwise to counter-clockwise. This can be helpful to fully relax the client.

Examples of Thai techniques that lend themselves to spiral rocking are:

Supine position: Hip and leg rotations, ankle and wrist rotations, palming knees, working the neck;

Sitting position: back mobilization with client's hands behind head, neck mobilization;

Prone position: gentle spirals in cobra position; and

Side position: hip openings, arm mobilizations, backward arm stretches.

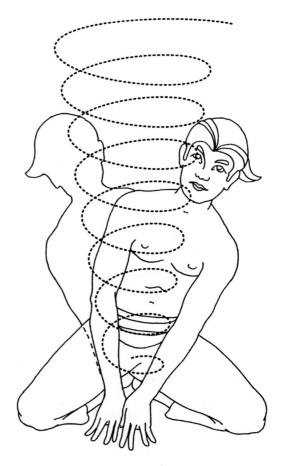

Work only within your reach and move your body positioning

When you work in Thai massage, it's important to stay as physically close to your client as possible. Physical proximity helps to maximize the use of your bodyweight, and it helps to keep your hara connected to the parts of your body that make contact with your client.

Don't stretch or reach too far when you work. When using your arms and hands to apply pressure, transfer your weight first to your shoulders, then to your arms and then out to your hands. Keep your shoulders straight but relaxed and then lean inward or downward.

Work only within your reach. A good way to determine the maximum range of your working area is to draw an imaginary arc with your finger on the floor (or above the client) ahead of you. Try it now. Imagine yourself, for example, working in supine position, doing some foot palming. You are kneeling and sitting back on your heels. Now fully extend an arm with a pointed index finger, and draw an arc beginning on one side of your waist and ending on the other side, in a half circle. Whether you are sitting back on your feet, or moving upward on your shins, or working from an even higher position on your knees, this arc is the maximum area in which you can safely work without having to radically change your body positioning.

Move your body throughout the course of a Thai massage session, so that you are close to the area you are treating. Try to stay directly on top of (or in front of) that particular area in order to apply your pressure as effortlessly and effectively as possible.

Don't overextend yourself. If you're uncomfortable with a technique or a sequence that you learned, and if it just doesn't feel right for you, then don't do it! Think of other ways to treat that area that would be less taxing on your body. And if you can't do that, then simply eliminate the move from your routine or sequence.

Protect your elbows, wrists, and thumbs

When performing butterfly palm presses, whether on the shoulders, or on the thighs or the back, keep the inner parts of your elbows facing each other, with the creases of your arms facing slightly forward.

Always keep your wrists at a comfortable angle. Maintain your bodyweight directly over your arms, and lean in to apply downward pressure. A comfortable angle should be around 80 degrees. Working beyond that angle may pinch nerves in your wrists or overstretch your ligaments.

Keep your arm rotation comfortable and sustainable. Shift the orientation of your body, whenever necessary, to keep your arms in a more comfortable position and to reposition your bodyweight.

When you're palm pressing, direct energy through your shoulders and arms into the heel of your hand, and then spread the pressure throughout the palm of your hand to broaden and soften the contact. If you direct the pressure to your hand without broadening it through your palm, it may feel intrusive and sharp to your client. Failure to spread the pressure can also result in injury to your wrists.

When you work the sen lines with thumb pressing, use the pads of your thumbs, about halfway between the top joint and the tip. Using thumb tips can result in a sharp or intense feeling for your clients. If your thumbs don't easily bend backward at the first joint, try to use less pressure at the tips, and spread the pressure inward toward the palm. Visualize the spreading of energy through the pads of your thumbs as you work.

When you are palm pressing, especially on the upper legs, keep your thumbs close to your other fingers, so they aren't isolated and vulnerable to injury. This is also a practical way to avoid coming too close to private areas between the legs.

Remember to keep your arms straight, your shoulders relaxed, and your elbows locked, whenever possible. Move from your hara, keep your back straight, and use gravity (not muscle strength) to apply pressure through your hands.

Keep your spine straight and your chest open

Always keep your spine in proper alignment, neither too rigid nor too loose. By engaging your core muscles as you move, you protect your lower back. This is especially true when foot-pressing thighs in supine or side position and when working the lower back.

Remember to keep your head up and your neck aligned with your spine. Eliminate or modify any moves that require you to bend forward while rounding your spine, whether from a standing or a sitting position.

If you need to bend forward, bend from your hips, and engage your hara before you exert pressure. For moves that require you to pick up your client's feet for a stretch, first kneel or squat as you grab their feet, then straighten your knees as you inhale and come to a standing position. Use the same strategy when you lift your client's back off the mat for a stretch. Keep your back straight and always inhale as you move into a more erect position.

Focus on the space between your shoulder blades. Keep your chest open, and your shoulders lowered and relaxed whenever possible. Correct posture helps to prevent kyphosis (rounding of the spine) and minimizes back strain and rotator cuff problems.

If you catch yourself drooping, slouching, raising your shoulders, or leaning forward, immediately straighten your back, take a deep breath, and continue your work. If you are unable to adapt your body to proper mechanics, discontinue those techniques from your repertoire that cause you to strain your body.

Keep hips and shoulders aligned

Keep your hips and shoulders in alignment

Keep your hips and shoulders facing in the same direction, and always try to move them together.

When executing spinal twists, such as the one in the photo, make sure to swivel your entire body from the hips upward, even if you keep your knee stiff against the client's thigh for stability. Work with synchronized breath, moving as you and your client exhale, and releasing or returning as you both inhale.

As a general rule, never apply pressure through your arms or legs if your hips are facing in another direction. Whenever you catch yourself doing this, immediately modify the movement by adjusting your body (or your client's body) into a posture with better alignment.

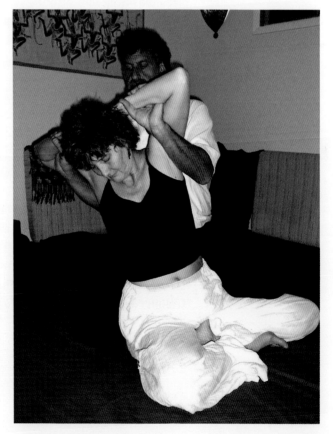

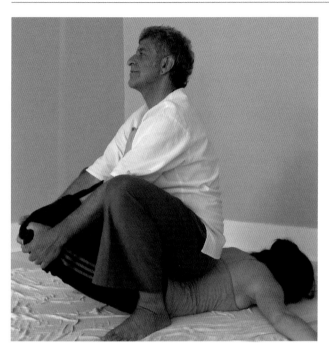

Support your
bodyweight

Support your own bodyweight

It's always best to support your own weight when working with your clients. If you allow your weight to transfer entirely to a client's body, you increase the risk of slipping, losing your balance, or hurting the client. It's generally more comfortable for your client to feel pressure only at the point of contact. Always be aware of the risks involved, especially with poses involving balance and suspension. Whenever you can, make modifications to poses, so you maintain a maximum amount of control and safety. If it feels unsafe, it probably is.

A few common Thai massage techniques that require the therapist to have good balance and to support his own bodyweight are: using feet to step on clients' legs in prone position; foot walking (stepping on feet); most types of gate openings ("blood stops"); and working back lines while sitting on the client's feet in prone position.

Let's take the example in the photo. The therapist's bodyweight is supported by his legs while he is squatting on the client's lower back and sacrum. The amount of weight that should be distributed is determined by the relative weights and sizes of the people involved. In this particular pose, since the therapist is larger and heavier than the client, he might apply only 30 percent of his bodyweight onto the client while supporting about 70 percent of his weight with his legs. If the roles were reversed, and if she were working on him, she would probably need to use 50 percent or 60 percent of her bodyweight to hold him against the mat while she executed this posture. The same would be true if she were opening wind gates at the femoral artery. A smaller person using palms, knees, or forearms to work these areas on a larger person needs to give more of her energy/weight.

By the way, keeping in mind what we discussed earlier about breathing techniques, which type of breathing might work best for the technique in the photo? That's right, oppositional breathing, with a synchronized ending!

Closing thoughts

In this essay, I've tried to describe some basic skills and concepts related to breath and body mechanics in traditional Thai massage. The concepts are fairly easy to grasp, but they require lots of practice before graceful mastery can be attained. Practice them first on your friends until you feel ready to integrate them in your work with clients. Try different ways of breathing that work best for you. Keep your back straight, and use your bodyweight not your muscle power. Practice safe. Practice happy.

Luk Pra Kob:
The Art of Thai
Herbal Compresses

BY BOB HADDAD

Most courses in traditional Thai massage focus on the execution of assisted stretches, acupressure, and a very basic discussion of *sen* line theory. If students are lucky enough to learn from an experienced teacher, they may also receive instruction about proper body mechanics, breathwork, and a general sense of how to flow gracefully from one technique to the next. But in most courses of study, even those that last for many months, the use of Thai herbal compresses is often overlooked or underemphasized.

After several years of studying *nuad boran* with a number of teachers and schools in Thailand and in the West, I was finally exposed to the wonders of *luk pra kob*. After a few months of rudimentary practice, I sought out teachers who used compresses in their treatments, and I began to experiment with different herbal mixes, wrappers, and application styles, but I had no idea how deeply this work would affect my practice.

Luk pra kob (or "Thai herbal balls" as they are sometimes called) can be purchased pre-made, or you can choose to make them yourself. If you live in a region where dry and fresh herbs cannot be purchased or easily shipped to you, you may have no alternative but to use the pre-made kind. Most commercially available pre-made herbal balls are imported from Thailand, and are made of dried herbs and rhizomes. They are wrapped in cheesecloth and have a distinctive long handle made of cloth, tied with cotton string or with thin strips of bamboo. In Thailand, however, many healers don't use pre-made luk pra kob, but prefer instead to make their own compresses from fresh herbs and rhizomes, as well as dried materials.

There are distinct advantages to preparing your own compresses. You can choose the quantities and types of herbal materials you want for each compress; you can use fresh, rather than only dried materials; and you can modify the ingredients of a compress for a particular client based on a specific physical condition, or perhaps to create a certain olfactory mood. In addition, you may direct your healing energy into an herbal compress as you prepare it for an individual client. Finally, your client may take home the compress after the session and use it as an herbal bath infusion. For these and other reasons, I choose to make my own herbal compresses.

Traditional Thai compresses have longer handles, requiring the compress to be held with a closed fist in vertical position, with the thumb on top. Rather than preparing compresses with long handles bound with string, I make them with shorter, rounded handles that fit more securely in the hand. The more rounded shape allows a therapist to hold it more securely and to use the compress with a greater degree of control. Because of the lack of a long handle, a small dry washcloth is needed to hold the top of the compress when it gets hot.

One of my teachers once showed me a method of placing herbs onto a sheet of cotton cloth and then sealing the bundle at the neck with a wide rubber band. This worked well, but after being steamed, the herbs stuck to the inside of the cloth, making it difficult and time-consuming to recycle the cotton wrapper. I further refined the rubber band approach by placing the herbs and roots inside a drawstring muslin bag first, which I then wrap with sheer cotton cloth. This allows for washing and recycling of the outer wrapping material, and provides a ready-made bath infusion to be taken home by the client for later use. Clients often love soaking in an herbal bath on the night of their Thai massage.

Mixing and preparing the herbs

Making a compress or a bath infusion can be an enjoyable part of the overall preparation for your sessions each day. If you have a very busy schedule on a particular day, you may choose to prepare several compresses the night before your sessions and put them in an airtight container in the refrigerator. Whenever possible, however, try to prepare your compresses each morning for the sessions you are about to give that day.

As you are preparing and mixing the ingredients, think of the client with whom you'll be working. Imagine that person's physical conditions, tensions, and difficulties. Consider ways you will work with them in your session. Take a moment to meditate, and direct positive energy into the compress you'll be using on that person.

Pour your dry herbal blend into a large mixing bowl, and get ready to add your fresh ginger root and any other fresh ingredients. It is best to not slice fresh ginger, turmeric, *plai,* lemongrass, or *galanga.* Instead, smash them against a flat surface with a heavy object such as a meat tenderizer or a rock, and separate them into small pieces with your hands so that the stringy fibers are exposed. If you use fresh leafy herbs, you should tear them with your hands, not cut them with scissors. When you are done with your preparations, mix the fresh pieces into the dry mix, and stir with your hands to distribute it evenly. Now you may begin to pack your compresses.

Making the compresses

For the wrapper you may use cheesecloth or any other sheer cotton cloth. I use cotton "shop cloths" – the ones used by car mechanics and industrial workers to clean their hands. These cloths can be easily found in major department stores and supply shops in the West, or you can buy them on the Internet. Make sure they are made with a loose weave, so that the herbal properties can pass through the cloth. Hold the cloth up to a strong light, and if you can see light shining through, it should be fine. Shop cloths are pre-cut to a reasonable size and they can be washed and used over and over again. You can also purchase sheets or rolls of sheer cotton or cheesecloth and cut them into smaller rags of your desired length and width.

If you decide to use muslin bags, place a generous amount of mixed fresh and dry herbs into the bag, add a pinch of camphor crystals if you wish, and tie the drawstring pouch with a tight bow. The muslin bags I use measure 15 x 20 cm – 6 x 8 inches. If you don't use muslin bags, you can place your herbal mixture directly into the center of the cotton cloth.

If you choose to make your own compresses with long stiff handles, you'll need a longer piece of cloth, a large amount of cotton string, and perhaps some small strips of bamboo. If you make them this way, or if you work with dry compresses imported from Thailand, you may also need a deeper steamer so that the taller compresses fit inside. If you want to assemble and disassemble your compresses quickly, however, and if you plan to use a domestic electric vegetable steamer, then try the shop cloth and rubber band approach. It works very well.

Bring the four corners of the cloth together with your hands, grab the neck of the bundle, and mold the herbal mix into a tight round shape. Use a wide rubber band to close the neck, and twist it around the neck two or three times to seal it tightly. Now create the small handle to hold the compress. Bring the four exposed flaps of cloth underneath the rubber band, and make sure they are tightly secured. Mold the new cloth "handle" over the top portion of the compress with your hand, and adjust the flaps as necessary so that you can grab the ball tightly. Make sure the rubber band isn't exposed, since it will become hotter than the cloth and it could potentially burn you or your client.

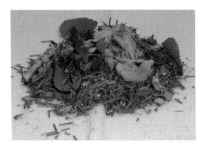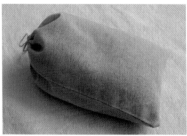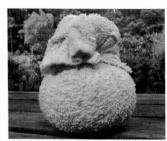

General recipes for herbal mixes are mentioned toward the end of this essay, as well as mixtures for herbal bath infusions. Whether you prepare your own compresses or use the pre-made variety, your clients will thank you for the warmth, steam, pressure and medicinal benefits that result from using luk pra kob.

General information about herbal compresses

Hot herbal compresses have a long history of use in Thailand and other parts of Southeast Asia. The earliest written records in Thailand are from the Ayutthaya period (14th–18th century), when Siamese soldiers returning from battle were treated with compresses to ease their mental states and relax their bodies. Today, in Thailand, herbal compresses are used in massage shops, spas, and among family members, using specialized recipes passed down through the generations.

There are many traditional Thai recipes for compresses. Common blends incorporate materials such as ginger, plai, turmeric, lemongrass, kaffir lime (leaves and the rind of the fruit), tamarind leaves, eucalyptus, galangal, and camphor. Salt is often added to open skin pores, and sometimes cinnamon or sweet herbs and flowers may be included. Knowledgeable herbalists and healers prepare their compresses based on the individual needs of their patients, but most of them also have a standard all-purpose recipe.

The herbal blend that I prepare is based on traditional ingredients, except that it doesn't use fresh kaffir lime leaves, tamarind leaves, and plai, which are hard to find and expensive in the West, or turmeric, which stains skin and clothing. In addition to a base of ginger, lemongrass, eucalyptus, and camphor, for example, you may choose to add a small amount of freshly picked herbs that are available in your region. Examples include peppermint, lemon balm, anise leaf, rosemary, lavender, and jasmine. Research the medicinal properties of each plant first, and make sure there are no contraindications for your clients' conditions. Add local herbs only in moderation, and make sure the majority of the mix remains true to Thai tradition.

Sick or sensitive clients can have a very relaxing and invigorating experience with herbal compresses, even if no traditional Thai massage is applied.

In this case, therapists commonly use several compresses to work the entire body, along the sen lines, and on the stomach, chest, back, arms, and legs. In Thailand, compresses are often used on pregnant women without any additional Thai massage treatment.

Inhaling herb-infused vapors during a compress session can induce deep relaxation. Many herbs have a balancing effect on the mind and help reduce stress. Materials such as eucalyptus, peppermint and camphor act as decongestants for the lungs and sinuses. Using hot compresses on the chest, throat, and sinuses can loosen mucus and open nasal passages.

The steamer

It's best to use an electric steamer, and one with a thermostat will give you extra control. Make sure you use a true vegetable steamer and not a rice cooker or a crock pot. A metal basket or plastic compartment has large holes in it and is positioned directly above the boiling water below. The herb bundles shouldn't come directly in contact with the boiling water, but they must become damp from the rising steam in order to be effective.

As water evaporates from the steamer, you'll need to replace it. Keep a large container of fresh water nearby, so you can replace the water several times during the course of your treatment. The lid should be firmly in position at all times, except when you move the compresses in and out of the steamer. Be careful to not overfill the steamer with water, since the boiling action might wet the bottom of the compress. A variety of electric steamers with thermostats are available in appliance and department stores, and on the Internet.

Application and warnings

Before steaming, sprinkle the outside of the wrapped compress with water or rice vinegar and massage the compress lightly to loosen the herbal materials and distribute the moisture. Steam for a minimum of 10–15 minutes at 93–107 degrees Celsius (200–225 degrees Fahrenheit). Don't submerge compresses in hot water because they'll become too hot to handle for the client and therapist, and also because much of their medicinal value will seep into the water. If a compress accidentally drops into the hot water in your steamer, make sure to wring out the water and dry the outside of the compress with a towel before reusing it, since it could easily scald your client's skin.

If you're doing a session where you'll be using compresses extensively, it's best to steam two at a time, so that the treatment can be conducted without interruption. Alternate them as necessary, and return one to the steamer as you remove the other. Use a dry wash cloth to grab a fresh compress from the steamer, and as you apply it to your client's body.

Always test a compress against your upper arm, neck, stomach, or face to make sure it's not too hot for your client. If it's too hot, use one of the cooling methods described in this article, or simply keep it out of the steamer for a minute or two.

Don't use compresses on clients within 24 hours of swelling, inflammation or bleeding, as the heat might worsen their condition. You can treat a swollen area 24–36 hours after the condition first appears, but be careful to use compresses that are warm, not hot, or to be safe, use pre-steamed cool or cold compresses. Take extra care if your clients have diabetes, paralysis, or varicose veins, and if you're working on children and older people, since their skin may be tender. Always test the compress on yourself first to make sure it's not too hot.

Advise your clients to avoid showering or bathing for at least several hours after an herbal session. This is so that the medicinal value of the herbs can remain on and under the skin long enough to be absorbed into the body. This is true even if you are applying compresses on top of clothing. Try to apply the compress onto bare skin, whenever possible. If you are working through clothing, make sure the client is wearing natural fabrics, such as cotton or rayon.

After the herbal session, a light stain may remain on skin and clothing, but it should come out in the wash with no problem. Turmeric, whether in fresh rhizome or dry powder form, may permanently stain clothing a dark orange color, so be aware of this if you use this powerful herbal medicine in your mixture.

Benefits

Thai herbal compresses are used to alleviate pain and inflammation by opening skin pores and transferring medicating heat to the muscles, joints, and energy lines. Compress therapy helps to harmonize and relax the body, to loosen energy blockages, and to speed the healing of scars, including those caused by childbirth. Compresses relax the muscles and stimulate blood circulation and energy flow. The powerful combination of heat and medicinal herbs helps to reduce aches, increase lymphatic drainage, and condition the skin. Medicinal herbs can effectively treat sprains, bruises, pain, and soreness, and they relax and loosen tendons and ligaments.

In Thailand, compresses often include antioxidants such as turmeric, a natural skin softener; tamarind, which hydrates and regenerates skin cells; kaffir lime leaves and fruit, a skin toner and blood circulation booster; and *plai,* (Thai ginger), which eases muscle and joint aches.

Storage

Herbal compresses may be used several times before they are discarded. Compresses may be refreshed by removing some of the used herbs and adding small amounts of fresh herbs, roots, and camphor as needed. To store overnight, wrap each compress in a small plastic sandwich bag after use, and store it in the refrigerator. If you or your clients use them as shower loofahs or bath infusions, make sure to wring them out completely before storing them in the refrigerator.

If you prepare your herbs from a pre-mixed dry base, such as the blends mentioned later in this essay, be sure to keep the dry herbs in an airtight plastic bag or container, and store them in a cool, dark place.

Herbs, rhizomes, and natural medicines

An extraordinary number of plants are used to prepare natural medicines in Thailand, and some of these are especially suitable for compresses. For Thai massage practitioners living outside Southeast Asia, access to some plants that thrive in Thailand is difficult. Nevertheless, good-quality herbal compresses can be made from natural ingredients that are available for sale and bulk distribution in many Western countries. The herbs mentioned below are a few of the most common Thai medicinal herbs that are used in compresses.

Lemongrass is a perennial herb that thrives in the tropics and subtropics. Thai lemongrass is known as *ta khrai* and is cultivated commercially throughout Thailand and Southeast Asia for culinary and medicinal purposes. The plant grows in dense clumps up to 2 meters (6 feet) in diameter and has leaves up to 1 meter (3 feet) long. The lower part of the stalk has a pale white color and contains the most pungent flavor. This part of the plant is used in Thai soups and curries. The entire stalk may be used to make teas, decoctions, poultices, and as a treatment for colds, fevers, coughs, and indigestion. It also is known to treat nausea, stomach pain, and vomiting. Among hill tribe people in Thailand, it is used topically for sprains, bruises and sore muscles.

As an aromatherapy oil, lemongrass is useful for treating headaches, and it works very well as an insect repellent. When it's mixed with a carrier oil and massaged directly onto irritated skin, it boosts circulation and speeds healing. If you live in the West and work with compresses regularly, it's easiest to work with dried lemongrass, since fresh stalks can be costly and hard to find. If you do use fresh lemongrass, make sure to crush the bulbs and stalks after you cut them, so that the herbal properties can be optimally released.

Eucalyptus (*yukhaliptat* in Thai) is native to Australia, and began to be used medicinally in Thailand only in the 20th century. It is increasingly used in Thailand to relieve sprains and sore muscles. There are several different species of eucalyptus, all of which have medicinal use. It is an extremely effective remedy for colds, sinus and lung problems, coughs, and asthma. Symptoms are relieved by inhalation of the vapors and topical application to the chest, throat, and the area under the nose. Eucalyptus tea is good for indigestion and fever, and the leaves are used topically on infections and skin burns. When steamed, the vapors of the herb open air passages and clean the sinuses and lungs.

The tree grows in many places around the world, and is readily available for herbal compresses in fresh or dried form. Note: Do not use the small round type of eucalyptus that is found in florists and supermarkets in the West, since the leaves are often treated with chemicals for use in floral bouquets. If you are fortunate to live in a zone where eucalyptus trees grow in the wild, you will be able to pick your own leaves. If not, you can use dried eucalyptus, which is available in bulk from herbal supply companies.

Camphor (*garaboon* or *kalaboon* in Thai) is a product that is distilled from the gum or resin of a type of cinnamon tree. The crystals that result are sold in powder form, or may be compressed into tablets for easy storage. Camphor is a strong decongestant, and is inhaled to treat colds, congestion, sore throat, coughs, sinusitis, and bronchitis. It is also beneficial for irregular menstruation, and eye and lung infections. Although camphor actually stimulates the brain and increases heart and blood circulation, it also reduces stress, anxiety, and insomnia. In herbal compresses applied topically, camphor crystals act as an anti-inflammatory, and relieve arthritis, sprains, and muscle pain. Add a pinch of crystals to the top of each compress before tying and steaming. Avoid touching your eyes and nose after handling camphor, and wash your hands thoroughly after contact.

Ginger (*khing* in Thai) is one of the most important ingredients in Thai medicine. As a topical application, it has strong antiseptic properties, and it treats bacterial and skin infections, acne, and parasites. Ginger is a powerful stimulant, and aids in digestion, control of flatulence, diarrhea, vomiting, colds, sore throat, insomnia, heart disease, acid indigestion, irregular menstruation, chronic back pain, and many other maladies. Common Thai ginger is called *plai*: a different variety than the ginger that is available in Western groceries, but the medicinal properties are similar. For Thai massage therapists living in the West, common ginger may be used with excellent results.

To prepare fresh ginger for compresses, smash the rhizomes with a hammer, meat tenderizer, or a hard flat object such as a rock. Once the roots are smashed and flattened, pull them apart into small fibrous pieces and mix evenly with your herbal mixture. Once hot, the ginger will help to maintain an even temperature in the compress. The fibers and juice of the ginger act as a transmitter of the combined medicinal properties of herbs and roots, and impart a fabulous aroma, which helps to calm the client's mind.

Turmeric *(kha min)* is an important herbal medicine and has been valued as such throughout the ages. Native to South Asia, it is known for its ability to reduce gas, ease diseases of the digestive system, and treat skin disorders such as rashes, sores, and insect bites. Scientific research has confirmed that turmeric blocks certain toxins from entering the liver and kills some types of bacteria. Turmeric is also known to arrest certain types of cancer, and is being used experimentally in some countries to treat cancer victims. Many cancer survivors are known to take turmeric in capsule form to ward off recurrences. In Thailand, turmeric is often used in cooking, herbal medicine, and herbal compresses. With its powerful curative properties, turmeric is one of the key ingredients in traditional Thai beauty treatments, and a wide variety of herbal soaps and skin products are made of this miracle root. Turmeric oil serves as an efficient moisturizer and has antiseptic properties to heal skin ailments.

Kaffir lime *(ma krut)* has various medical and culinary uses in Southeast Asia. The leaves have antioxidant and anti-inflammatory properties and are believed to cleanse the blood. In Thailand, kaffir lime extract is used as a natural deodorant, and leaves are added to shampoo since they clean the scalp and hair and are believed to reduce hair loss. Traditionally, fresh peels and dried fruits have been used to relieve nausea and dispel gas. The leaves grow with two opposing sections joined at the center. Sizes vary, but the average individual leaf is approx. 2 inches long. Harvesting is done by hand; it's a time-consuming process because the branches have thorns. The leaves impart an unmistakable, refreshing taste that is essential to many Thai soups and curries. For use in cooking, kaffir lime leaves freeze well in an airtight container.

Other ingredients commonly used in compresses

Plai *(prai)* is a type of ginger that is widely used in Thai traditional medicine for topical treatment of sprains, contusions, joint swelling, muscular pain, abscesses, and similar inflammation-related disorders. Plai oil has long been used by Thai healers to ease joint and muscle pains, and it is used as a natural moisturizer to tone and soften the skin and condition the scalp. The ground fresh rhizome is used in traditional Thai massage as a muscle relaxant and may be applied as a poultice or steamed in a compress. The flesh is dark yellow-orange, and it can stain clothing and skin temporarily.

Salt is sometimes added to Thai herbal compresses. It is an important ingredient in herbal bath infusions, as it cleans and opens skin pores, thereby facilitating the transfer of medicinal properties. Known as *klua (glua)* in Thai language, it softens the skin and works as an exfoliant for dry skin cells. Salt eases muscle aches, and relieves sunburn, rashes, and skin irritations. You may add small rocks of sea salt or large flakes of kosher salt to your compresses and bath infusions.

Tamarind leaves and flowers are used in compresses and poultices in Thailand to address swollen joints, sprains, and boils. The tree is native to Africa and probably reached Asia thousands of years ago. Known as *ma kaam* in Thai language, dried or boiled tamarind leaves reduce inflammation and treat skin disorders. There are many other medicinal uses of the fruit, seeds, and bark of the tamarind tree.

Peppermint leaf (*saranae* in Thai) is considered a hot and aromatic herb in Thai medicine, and is a common treatment for stomach pain, nausea, and indigestion. The aroma is delightful when steamed in compresses, and the vapor treats nervousness, insomnia, and stress-related conditions, such as exhaustion and headaches. Inhalation of vapors can calm coughing and relieve asthma. Peppermint grows easily in almost all soil conditions. If you're fortunate to have a garden at home, consider growing your own peppermint to use in compresses, and to make hot or cold tea. Whenever you use fresh herbs, always rip the leaves with your hands.

Galangal or galanga (*kha* in Thai) is a relative of the ginger plant. The flavor is considerably stronger than that of common ginger, somewhat similar to mustard, and it has a rich aroma. It was used traditionally to cure skin diseases, and is now used in spa treatments as an ingredient in body wraps to soothe and nourish the skin. The pale yellow skin of galangal is striated like snakeskin and has pink-tinged tips, but the interior is cream-colored. Slices of galangal are often added to soups, and it's an important ingredient in Thai curry paste.

How to use herbal compresses in Thai massage

Herbal compresses may be used during the course of a Thai treatment in several ways. It's common to use them during a session whenever we find blockages that need softening before manual techniques are used. Compresses may also be used to welcome or calm the client before beginning an otherwise "dry" Thai session, or they can be used only at the end of a dry treatment, as a final technique for relaxation and integration.

Compresses during the Thai massage

An effective way to use compresses in a Thai treatment is to integrate them into a regular Thai massage session. Prepare your compresses, and steam them for at least 15–20 minutes at medium heat before you start using them. During a session, place the steamer so that it is within easy reach as you progress up and down the body during your normal routine. In order to accomplish this, you may have to place the steamer on a tray of some sort, so that you can slide it easily on your floor surface. Food trays or cutting boards work well, and you may also need an electric extension cord. Maintain the water level in the steamer, and adjust the thermostat as needed during the session.

Begin your Thai massage treatment as usual, at the feet, and continue your sequence until you find a spot where you sense holding or tension. Reach for a compress with your free hand, test it on yourself first, and then begin to apply heat, pressure, and herbal medicine into the blocked area. Work directly on the blockage while supporting the body part either on the mat or against your body somehow. Once you feel the area has responded to your work, return the compress to the steamer, and continue with your palming, thumbing, or other Thai techniques. Repeat this pattern as necessary during the course of the entire session. At the end of the session, you may consider using the compress for a longer duration on the neck, head, and face.

Compresses before or after the Thai massage

Compresses may be used on a client's entire body either before or after a regular (dry) Thai massage session. Work the sen lines with your compresses in supine position by starting with the feet, proceeding up the legs, and working the inside lines to the groin. Then work the outside lines of both legs. Proceed to the abdomen, crossing the chest and up to the shoulders. If you work in prone position, start again from the bottom, working the backs of the legs, the buttocks, the lower back and hips, the main back lines, then the shoulders, neck, and arms. Stay on the lines as much as possible throughout your entire routine, and hold the compresses for a few seconds in each place before moving onward along a sen line.

Using compresses before a Thai treatment is a wonderful way to welcome your client and to warm up and open the body. Using them after a Thai treatment provides a soothing, peaceful closure.

Refining your work with herbal compresses

Once you learn the basics of using Thai herbal compresses (medicinal properties, mixing and preparing compresses, and basic handling techniques), then you begin the real learning curve: working with them skillfully and in a flowing fashion during a Thai session. Here are some issues to consider when using compresses during a Thai massage session:

- How to transition gracefully from a "dry" Thai massage technique to a "wet" compress technique;
- Handling the steamer with one hand while maintaining client contact with the other hand: (removing and returning compresses, adding water, and changing thermostat temperature);

- Maximizing use of the heat and vapors each time you remove the compress from the steamer;
- Remembering to test the compress on yourself at regular intervals to avoid burning your client;
- How to master the various active and passive compress techniques outlined in this essay, and how to know when to use them.

General guidelines

Regardless of where on the body you apply your compresses, consider the following general guidelines:

- Work slowly, but be very careful to not burn your clients by holding the compress against their skin for too long. When you remove a hot compress from the steamer, test it first on your skin first, before applying it to your client. If possible, test it on the same area of your own body. Keep in mind that men generally tolerate hotter temperatures on their skin than women.
- In most cases, begin on the left side for women and on the right side for men. Generally, you should work on both sides of the body, even if symptoms appear only on one side.
- On arms and legs, consider working medially, toward the center of the body, as you continue your work upward on a client's body. An exception to this general rule is when you encounter a blockage that is near the end of an extremity, such as on the forearm, wrist, hand, calf, ankle, or foot. In this case, you can try to dissipate the blockage outward, instead of pushing it inward toward the center of the body and then upward. *Lom* (energy) flows in both directions through the sen lines, but as with general Thai massage, it's a good idea to work compresses beginning at the bottom of the body and ending at the top of the body.
- If you prepare your own compresses with short, rounded handles, make sure to have a few dry washcloths nearby. When you need to remove a hot compress from the steamer, do so with a dry washcloth in your hand. This minimizes transference of heat to your hand as you work.

Active techniques used with compresses

Tapping

Rapid, light tapping along the body is an excellent way to cool down an extremely hot compress. The medicinal components of the herbs are transmitted partially through the heat, so tapping and dabbing allows you to make use of the compress as it cools to a more practical temperature. Make sure you first test the compress on a similar area of your own body before you

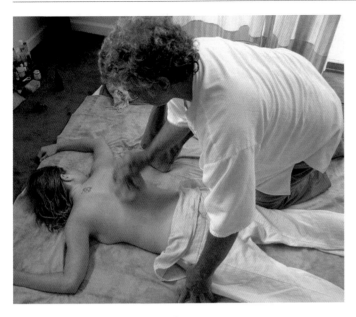

Rapid tapping is stimulating and helps to cool down a hot compress

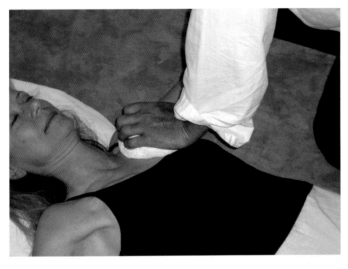

Pressing, using the compress as an extension of your hand

make contact with your client. Tap lightly and quickly to release vapor and to warm up an energy line before you go deeper with the compress or execute Thai massage techniques.

Pressing

A common way to use compresses is to press them onto the body, using light to moderate pressure. The compresses should be in a medium-hot state. Apply directly onto light clothing, or to bare skin, which is preferable. Take hold of the compress, position yourself so that you use your bodyweight and not your arm muscles, and press into the area. Hold it for a second or two, and release slowly before moving to the next area. This technique is good for the legs, abdomen, chest, arms, shoulders, and back.

Mobilizing a body part around a compress

In some cases you can move the client's body around a compress that is not too hot, rather than simply pressing it against the body. This is an especially good idea whenever you can use the client's bodyweight to sink into the compress, such as in the neck sequence below. Gently support the head, and roll it slowly from side to side. Then slip in the compress, holding it in one hand and supporting the other side of the head with your other hand. Always be ready to lift the head away from the compress if it becomes too hot. Move the compress incrementally from one side of the neck to the other, while gently rolling and lifting the head and allowing it to sink into the compress. Switch the compress to the other hand, and repeat on the other side. Finally, place the compress against the occipital

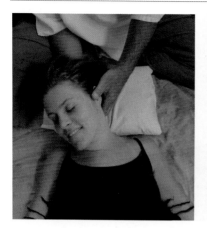 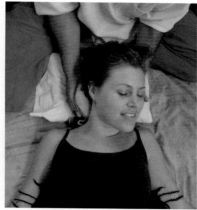 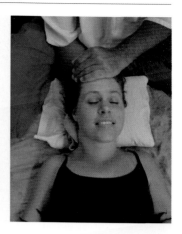

ridge, and while holding the client's forehead, bend the head backward over the compress. Repeat the whole routine as many times as you wish. Be careful to not burn your client.

Mobilizing the body around a compress

Rolling

This is a traditional Thai way to apply compresses. Start with one end of the compress on the body. Keep your wrist flexed upward to begin, and then apply a rolling movement by lowering your wrist and raising your elbow. Begin working at the end of a sen line and work upward (or downward) on that line using this rolling motion. When using this technique, roll in one direction for as long a distance as possible.

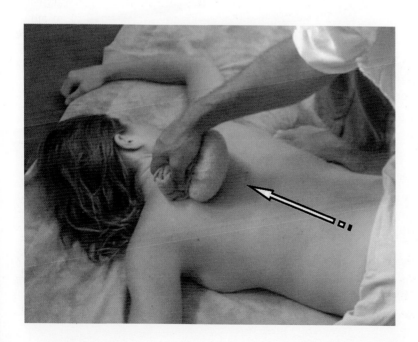

Rolling with a compress

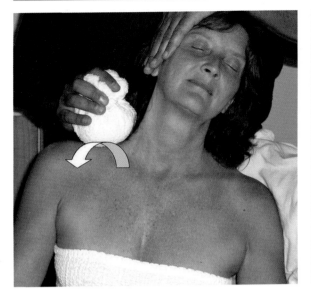

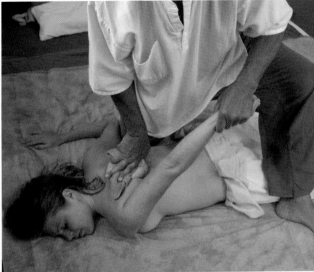

Stretching and rolling

Stretching and Rolling

You can use a hot compress as an aid in stretching techniques, especially for the neck, shoulders, arms, and legs. Traditional forearm rolling movements can be carried out with compresses, too. Instead of rolling the shoulders with your forearm, use a rolling compress. The neck and adjacent shoulder can also be stretched with a compress in final supine position, or in prone position.

Chopping

Good for working the back lines, use the compress in a percussive way, quickly striking the back, and working up and down the back lines and outward to the shoulders. This is usually done in a seated position, with the client bent forward, palms on the ground, but it may also be done in prone position. In addition to the stimulating effect of the chop itself, this is a good way to cool down a very hot compress. In fact, it's best to use this technique with a very hot compress. Don't press or hold the compress against the skin. Make sure your contact lasts only as long as the chop itself.

Passive use of compresses

Inhalation

You normally need to raise the temperature of the steamer in order to prepare a compress for inhalation. In Thai massage, we generally work the head and face at the end of a session. When you are almost finished working the body, and you're getting ready to start working on the head, raise the thermostat so that the water begins to boil vigorously. After a few minutes, the compress should be too hot to handle, but it will be perfect to use as an inhaler.

Turn your client's head to one side, place the steaming hot compress on the mat alongside her face, and encourage her to inhale the medicinal vapors. You may gently tap the compress to release more vapors. After a few seconds, move your client's head by supporting her neck from underneath and twisting it gently in the other direction. Switch the compress to the other side of the mat, and repeat the inhaling action.

When working on the face, if the compress is not too hot, hold it directly underneath the nose and then move up slowly, gently pressing the point of the nose upward. Then work up the bridge of the nose, and apply pressure under the forehead ridge. Repeat this technique as often as you like, while encouraging your client to inhale the vapors.

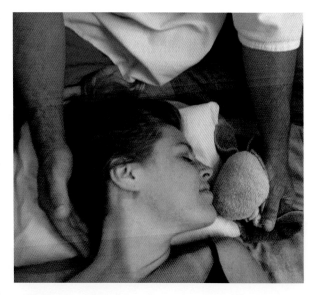

Inhalation of vapors

As pillows

A compress that is slightly warm can be ideal as a head rest. Place it under the middle section of the person's neck, and allow the head to drape over the compress. Keep in position for as long as you are able before removing it to the steamer, or until the session is finished.

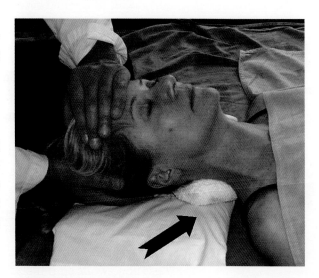

Compress as a pillow

As warmers

Warm compresses can be used to passively warm important areas of the body. When the client is lying on her back, and you, for example, are working behind her, place a medium-warm compress on her *hara*, the area slightly below the navel. Continue your work on other parts of the body, and occasionally, reach down and move the compress a bit higher up the center of the rib cage. Continue in this way, following *sen sumana* up to the neck. If time allows, you can repeat this pattern, working from the hara to below the jaw. Compresses made from old socks are especially conducive to working sen sumana, since the tubular shape fits nicely as you slide it up and down the chest groove.

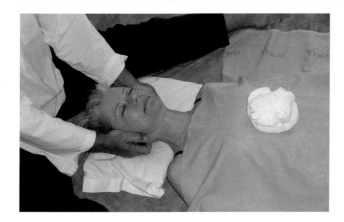
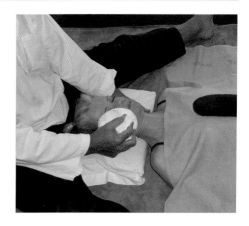

Compresses as
warmers

Reusing compresses

Thai herbal compresses can be reused throughout the day from one client to the next. Just keep them in the steamer on the "warm" setting all day long, and check your water level every few hours. If you are using compresses for light duty, as an occasional accompaniment to your Thai massage sessions, then they can even be used from one day to the next, as long as they are kept in the refrigerator in an airtight plastic bag or container in between daily sessions. If you use the compress on more than one person, it can be helpful to add a small amount of new herbs, a few pieces of fresh ginger, or an extra pinch of camphor. To do this, open the drawstring of the muslin bag, remove some of the ingredients, and mix a handful of fresh herbs into the already moist materials. For each new client, however, always replace the outer cotton covering. If a compress has been used in a session where there has been a severe reaction of some kind, especially an emotional release, it's best to discard the compress and never use it again.

If you prepare the herbs and roots in a small muslin bag, as previously discussed, you can give your clients the recently used compress to take home, so that they can use it as a bath infusion or a shower loofah. At this time, you may choose to refresh the contents of the muslin bag with a handful of fresh herbs or a few drops of essential oil. Instruct your clients to wring out the compress after each use and to store it in a plastic bag in the refrigerator. The herbal sachet can be used several times, thereby extending the use of the herbs and their healing benefits. After it is used once as a bath infusion, it will lose many of its medicinal properties, but it still may be used afterward as a shower loofah. Once in the shower, rub the compress bag against a bar of soap and use it to scrub the body.

Using cold compresses

An often overlooked but important way to apply compresses is when they are cold, not warm. The compresses must first be steamed for 15–20 minutes in order to release the medicinal properties in the herbs, and then they can be refrigerated or iced. After they've been thoroughly chilled, they may be applied onto ligament or tendon sprains, hematomas, hernias, contusions, and other injuries that may benefit from cold therapy, including headaches and neck pain. Apply cold compresses only to the specific site of the injury. Cold compresses generally reduce swelling, and can help to dissipate stagnant or blocked energy. Cold compresses can be left on the injured area for sustained periods of time, while the practitioner attends to other parts of the body during a session. Return the cold compress to the refrigerator, or if you wish to use it continuously during a session, place it on a bowl of ice that is covered with plastic wrap.

Sample routines for Thai herbal compress therapy

Below are two sample routines to treat clients with specific conditions, namely shoulder/neck pain and general stress. These routines demonstrate how compresses may be used in order to address a client's individual conditions.

For neck and shoulder pain

Apply compresses with a firm, slightly rolling pressure. If the client is in seated position, support her back with your leg or abdomen as you work. You may also work the neck in final supine position. If the compress is extremely hot, you can begin by tapping or lightly chopping along the indicated areas. Once the compress has cooled down, you can proceed with deeper pressure.

It is often helpful to move the client's neck gently from side to side, and from front to back, as you work. Secure the forehead with the palm of one

Some neck and shoulder points

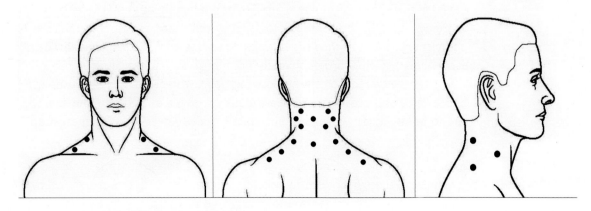

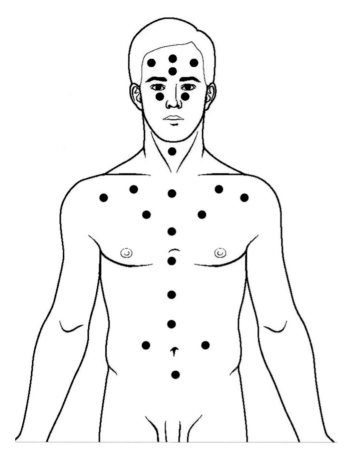

Stress and
anxiety areas

hand, and apply a compress with the other as you slowly mobilize the neck clockwise, counter-clockwise, forward and backward.

For general stress and anxiety

Work the stomach either with direct pressure downward, or by pressing downward and then rolling toward the navel. Press downward as your client exhales. Hold the pressure for as long as the heat allows, and release as your client inhales. Once the stomach is relaxed, work upward on sen sumana, and outward on *sen kalathari* to the shoulder sockets. Work back to sen sumana, work downward slowly to the hara, then ascend all the way to the throat, just below the chin, and then upward onto the face. Allow your client to breathe in the vapors as much as possible. Test the compress on yourself, as needed, to insure that it's not too hot, and to know how long to hold it before moving to another spot. Visualize the sumana and kalathari sen lines as you work. When pressing on the abdomen and chest, always work with the client's natural breath as much as possible.

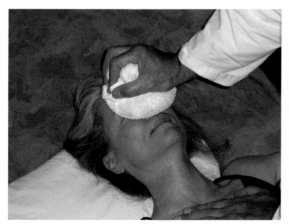
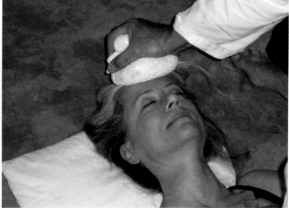

Herbal compress recipes

All-purpose herbal blend

The all-purpose mix that I prepare and use with my clients and students is based on Thai herbal materials that are readily accessible in The West.

Ingredients	
lemongrass (2 parts)	peppermint (1 part)
eucalyptus (2 parts)	dried galangal pieces (½ part)
dried ginger pieces (1 part)	camphor
ginger powder (1 part)	fresh ginger

For each compress, mix approximately 50 percent volume of freshly smashed ginger into the dry blend proportions above, then add a pinch of camphor crystals. You can also add some salt to the mixture, if desired.

Here are some other compress blends you might try:

Decongestant blend Good for clearing congestion in lungs and sinuses. Spend extra time working on the chest, lung area, upper back, and throat:

Ingredients	
eucalyptus leaves, fresh or dried	kaffir lime leaves, or fresh lime rind
fresh ginger root	cloves
	camphor crystals

Relaxing blend This sweet-smelling mix is good for general relaxation and to relieve stress:

Ingredients	
peppermint	rose petals
ylang-ylang flowers	lemongrass
jasmine flowers	salt

Skin cleanser Good to cleanse the skin, open pores, and care for insect bites and superficial cuts and wounds:

Ingredients	
eucalyptus leaves	salt
galangal root (fresh or dried)	lemon, lime or orange rind
turmeric (fresh or dried)	citrus essential oil

Stimulating blend Good for energizing and lifting spirits:

Ingredients	
fresh ginger root	cinnamon sticks (small pieces)
lemongrass (fresh and/or dry)	camphor crystals
peppermint	

Herbal bath infusions: procedure and recipes

If you have never experienced a Thai herbal bath soak, you're missing out on one of life's simple pleasures. Herbal bath infusions can be made fresh, just for the bath, or they can be prepared using a warm compress that just came out of the steamer after a Thai massage. You will need to place the herbs, roots, and flowers in a tied muslin bag. Use large muslin bags, so that the herbal mixture can move around freely inside the tied bag. Use a generous amount of herbs and rhizomes, and fill the bags to about ¾ of their volume capacity. If you're using fresh herbs that haven't been pre-steamed, be sure to soak the sachet in the tub for a few minutes in extremely hot water. Before soaking in the bath, first take a shower to remove surface dirt, sweat, and oils from your skin.

To prepare the bath, follow these guidelines:

Place the sachet directly under the faucet and allow only hot water to run directly over it. Use the hottest water you have available, and allow it to run slowly over the sachet until the tub is filled to approximatey ⅓ of its volume. Close the bathroom door as the tub is filling, so that the medicinal vapors remain in the room. Return in a few minutes to see how things are going. Stir the water, and squeeze the herbal bag a few times so the tinctures are released into the water. If the infusion is too hot for your hands, press the bag against the side of the bath tub with another object to release the herbal properties. Stir the bath again, and continue to fill the tub with more hot water, or mix in some colder water, so the next ⅓ of the tub will be close to the temperature you desire for the bath. Use as much hot water as possible, even if you must wait for the water to cool to your optimal bathing temperature. Prepare the bathroom with anything else you might desire, such as candles, a glass of water, or a cup of herbal tea.

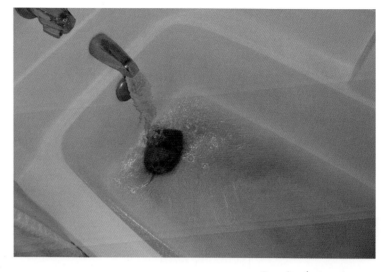

Running hot water over an herbal bath infusion

The all-purpose herbal blend for compresses mentioned previously makes an excellent bath infusion, but I find it interesting and fun to modify ingredients and herbal properties for specific types of results. In addition to the dry and fresh herbs and roots, you can always add a few drops of complementary essential oils or extractions to the bath water.

> Remember to shower and scrub your skin first before taking the bath. Place the herbal pack under hot running water and slowly fill your tub. Soak for 10–15 minutes at the hottest temperature you can bear. Once in the bath, you can continue to squeeze the infusion into the bath water, and you can also squeeze the warm tinctures over your face and head. Don't use soap; just rub the muslin bag over your body as you soak. Pat yourself dry after the bath and don't apply creams or moisturizers. Let the herbs work their magic.

Cleansing and detox bath

Ingredients	
galangal (30%)	kaffir lime (10%)
lemongrass (30%)	pandan extract
ginger powder (30%)	

This recipe can help to revitalize the mind and cleanse the body. In a muslin bag, place 5–6 slices of dried or freshly smashed galangal (or a handful of small pieces of dried galangal), a handful of dried lemongrass, 6–8 ripped kaffir lime leaves (or a tablespoon of kaffir lime power), and a generous amount of ginger powder. Then add a few drops of pandan extract to the sachet and tie it closed with a bow, or add the drops directly into the bath water if you like, and proceed from above.

Invigorating bath

Ingredients
lemongrass (20%)
peppermint (20%)
eucalyptus (15%)

fresh ginger (20%)
cloves (10%), salt (10%)
rose petals (5%)

Use dried and/or fresh lemongrass, peppermint, eucalyptus, and rose. If fresh, make sure to tear and crush leaves and petals. Smash and tear the ginger root into small pieces. Crush fresh cloves to a thick sand consistency in a mortar and pestle, or if not available, use clove powder.

Relaxing bath

Ingredients
lemongrass (20%)
rose petals (20%)
lavender (20%)

ginger (20%)
lime or lemon rind (5%)
liquefied honey (10%)
salt (5%)

Use fresh and/or dried herbs and roots (if fresh, crush and tear as indicated above). Cut the rind off the fruit, including the pith (the white flesh directly under the skin), or grate it. Place all herbs, roots, and fruit in a muslin bag, but blend the salt and liquefied honey directly into the bathwater.

Final words

I hope this article serves as encouragement for those Thai therapists who do not use luk pra kob with their clients, and that it offers new ideas for those who already do. Thai herbal compresses are an important part of traditional Thai medicine, and they greatly complement the practice of traditional Thai massage. Happy compressing!

Self-Protection Techniques for the Thai Therapist

BOB HADDAD

As beginners in traditional Thai massage, we follow the initial sequences that we were taught by our first teachers. Sequences are important when we first learn Thai massage, but they become less relevant as we sharpen our intuition, focus on the human energy system, and learn to listen to the body. As we mature in our practice, we learn to respond to what we sense our clients truly need, and the more we practice, the more aware we become of our clients' energies. Our intuition sharpens, and we learn how to work more effectively in order to diminish or eliminate blockages in the *sen* lines. As we become better at releasing this blocked energy, it becomes more important to protect ourselves as we work.

The Buddhist principle of *metta,* or loving-kindness, is a cornerstone of the healing power of traditional Thai massage. As we work, we send love and compassion to the person we are touching. Because of this, it is important to keep an open heart. But when we facilitate or witness physical releases of tension and stress, and emotional releases of grief, sadness, or anger in our clients, then our heart energy must become more self-serving. It is important to not ingest the "negative energy" that our clients release as we work. To accomplish this, we can strengthen ourselves by visualizing and holding in place a shield of protective armor, and by engaging in one or more techniques described in this essay.

As experienced practitioners of *nuad boran,* we must understand the value of preparation before we work, and the need for self-protection during each session. It's also important to know when and how to detoxify ourselves after a stressful session. The techniques and practices described in this chapter may be helpful tools as you progress in your work as a Thai massage therapist.

Preparing for the session

Preparing for a Thai session is an important step in the therapeutic process, both for yourself and for your client. Both the therapist and the client should avoid eating heavily for at least 1–2 hours beforehand. For the same amount of time prior to the session, both parties should avoid consumption of foods that can bring about edginess, such as sugar, caffeinated coffee or tea, and soft drinks. Remove all jewelry before a session, and try to wear loose clothing made only from natural fabrics.

Focusing on the client

Make sure to take at least a few minutes to focus on the client you are about to receive into your space. For returning clients, review their session logs and recent treatment history. Remind yourself of any physical restrictions that are indicated in their health history form, review their personal likes and dislikes, and read through your logs from the previous one or two sessions to see what you did and how you felt the client responded to your work. Take a moment to think about what you might do today with this person, based on your previous work and based on their current mood and energy. For new clients, present a brief verbal introduction to traditional Thai massage, and make sure they feel comfortable and welcome from the moment they walk through your door.

Physical and spiritual preparations

Yoga

Before your client arrives, and after you have reviewed your client information, take some time to prepare yourself on the physical and spiritual planes. Take note of any tensions you are carrying in your body and address them by stretching and doing yoga. Performing 5–10 minutes of yoga before a session is often enough to help you physically relax and bring about focus. Concentrate on those poses and postures that address your specific weaknesses. We all know where those points are in our bodies. Bring awareness to them as you warm up your body, and try to feel strengthened and at peace.

Reusi dat ton

If you prefer to stay within the traditions of Thailand, you can practice *reusi dat ton*. This type of stretching and focused breathing was practiced by Thai ascetics who lived in caves and mountainous areas of Thailand hundreds of years ago. These days, basic reusi dat ton courses are taught in Thailand, and there are several books and other written materials on the subject available in print and on the web.

Meditation and centering

A short period of silent meditation can be very helpful in strengthening the protective energy layer that is believed to exist outside the edge of our physical bodies. Centering can be achieved through meditation and breath awareness. If you're centered and focused as you work, it will be easier to distinguish between your own energies and the energies of your client. If at any point during a session you feel that you have absorbed an external energy, bring breath awareness to that point. Inhale with the intent to purify yourself, and exhale with the intent to purge the negative energy.

Pranayama and breath awareness

Indian Ayurvedic breathing exercises (*pranayama*) can also be extremely helpful in preparing for your session. Long ago in India, pranayama was developed as a self-healing art to induce states of meditation, relaxation, and inner strengthening. Two important pranayama exercises are presented here. They may be used by the therapist prior to a session, and can even be recommended as homework to clients who have shallow breathing patterns.

If you don't have the time or the physical space to engage in drawn-out pranayama exercises, then any type of protracted deep breathing can be useful in preparing yourself for a session. Sit in cross-legged position, or lie on your back. Stay still, and take long deep breaths into your body. As you breathe in, notice any places where you feel tension or unrest, and as you breathe out, imagine that tension is leaving your body through the force of your exhalation.

Preparation checklist

Before your client arrives, it may be good to keep these things in mind:

- Do yoga exercises that strengthen your *hara*.
- Practice meditation or breathing techniques to bring about a strong sense of self.

- If working with a sick or emotionally stressed client, consider a self-protection exercise such as "prana eggs," described later in this essay.
- Review your client's session logs.
- Wash yourself well.
- Take a moment to focus yourself before you touch your client.
- Be ready to engage in a self-protection technique when and if your client has a physical or emotional release.

Protecting the Thai therapist's energy system

As a Thai massage therapist, you are involved with intensive energy work, so it's important to take great care to prevent your clients' energies from entering your system during the course of a session. When you give a Thai massage, you act as an agent for the release of your patient's tension, stress, and anxieties. If you don't maintain a strong sense of self and take the necessary precautions, these negative energies may easily enter your own body, thereby bringing about tension, headaches, stomach problems, or even prolonged illness. It is no secret that many Thai massage therapists and teachers have become seriously ill from their clients' energies, or from their inability to prevent external energies from entering their systems. Sometimes the deeper we go in our work, the more difficult it is (and the more important it is) to protect ourselves. When we work in nuad boran we should work with great compassion and metta, but this doesn't mean we should allow ourselves to be vulnerable!

Protecting yourself before the session

Washing and cleansing

Make sure your session room is clean, and that there are no lingering odors or residual energies from the previous session. If there are, open a window or cleanse the room as mentioned previously. It's important to wash your hands and feet before each session. If possible, take a shower. If you are congested or have allergies, consider cleansing your nasal passages with a *neti* pot and warm salt water. You may also brush your teeth. Make sure that your client washes her feet, or even better, wash them yourself with some warm water and peppermint oil.

Prana eggs

One of the most powerful visualization exercises you can perform before beginning a Thai massage session is called "Prana Eggs." The objective of this exercise is to surround yourself in a field of protection, and to minimize the transference of your client's energies to your energetic field. Allow a minimum of 10–15 minutes for this exercise:

Outer egg: Lie on your back with your head preferably pointing north to make use of the polarity of the earth. Use your mind like a pencil. As you inhale, imagine drawing half of an oval on the right side of your body, beginning about 6 inches below your toes and ending 6 inches above the center of your head. As you exhale, draw the other half of the egg on the left side of your body, starting at the head and ending below the toes. Imagine that you are lying now in the middle of a large protective egg. Repeat this sequence with coordinated breathing nine times. This part of the exercise protects you from negative external energy influences.

Middle egg: Then start directly at the toes, and on the in-breath, draw the oval closer to the body, intersecting the head. As you exhale, close this new egg on the left side, running from the head and touching the toes. This part of the exercise creates self-confidence, equanimity, and balance. Repeat this cycle nine times.

Inner egg: Finally, draw a small egg starting at the pelvis and ending at the "third eye" in the middle of your forehead. Visualize drawing the oval up on the right side as you inhale, and down on the left side as you exhale. Repeat this part nine times. After the exercise, remain on your back in *savasana* (corpse) pose for a minute or two, and visualize a field of protection around your body.

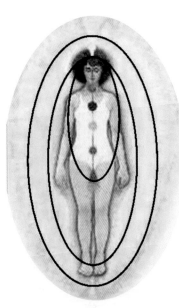

Prana eggs

Prana eggs provides you with a strong protective energy field, and allows you to be fully relaxed before you begin your session.

Breathing exercises before the session

As Thai therapists, it's important to be relaxed with our breath and energetically composed before we begin working with clients. Focused breathing can be attained through meditation, yoga, reusi dat ton, and pranayama. Many breathing exercises are done in the typical sitting meditation pose, but effective deep breathing exercises can also be done in supine position, lying comfortably on your back.

During deep breathing exercises, we charge the blood with extra oxygen, and by extension, we also take in more *prana* (energy), which is equivalent to *lom* in the Thai medicine system. I have found that deep breathing exercises can be very helpful when used in conjunction with traditional Thai massage. It can be helpful to prepare for a Thai session or to de-stress from a difficult session by saturating the body with fresh lom. Here are two basic exercises to consider.

Contiguous breathing

Description: This exercise incorporates three levels of breathing: from the abdomen, through the chest, and into the collarbones. The three parts are meant to flow sequentially from one area to another, as one complete breath.

Technique: Begin by exhaling slowly through the nose. At the end of the exhalation, pull the abdomen in slightly. Then begin to inhale by slowly releasing the abdomen and allowing it to expand. Continue your inhalation as you direct the air to expand your rib cage, and then, as you continue to inhale, allow your upper chest to expand until your collarbones rise slightly. Avoid lifting or tensing the shoulders. To exhale, reverse the order of the inhalation. First release your collarbones, then contract your chest, and then your stomach. Each section should flow into the next, in one continuous breath.

Total time for this exercise is 3–5 minutes. It can be practiced lying down or even sitting or standing, and may be done at anytime during the day.

Sectional deep breathing

Description: I developed a variation of the above exercise that is very effective and brings about a deep state of relaxation. I use it to prepare for a Thai massage session when I feel I need extra composure and protection, and I also do it whenever anxious. Whenever I experience insomnia, it usually puts me right to sleep. If, during the process of a Thai massage I notice that my client is restless, or if his breathing is shallow and soft, I may sometimes guide him though this exercise in a soft voice while I am positioned near his middle section in supine position. For people with extremely shallow breath, it can be helpful right before doing deep stomach work. I find that it brings about expansive breathing and a sense of relaxation and surrender.

Technique: Lie on your back and imagine that your upper body is divided into three sections; your abdomen, your middle chest/rib cage, and your upper chest from the sternum to the neck. Now take a deep breath, and as you do so, notice which one of these three sections inflates most deeply. Are you predominantly a belly breather? Or does your middle section or upper section inflate the most as you breathe in? Do you breathe mostly into your middle chest or into your upper chest? Once you understand your dominant breathing zone, take a moment to relax before you begin the exercise.

First, take a few deep breaths through your nose, and try to inflate only your dominant breathing zone. In other words, if you've determined that you breathe mostly into your belly first, breathe only into your belly. Breathe slowly and fully into your dominant breath area, pause for a moment in a state of rest, and then exhale slowly and fully only from that area of your body. Pause again after your exhale, and take another breath into that same section, so that you understand the feeling associated with directing air into and out of that area only. Now choose another zone, and repeat the process of acquainting yourself with the sensation of breathing only in and out of that area. Finally, breathe in and out of the remaining area once or twice to get acquainted with it.

Now change a different section every time you breathe. Constantly change the order, and try to not think about which section you will inflate until the very last second before you change zones. Breathe in and out through the belly, then the collarbones, then the mid-section; in and out through the mid-section, then the belly, then the collarbones; in and out through the collarbones, then the belly, then the mid-section, and so on.

After you play with your breath in this way for at least 3–4 minutes, and when you feel you are ready to close the exercise, take a full and complete breath into all three sections at the same time. Take note of how expansive this feels, and what it is like when we breathe fully into our entire upper body. Take several more complete breaths, languishing in the relaxation that this complete breathing brings. You may feel tingly and experience a deep calming sensation. Slowly wind down the exercise, remain in resting position for a few more sections, and then, when you are ready, slowly come to a sitting position.

Protecting yourself during the session

Washing during the session

It may sometimes be helpful to wash your hands during a session. If, for example, you have just facilitated or witnessed a major release of energy, tension, or emotion from your client, it may be wise to wash the part of your body that was in contact with that person at the time of release. Obviously, we can't excuse ourselves to wash after every reaction our clients may have. But if you have a strong premonition that you may have been affected by your client's release, then by all means, take a moment to cleanse yourself before you proceed. If a bathroom is nearby, excuse yourself and quickly wash your hands with soap and cold running water. Sometimes I time my washing to go along with a client's requested bathroom break, but whenever I feel the need to wash for any reason, I excuse myself and quickly wash myself.

Ajahn Pichest Boonthumme always keeps a bowl or cup of water nearby with a piece of sour tamarind in it. The antiseptic water is acidic and is believed to be a major cleansing agent for "bad energy." Water with lemon or lime juice can also be effective. If you can't remove yourself physically from the room, you might keep a bowl of water and a washcloth nearby, or spray yourself with a neutralizing solution. Neutralizing solutions are made by combining essential oils or extracts with a transmitter, and some water. See the "clearing energy" section ahead for a few recipes for neutralizing solutions.

Visualization techniques

A number of visualization techniques may be helpful for self-protection during a Thai massage session. Here are a few:

- A simple but important way to maintain strength is to focus attention on your hara. When your client becomes stressed, upset, or emotional, bring more attention to your hara, and imagine it as strong and unwavering. If necessary, you may even touch it lightly to bring focus to that area as you continue to work with your client.
- Utilize a "mental wash" when you sense something is uncomfortable or negative in your client. To do this, imagine clean fresh water running down through the top of your head and then continuing through your entire body. The water should be at a comfortable temperature, and it should run through your body from your head to the bottoms of your feet, where it exits. As the water passes through you, imagine it cleaning each section of your body, including particular areas or organs that you feel need to be cleansed.
- Visualize a strong, mental shield of positive energy around your body, and hold it there. Imagine gathering all the energy from different areas of your body and bringing it together slightly outside your body to form a protective shield. Now flood the shield with sunlight or golden light, and imagine that this boundary is permanently in place around you as you work.

Burning energy at the source

One way to prevent or minimize unwanted energy from entering your system is to imagine "burning" it at the source. As you feel or sense energy, shaking, or tension emerging from your client's body, while you're palming, for example, imagine a bright flame of fire between your hands and their body. As the energy comes out, visualize that it is being burned at the source, and that there is no way it can enter your body.

Acting as a conduit

An alternative to burning the energy at the source is to imagine it entering through one side of your body and exiting the other side. If you are facilitating a release using your left hand or foot, for example, imagine that the energy is entering your body there and exiting through your opposite hand or foot. If you're in a sitting position using one hand, extend your other hand, palm upward, and imagine the energy running through your body and exiting through your outstretched hand. If you're in a standing or kneeling position and both hands are engaged, move or lift one of your feet, and imagine the current exiting through the sole of your foot. Be creative with this technique, but make sure you focus on the exit point, and that you imagine the energy completely leaving your body.

Utilize resting poses when necessary

During periods of emotional release, it can be important to engage yourself and your client in a resting pose; a technique or posture that requires little or no movement. Silence and stillness are often necessary for a client to calm down and for the therapist to stay relaxed and focused.

In supine position, if an emotional release is emerging, you may gently rest your hand on your client's heart and remain still. Establish a protective shield around your body, try to be as "empty" as possible, and wait. You may also gently work sen sumana with two fingers of one hand. This requires very little effort on the part of the therapist, and can be quite calming for the receiver. More information on resting poses can be found in the earlier essay entitled *Care and Feeding of Your Thai Massage Practice,* but only you can determine when and how to modify or stop your work when a short break is needed.

Protecting yourself after the session

Washing

I can't overstress the value of post-session washing. Use cold or room temperature running water and plenty of natural soap. Make sure the water runs freely over your hands, and keep your fingers pointed downward as you wash. If the session was stressful or emotional for your client or yourself, try to take a vigorous shower as soon as possible after the session. After a difficult session, if I know that a particular client always takes a lot of time to emerge from the treatment room, I sometimes take a quick shower and then I return to say goodbye to the client.

If running water or a shower is not available, use salt water or water infused with something tannic, like sour tamarind, or the rind of lemons or limes. You can keep a bowl or jar of liquid nearby, and pour it over your hands and arms, and brush it across your face and your head. With all post-session washing, the sooner you do it, the better.

Physical de-stressing

Deep yoga stretches, such as sun salutations, back bends, plows, and cobras, can be very effective for the therapist immediately following a session. Try to always incorporate deep inhalations and exhalations into your exercises, and imagine bringing clean energy into your body with your inhale, and releasing the stale energy with your exhale. Any kind of forward or backward bending can be helpful, and even dangling your back on an exercise ball while expelling air deeply as you do sit-ups may result in energy release.

If you feel unwanted energy residing in a certain part of your body, such as your stomach, chest, back, or arms, focus on those parts of the body as you do yoga and utilize creative visualizations to attempt to expel the negative energy. If your client had a strong emotional response in her session, or if you sensed an energetic release through her body, or if you feel you may have absorbed negative energies from your client in any other way, consider doing one or more of the post-session exercises described on the next pages.

Clearing energy

Even if the therapist hasn't directly absorbed energies from a stressed client, the mood of your practice room can be altered by lingering, stale energy left over from your client's session. Open a window (two if possible for cross-ventilation), and let the room breathe a bit. Light a fresh candle at your altar, change the sheets and pillowcases your client was lying on, and make a deliberate effort to bring new, cleansing energy back into your room.

Neutralizing solutions can help clear the energy from the session room after a deep or stressful session. You can prepare your own solutions using an essential oil, a transmitting medium such as alcohol or witch hazel, and some water. My favorite blend is to mix equal parts of rosewater, witch hazel, and water. Another effective blend can be made by combining clear grain alcohol such as vodka or gin with some water, and adding as many drops as needed of a cleansing essential oil such as cedar, sage, lime, lemon, or peppermint. You may use sour tamarind soaked in water or diluted lime juice, plus a bit of alcohol. No matter which combination of essential oil and transmitting agent you choose, send healing energy into the room as you spray high into the air after your client has left. Imagine the negative energy being lifted as you treat the room.

Kaya kriya

The *kaya kriya* exercise is a wonderful way to release negative energies and to detoxify after any Thai massage session, but it is especially effective after a difficult session, that is, whenever you work with someone who is holding a lot of tension or going through difficult times or emotional or physical stress.

This traditional yoga kriya was popularized for use in Thai massage by Asokananda. The routine is comprised of four parts, and each part should be done seven or nine times to ensure deep relaxation. In Thailand, odd numbers are believed to be more auspicious than even numbers.

Lie on your back, preferably with your head pointing north. Open

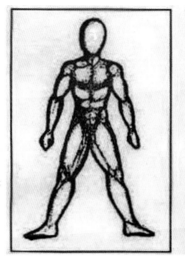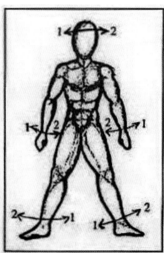

Kaya Kriya

your legs, and keep your arms away from your body, as in the illustration below.

Remember, each of the four sections should be done seven or nine times in succession.

Part 1: Inhale only into the lower part of your lungs, near the diaphragm, and turn your feet and legs inward with as much pressure as possible. As you exhale, roll your feet and legs outward again.

Part 2: Breathe only into the middle part of the lungs, at the mid-chest, and roll your arms and hands outward with strong pressure. Your back may slightly lift off the ground as you inhale and hold your breath. When you exhale, roll your arms and hands inward again.

Part 3: Breathe into the upper part of your lungs, near your breastbone. Turn your head to the right as you inhale, and then to the left as you exhale.

Part 4: Now take a full deep breath as you perform all of the above movements at the same time. Repeat many times. It can be confusing at first, but it becomes easier with practice. After you complete this final section, return to your normal breathing pattern, and stay relaxed on your back for as long as you like. You will often feel a powerful release of tension.

Additional post-session exercises for Thai therapists

Although the kaya kriya is an efficient way to de-stress and purge negative energies, completion of the exercise requires a private space and a fair amount of time. Since you may not always have the space and/or the time necessary to perform a full kaya kriya, do whatever you can right after the session, and then follow through with a more vigorous de-stressing later in the day, at a more convenient time. Here are some other ideas for cleansing and detoxifying yourself after a difficult session.

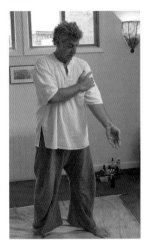 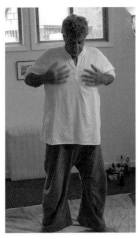 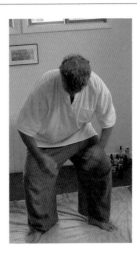 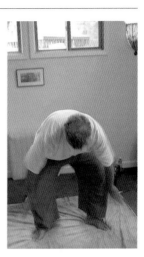

Brushing and
breathing

Brushing and breathing

This exercise involves "brushing" the stressful energies from your body. It can be done as soon as you leave the treatment room, even as the client is still resting or getting dressed. First wash your hands. Then, using the outstretched palm of one hand, vigorously brush the other side of your body with a downward sweeping motion. With every downward stroke, rotate your wrist slightly away from your body, and vigorously sweep away negativity from your energetic field. You can begin at your head and then work downward to your face, neck, shoulders, arms, and hands on one side of your body. Then work your chest and lower back with both hands. Start again from the top of your head on the other side of your body until you reach your groin. Then finish the rest of your body with two hands at once, covering the front of your body, your legs, and as much of the back of your body as possible, until you end at your feet.

This exercise can be even more powerful if you combine strong exhales with every downward stroke. Keep your cheeks slightly rounded, and exhale deeply with every brushing stoke. Imagine that you are removing traces of bad energy, both with your hands and with your breath.

Rapid diaphragmatic breathing

This a classic pranayama exercise, in which only the abdominal area moves and the chest remains still. Make sure you don't slump your posture because it's easy to strain your chest muscles if you're in the wrong position. Sit on the floor in half-lotus posture. Place your hands on your knees, and make sure your body is straight, but relaxed and not stiff.

The exercise is composed of a series of rapid breath expulsions, which are done in quick succession. After every breath expulsion, the air naturally flows back into your lungs, and you immediately proceed naturally to the next expulsion.

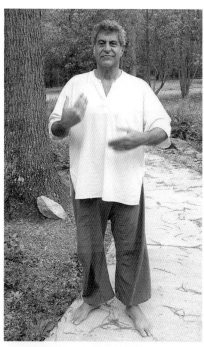 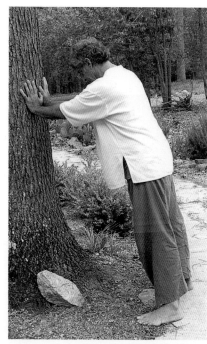

The first few times you do this, place a hand on your abdomen, so that you can feel how it contracts as you forcibly exhale. Quickly and forcefully contract your abdomen by snapping it inward, and allow the air to forcefully exit through your nose. Your abdomen will relax very briefly between contractions, and before the air automatically flows back into your body. Make sure your shoulders don't bounce up and down, and that only your abdomen moves during the exercise.

Take at least fifteen breaths, as described above, in rapid succession. You may do more expulsions, as long as you don't get too dizzy or bring about excessive strain to your system. You can easily feel light-headed after this exercise, so make sure to relax and reintegrate yourself before you stand up.

Shaking and draining

This is a Chinese *qi gong* exercise that may also be helpful. To clear yourself of negative energies following a difficult session, vigorously shake your hands for 30–45 seconds while you focus all your energy on your hara. Imagine the negative energy rising through your body and gathering at your hands as you shake them. As you are doing this, take deep, prolonged inhales, and long, protracted exhales. After a minute or two, your hara and your hands will become warm. Then immediately place your outstretched hands on a rock or a brick wall, or a tree, or a drainpipe, or anything that runs directly into the ground. This allows the "sick" energy that just surfaced through your body to drain into the ground. Try to sense the energy exiting your body as you make contact with the drain that is connected to the earth.

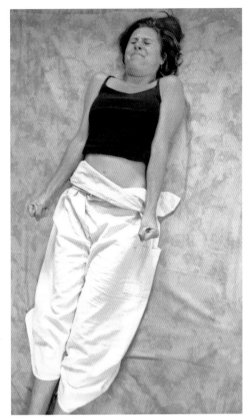 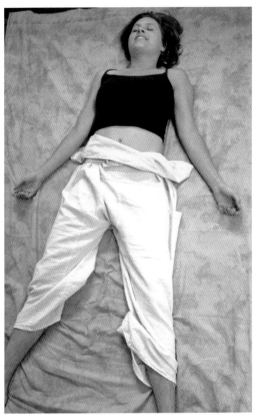

Tighten and release

Tighten and release

This exercise is helpful for tension release if you don't have a lot of time after the session. As you inhale, tighten all the muscles in your body with maximum tension. Squeeze them as tightly as possible, with all your strength. Hold your breath as you maintain the tension for a few seconds. Exhale, and then completely release all the tension, as you allow your body to unfold on the mat. Repeat this cycle at least five times, even more if desired, and then resume normal breathing.

Sun / Moon visualization

This is a creative visualization intended to restore peace and balance. Do it after you have engaged in any of the more physical exercises for tension release mentioned above. Inhale slowly, and imagine golden sunlight entering the toes of your right foot, moving up the side of your body, and leaving your head. After you finish inhaling, hold your breath for a few seconds. As you exhale, imagine a silvery moonlight moving downward from your head, down the left side of your body, and exiting through your toes. Repeat this visualization until you feel a deep sense of relaxation, at least seven to nine times. Then continue to breathe normally.

Meditation

If you have time, and after you have done one or more de-stressing exercises, you may take a short period to meditate silently, in order to balance yourself further and bring new healing energy into your system. Any type of silent, focused meditation will do. Remember to utilize as much breath awareness as possible while you meditate.

Protect yourself

I hope that this essay helps to bring about a greater awareness of the need for self-protection among traditional Thai massage therapists. With a little bit of practice, the concepts and techniques presented here can help you protect yourself against outside energies, and can fortify and maintain your own energy system so you can be a more effective healer.

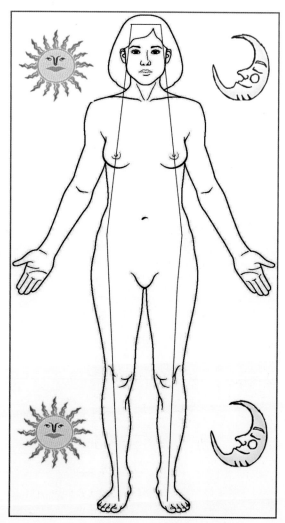

Sun and moon visualization

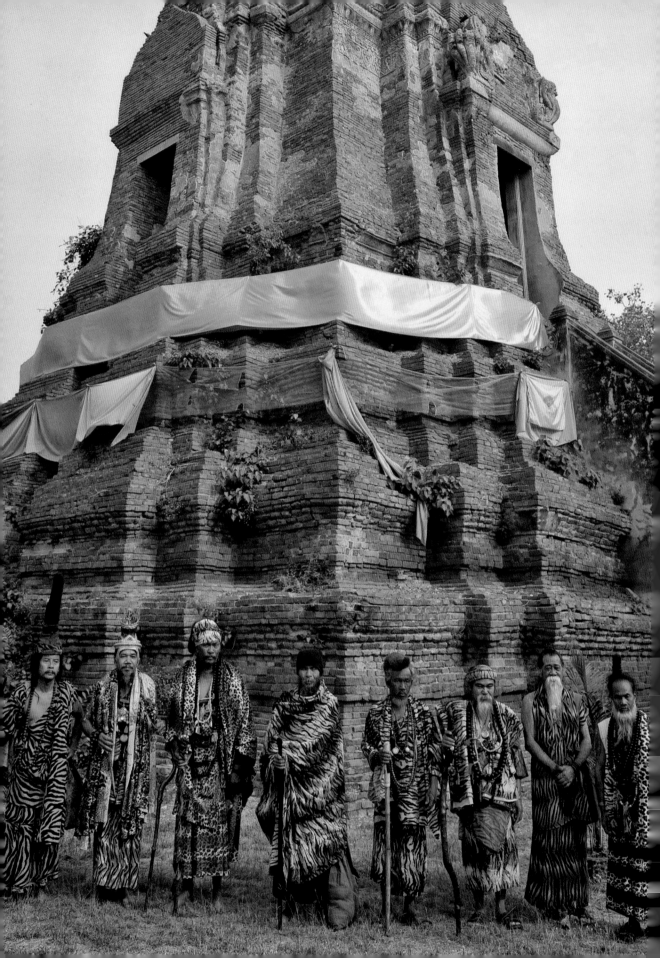

Section 3

Spiritual and
Cultural Connections

The Art of Tok Sen

JOEL SHEPOSH

The Thai healing technique known as *tok sen* evolved in what is now northern Thailand, though its origins probably lie outside the Thai traditional medicine system. Tok sen has been part of the Lanna Thai healing tradition for centuries, when Burma controlled the present-day provinces of Chiang Mai, Chiang Rai, Lampang, Lamphun, and Mae Hong Son. Since territorial borders have changed over the years, it is not clear if the tradition began in the Lanna kingdom or in Burma (current-day Myanmar).

Even though tok sen's beginnings are shrouded in mystery, there can be no denying that it is thriving. In recent years, it has become one of the most popular healing arts in Thailand's northern provinces of Chiang Mai, Chiang Rai, Lamphun, and Lampang, and also in neighboring Myanmar and Laos.

The name tok sen is interesting. Tok (ตอก, pronounced "dtaawk") is a verb that means "to hammer" or "to apply with force." Sen is the Thai word for string, thread, cord, or route, but in Thai medicine it refers to the energy pathways that travel through the human body. There are ten main sen lines in the body (*sib sen*), and it is through these lines that the wind element called *lom* travels. In tok sen, the practitioner uses a wooden hammer (ค้อน, pronounced "khawn") to tap a chiseled wooden stick (ลิ่ม, pronounced "lim") along sen lines and pressure points on the body. Although tok sen literally means "to hammer the sen," there are parts of some sen lines that should never be tapped. Conversely, there are areas outside the sen lines that should be tapped.

A variety of sticks and hammers

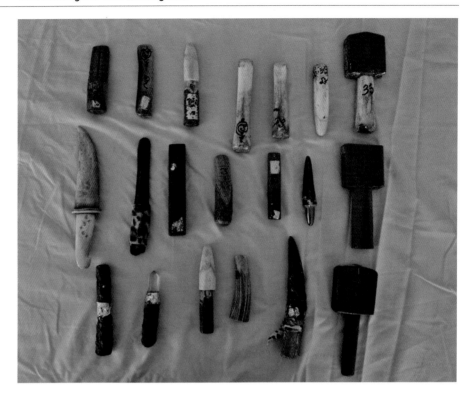

Tok sen tools

The hammer and stick used in tok sen are carved from wood. Ideally, the wood should be from a tree that was struck by lightning, because it is believed that this wood contains more power. Any type of wood may be used, but the tamarind tree seems to be preferred. Wood from a home may also be used, as long as the wood is taken from the walls or roof, and not from the floorboards.

The hammer has a rectangular head measuring approximately 10 x 5 centimeters (4 x 2 inches) that is attached to a 15-centimeter (6-inch) handle. The stick measures approximately 15 centimeters long by 5 centimeters wide/round (6 x 2 inches). The hammer and stick are carved by hand, and special incantations and spells are performed before, during, and after the carving process. Most practitioners in Thailand have their tools blessed by a monk or a teacher, and all tools are kept in a safe, respectful place when not in use.

There are many variations in the sizes and shapes of the hammers and sticks. Some hammers have rectangular or cube-shaped heads, others have shorter or longer handles. Some sticks have a round tip, some have a flat tip, and some have a wedged tip; some therapists even attach a crystal to the tip of the stick. And while the traditional material is "thunder wood" (wood from a tree struck by lightning), the stick can also be carved from bone or ivory, but only if the animal died from natural causes.

Ultimately, the tools must be easy and comfortable to use. As a natural extension of human hands, they should allow the therapist to control the weight, placement, and rhythm of his work.

It is common for a tok sen therapist to use several sticks during a session. A round or flat-tipped stick is suitable for tapping on most of the body. The wedge-tip stick, however, is especially useful for tapping between the bones on the back of the hand and on the top of the foot, and for working the five lines on the palms and soles.

Usually a beginner will learn and practice with the style of hammer and stick that his teacher uses. In most cases, the student keeps the hammer and stick that he used in class. Over time, a therapist will add to his collection of tools, and by experience, he will know which tool to use for which client, and on which part of the body.

Tok sen treatment

As with traditional Thai massage, a tok sen treatment can be either relaxing, therapeutic, or both. A typical relaxing session includes tapping along lines and points on the legs, feet, arms, hands, back, and neck. A therapeutic session would add focused tapping in specific problem areas.

The treatment takes place on the floor. The client wears loose, comfortable clothing, and receives treatment in all four basic positions of traditional Thai massage: supine (face up), prone (face down), side-lying, and seated. Many schools and teachers in Thailand prefer the common face-up, side-lying, face-down, and seated sequence, while other teachers encourage variation, as long as the techniques are well executed.

A stand-alone tok sen treatment consists of palm-walking a section of the body, and then tapping with the hammer and stick on sen lines and points. It is possible to tap along a specific sen line from its origin to its end, but it's rare that a therapist would tap along the entire length of any of the ten major sen. Instead, the therapist taps along the familiar lines found in a Thai massage session: outer and inner legs, outer and inner arms, palms and soles, backs of the hands, tops of the feet, and the back of the body.

There is no rule for the direction of the tapping. Just like the "thumb-chasing-thumb" technique in Thai massage, the tapping may be done either proximal to distal, or distal to proximal. A typical pattern might go like this:

- Palm-walk to warm up the area
- Tap along a major sen line
- Tap along the minor (diagonal) sen line
- Tap on selected points along that line
- Palm-walk to cool down the area

Tapping on selected sen points is optional, and to be effective, the therapist must know the exact location and function of each of the pressure points. Unfortunately, general knowledge of Thai sen points is not as widespread in Thailand as it is, for example, in traditional Chinese medicine.

A small amount of herbal oil may be applied to the body. One herbal oil recipe mixes goat and antelope oil, sesame oil, jungle butterfly, peppers, cardamom, python bone, and camphor. My teachers say this mixture helps the effectiveness of a tok sen treatment, but they haven't offered an exact explanation.

After the session, the therapist might brush the body with a leaf dipped in *nam mon* (blessed water). This is done to remove any remaining unseen oil residue and to help cleanse and purify the area.

Before the session begins, the practitioner interviews, evaluates, and observes the client to determine if there are any pre-existing conditions, and if there are any contraindications to receiving tok sen. Contraindications include broken bones, any metal in the body, high blood pressure, certain skin conditions, and pregnancy. Use caution if the client has diabetes, edema, or fever.

While most areas of the body may be treated with tok sen, avoid tapping on specific areas, including:

- The face and scalp
- Directly on bones
- On or around any joint
- At the distal anterior forearm
- On the chest

Ajahn Bundit Sitthiwej works the back of a client in prone position

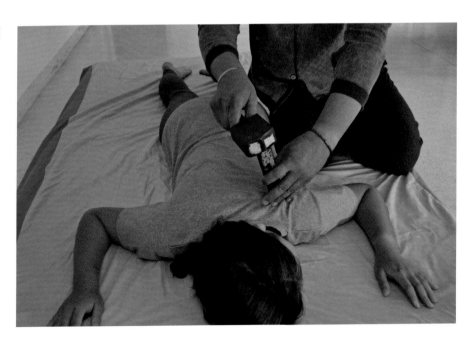

Tapping on the abdomen and neck may be done, but only very lightly and with great attention.

A tok sen treatment can last anywhere from one to several hours, and it should not be painful to receive. Pain can occur if the therapist is not mindful, or if he taps in any of the forbidden areas.

Spells, mantras, and maintaining a calm mind

Before starting a treatment, or at the beginning and end of their workday, the tok sen therapist pays respect to the Father Doctor by chanting the mantra *(Om Namo Shivago...)* and by offering incense and flowers to a statue or image. There are also spells specific to tok sen that a therapist may use before a session. One such spell is from Ajahn Sompong from Chiang Mai. It is in Pali, and he says he cannot offer a specific translation, but that the prayer asks for help from teachers and the Buddha, and for guidance and protection in order to "release the bad things from the body and have good things and good health for your client." Ajahn Sompong learned this blessing from his teacher, who learned it from his teacher, and so on. Holding the hammer in one hand and the stick in the other, the therapist sings the short three-line chant, which is not reproduced here because it is not appropriate to do so according to Thai tradition.

Then the therapist blows on the part of the stick that will come in contact with the client, and taps the hammer and stick together three times. This ritual is repeated three times. Once this is done, the hammer and stick are now considered ready to use.

Before beginning the treatment, the therapist must have a calm, clear, and strong mind, and that focus must remain constant throughout the session. The therapist must be very clear at all times how and where to place the stick, and the correct amount of force to apply with the hammer. It is therefore imperative that the therapist develop and cultivate tranquility and insight through a consistent and regular meditation practice. In Theravada Buddhism, this is accomplished through the practice of samatha-vipassana meditation.

The tapping technique

For many years, tok sen was taught in the traditional system of learning based on teacher-apprentice relationships, and as a result, few written materials exist. It is therefore difficult to know for sure if there is any single authentic style of tapping.

Nowadays, one teacher might instruct the student to divide a sen line into segments and then to tap a pattern of 1-2-3, 1-2-3, 1-2-3 on the first portion of

Working the back
lines in sitting
position

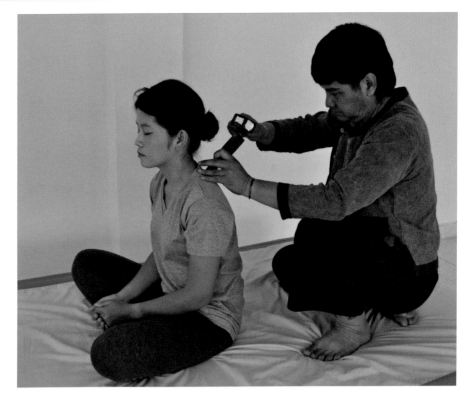

the line. Then the tapping sequence would continue at the next portion of that line, and so on. Other teachers prefer a tapping pattern of 1-2, 1-2, 1-2 on each segment. And yet another teacher might work in single, double, or triple taps from the beginning to the end of an entire line.

Some teachers say tapping is done in only one direction; while others say it is fine to tap in both directions. Regardless of the style taught, there are common rules that the therapist must follow, namely:

- The stick must always be placed one finger width away from any bone.
- The tapping must be constant and steady.
- The therapist must control the stick placement and tapping pressure at all times.

Conditions that can be helped by tok sen

Whenever I have asked my teachers which conditions were traditionally treated with tok sen, they have frequently answered my question with the phrase, "In the old times in Thailand ..." The consensus of my teachers is that "the old times" is a period in Siam roughly 100–500 years ago. During that time period, they say, tok sen was used to treat sore muscles, joint pain, pinched nerves, diseases associated with specific sen lines, paralysis, and diseases from supernatural causes. Nowadays, folk healers in northern Thailand still treat these and other conditions, using tok sen combined with other elements of the Thai healing tradition.

How does it work?

The light and rhythmic tapping along sen lines and points may work in a number of ways. The vibration caused by the tapping is believed to clear blocked energy along that line. The tapping's physical effect tends to soften the muscles. Tapping along a sen line may help conditions associated with that particular line, just as tapping on a specific point can produce a certain therapeutic effect. Finally, there is the hypnotic effect from the constant and steady tapping that helps to relax the body and mind of the receiver.

One of my teachers, Bundit "Billy" Sitthiwej, explains it this way: "The body is 70 percent water. The tapping makes waves, and it makes the bad things go away."

Study and practice

The basic techniques of tok sen can be learned in a two- or three-day class, and there are a number of schools and master teachers in northern Thailand that offer courses of study. As stated earlier, since there is no one, single authentic style of tok sen, it's possible for a student to learn different approaches with different schools and teachers. Another good way to learn is to learn by receiving. This is especially easy in Chiang Mai, where one can receive tok sen at street markets, massage shops, schools, and clinics.

While tok sen techniques may be easy to learn in just a few days, it takes years of practice to fully master the essence of this fascinating healing tradition. Controlling weight and pressure, maintaining a steady rhythm, correctly placing the hammer and stick, and developing and maintaining calmness and clarity of mind are all required for advanced practice.

Tok sen can be a wonderful accessory technique for the Thai massage student and therapist. As more schools and teachers offer courses, it will continue to spread in Thailand and around the world. If you have a chance, try a tok sen session. You will probably be glad that you did.

Memorial for Chaiyuth

BENCE GANTI

On 31 January, 2004, around 3 p.m., Chaiyuth Priyasith died at a traditional healers' dance in a village near Chiang Mai in northern Thailand. I had spent a little more than two weeks studying with him as a Thai massage student, and here I was, along with my fellow students, witnessing his death. I felt as if I'd been thrown into a natural flow of events that I couldn't even comprehend. After some time, I felt a need – a duty – to write about the day of his death and the events that led up to it. This is a memorial for someone who touched the hearts of many Thai massage students around the world.

A few days before his death, his students had asked him about the meaning of his name. He answered: "*chai* – winner; *yuth* – strategy." The issue of death had already been in the air in a gentle way during previous days. On one hand, the avian flu was a hot topic in Thailand, not yet threatening Chiang Mai but constantly being reported in the news. But more than that, Chaiyuth had also mentioned his possible death to us during class. One day he said, "When I die, I will not be reborn again. I will be a healer spirit so I can be in many places to heal, not just one." At that time we thought he was speaking about his death in a general way – after all, he was only in his early sixties. He looked well, with elastic skin, and he appeared much younger than his age. Through his movements and expressions he also conveyed youth.

Chaiyuth usually gave 1–2 sessions a day, each lasting 2–4 hours. In addition, he formally taught us each morning for several hours, and, almost every day, we would join him in "the dance," where he danced intensively for another few hours. Chaiyuth loved the dances as much as he loved giving massage and teaching. There was one common denominator in these three activities: his devotion to his spirit teacher, the father doctor of Thai massage, Jivaka Kumar Bhacca. Chaiyuth said that he maintained continuous personal contact with Jivaka, and that he channeled him during his Thai massage sessions. Chaiyuth referred to him simply as "my teacher," and said that his spiritual dances were directed to Jivaka as an offering. He brought his students to the dances in order to intro-

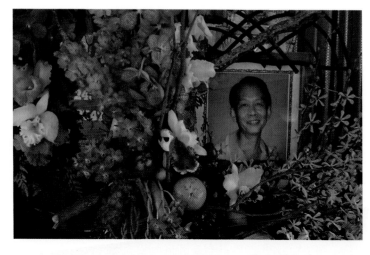

Chaiyuth's photo as it appeared on his coffin

duce them personally to Jivaka, and because "dancing opens your mind." The words he used to speak about Jivaka, the way he carried out his Thai massage sessions, the care with which he prepared his dance costume each day, and the dance steps and movements he used seemed permeated by a special kind of respect, sacredness, reverence, and humility.

Chaiyuth told us one day that he never wanted to teach large groups, even if he could make more money. He said he preferred to teach 3–4 people at a time. He often criticized the way people do Thai massage today, and the way many schools were oriented to making as much money as possible. "Everywhere relax, relax, just relax, but no healing."

Rather than take notes and photos, Chaiyuth encouraged us to memorize and internalize the movements, according to the traditional Thai way of learning and practice. It was hard for me not to take notes, especially by the third day, when everything seemed too much for me to memorize. The most effective learning took place on those occasions when we worked in steps. First, Chaiyuth would demonstrate a movement on us, so that we could feel it from inside. Then we would practice on each other while he observed, so that he could correct us from the outside. Finally, we would practice on him, so that he could feel if we were performing it correctly.

The last day of class

On January 31, we started class at 6 a.m., earlier than usual because we had planned to leave for the spirit dance around 10. That morning in class, Chaiyuth taught abdominal techniques. At one point a Greek woman appeared. She said she had a girlfriend who was sick with a severe bladder inflammation, and she asked if she could bring her to be treated by Chaiyuth. Chaiyuth told her, "Okay. Come now."

We finished the morning session at 9:30 a.m. that day. Usually Chaiyuth would take a one-hour break to prepare for the dance and to pack the dance robes, so I returned to my guest house to pick up a few things. When I got there, I saw a group of foreigners chatting in the garden, and I also noticed Tim, who sometimes came with us to Chaiyuth's dances. I assumed that these *farang* had just arrived at the hotel and were waiting to check in to their rooms, but when I asked Tim who they were, he replied that they were coming with us to the dance. Usually only three or four people attended the dance ceremonies, but here were twelve more people.

I immediately returned to Chaiyuth and told him there would be fifteen farang coming that day, and I asked if we should go in cars rather than by bike. Surprised by the number, he answered, "Fifteen?" Then he laughed. "Car okay. No problem."

In the meantime, the Greek woman arrived with her ill friend while Chaiyuth was in his kitchen. I asked him if I could watch the session, and he agreed. I had never seen Chaiyuth give a full session, and I was eager and curious to see what he would do with this woman. I wondered how Chaiyuth could heal physical problems like bladder infections that are not typically treated through Thai massage techniques, nor taught to students in normal courses of study. I reasoned that Chaiyuth's elevated sense of intuition and sensitivity, along with Jivaka's intercession, allowed him to heal many kinds of problems, even those beyond the limits of normal therapeutic massage.

At the outset, he made it clear to the lady that his teacher, not he, would be conducting the healing session today. He asked her if she believed in this, because she could only be cured if she believed. She replied affirmatively. He started with a stomach massage, similar to what we had done in class that morning. It was a long-lasting, deep, and thorough abdominal massage. I thought that when he finished with her stomach the healing session would be completed. But then he began working the arms, the back, the legs, and the head, and finally he finished with some long, flowing postures, with his eyes totally closed.

We didn't know that this would be the last healing session he would give before he died. The session lasted about 90 minutes. Meanwhile people were patiently waiting and gathering in Chaiyuth's garden. By the time we exited the healing hut, the garden was full of people from all over the world. They were chatting quietly underneath the lush trees, the shadows playing with the sunlight, casting stripes of light on the ground and chairs and on the small fountains in the garden. The atmosphere was peaceful, respectful, silent, and gentle, but you could feel the curiosity and excitement about the ceremony we would shortly be attending. Many people would be meeting Chaiyuth for the first time, and some had just arrived in Thailand, being referred to Chaiyuth through friends. Some weren't even familiar with traditional Thai massage.

Soon we left the garden and got into a *songthaew* that someone had hired for us, along with a driver. We sat on the seats and the floor of that little white truck, and some of us were even standing outside on the back of the vehicle. Two people went by motorbike, and so did Chaiyuth, with a student on the backseat. First, we stopped as usual at the vegetarian restaurant close to Suan Dok Gate. After lunch, we continued to the flower stalls at Warorot market. As always, we bought many flowers: three garlands to put around our necks, and yellow flowers to decorate the big drum that was

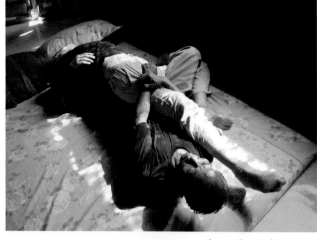

Chaiyuth working on a woman in his treatment room, a few days before he passed away

played at the dance. It was a bright and sunny day, and we headed out of Chiang Mai in a southeasterly direction. We drove through the countryside, effortlessly navigating the route, and arriving at our destination in a very short time.

Spirit dances are always held at a different place, and always at the home of someone from the healing dance community. Each host organizes a party and invites whomever he or she wishes. For today's event, an invitation card was provided with the address, and as we got closer, we began to see red flags marking the way on the roadside. We arrived at an area that was filled with cars and bikes, and it looked like this would be a big gathering. Chaiyuth parked his bike at the back of the lot, and we jumped out of the songthaew and began to gather in a loose line in front of a long path that marked the entrance to the venue.

Arriving at the dance

On our way to the dance area, we came upon an offering plate. At the entrance to the garden, guests were welcomed by receiving a huge plate with water and floating flowers. We were to take it into our hands, lift it, and say a prayer. It was such a wonderful way to enter the dance garden: a gentle reminder of the need for spiritual awareness. Thai people understand the importance of creating a spiritual atmosphere with the integration of small ritual acts into the events of daily life.

It took a few minutes for all of us to say our prayers and reassemble at the entrance to the garden. While waiting, I had a chance to look around and explore the site. It was a wonderful Thai village setting, with tropical vegetation. Bright midday sunlight played among the trees and bushes surrounding the house and the dance floor. The dancers were dressed in brightly colored traditional robes and headdresses. They were already dancing under a tent roof, which had been set up in the garden of the host's home.

The dance area was filled with more people than usual. The band was larger than most, and included both Western instruments and traditional Thai folk instruments. The dancers were dressed in all shades of Thai silk – red, blue, purple, green, and white – and they sported scarves, headresses, and ornate necklaces. Men and women alike wore dance skirts. Around the dance floor were many tables and chairs, where non-dancers, mostly villagers, family members, and friends, were sitting. They were nibbling on peanuts and crackers, sipping local sweet wine, homemade Thai whisky, soft drinks, and coconut water from freshly cut coconuts.

The featured dancers were all healers of some kind. Chaiyuth said they all had guiding spirits. Each had his or her own way to heal, and some were shamans and intuitive readers. Their common link was that they were guided by spiritual forces, and this event was an opportunity to make offerings to the spirits through sacred dancing. The host family had a huge altar adorned with flowers, incense, candles, and offerings of food and drinks. Ordinary people were spectators, and the invited healers were the only ones allowed to dance during the central part of the ceremony. During the course of the afternoon, a good number of them fell into trance, or otherwise became possessed by their spirit guides. I saw several healers writhing at their tables before and after they danced. I asked Chaiyuth about it, and all he said was, "They spirit."

Chaiyuth was chatting and laughing with some local friends, and he asked some other Thais to show us the way. Some of them quickly and graciously arranged a few tables for us. We put down our bags, and those who had brought special clothes for the dance put them on. We took out the flowers and put them around our necks, and also brought some to the dance floor to offer to the band. We attached yellow garlands to the big drum. Then we,

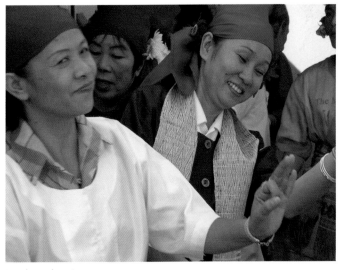

Healers dancing at the spirit dance that day

along with other visitors, were allowed to dance.

One dancer came to greet us. Another gave us invitation cards for the next party. Others brought local cigars and whisky to share with us. Some people were smiling at us, and others had more serious expressions. Some dancers encouraged us by showing us basic movements, while others observed with a more dubious look. It seemed to me that some of them were friendly toward us, some were ambivalent, and some weren't particularly happy that we were there. In any event, the vivid colors, the undulating crowd, and the loud, rhythmic music set the stage for what would be a very special event.

During all of this, Chaiyuth was putting on his ceremonial clothing back near the tables. Every movement he made was like a meditative prayer. He would slowly withdraw each piece of clothing from his small suitcase, and place each item on his body, one after the other, in a slow, methodical manner. With each item of clothing, he would softly recite prayers to Jivaka, sometimes sending his prayers to the item by blowing with his breath.

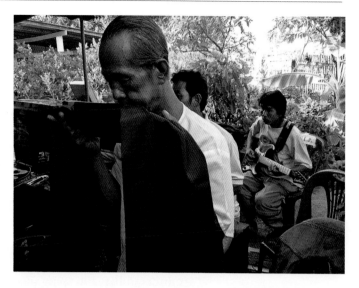

Chaiyuth praying to Shivago over a red silk shawl before approaching the dance floor

After he finished dressing, he remained seated at the table with closed eyes, looking very prayerful, and he began to be drawn into the music. Whether he was relaxing at home, giving a Thai massage, teaching his students, or at a spirit dance, Chaiyuth's mood was always one of humility and prayer mixed with gentleness, relaxation, and good humor. I felt sometimes as if he were constantly praying. He lived within his own peaceful space, and it followed him wherever he was. His energy field was silent, strong, and modest, and it could be revealed only to those who could stop, be still, and pay attention.

After some time he walked toward the dance floor. I remember his face. He approached very slowly and looked deeply at his students. He was gently smiling, and he displayed an expression of fulfillment. He greeted the band, put a flower on the drum, and started to dance. Chaiyuth danced differently than the others, with freestyle spiraling and rotating movements. He didn't restrict himself to the basic movements and the typical hand gestures that most everyone else used. He had his own perfectly unique style, what he and others called "the snake dance." I'd heard that some people didn't appreciate his strong movements, while others were attracted to his power and always smiled and followed him as he moved. That day the band members seemed very attracted to his presence, especially the drummer.

An extraordinary chain of events

It was while sitting at our table that an extraordinary and surreal chain of events unfolded before us, one that shook the roots of our minds and hearts. I saw from the corner of my eye that Chaiyuth was coming toward us. I began to pour water from a plastic bottle into my glass, and I felt the table move slightly when he sat down. Thirty seconds later, while holding the glass of water in my hand, I turned my head toward him and couldn't believe my eyes. Chaiyuth was lying face down on the ground beside his seat. He seemed paralyzed and he wasn't moving at all. Time stopped, and everything froze around us. Then he began to rattle and shake, as if he wanted to cough something up and expel it from his chest. He began to snort into the dry earth with an unusual type of sound.

It all happened so quickly – in the space of seconds – that we remained stuck and frozen. No logical, rational response came to mind. We were stunned and didn't know what to do, or whether we should do anything at all. He continued making strange sounds, snorts, and grunts that came out of the deepest part of his body. Only a few days before, we had seen a woman in red garments making this same rattling sound. She was sitting at her table after a round of dancing, and surrounded by family members. I had asked Chaiyuth about it, and he had said, "Spirit! Say goodbye to spirit." I assumed that the lady had been possessed by a spirit, and that the spirit was leaving her body after the dance. Now the very same thing was happening to Chaiyuth, lying on the ground before us. The half of his face that I could see from my seat was not of this world.

A Canadian woman who was at the event later told me that she was watching his face right before he fell. She said Chaiyuth had a peaceful, gentle expression on his face, and that he slowly closed his eyes, lost the color tone of his skin, and simply surrendered to the ground.

At first I didn't think he was suffering or dying. I found myself watching him, as if he had simply become possessed. The Thais remained sitting or standing, and some were calmly watching Chaiyuth in this state. This might have been a familiar scene, an after-effect of a person who had just emerged from a deep spiritual trance. But none of us had ever seen Chaiyuth possessed in this way before, and after a few more seconds of watching, a thought germinated in the back of my mind. What if he's dying? I confronted my own feelings and convinced myself that I shouldn't be thinking that way. It was probably a passing possession, and he would emerge from it soon.

Suddenly Terry appeared, and after a few moments of watching worriedly, she began to intervene. She squatted down and lifted Chaiyuth from the ground. His face was gray with dirt, and completely stiff and expressionless. A deep, raw fear arose within me, reinforced by an instantaneous understanding that spirits have the power to take our lives in one second, and that engaging with spirits who hold enormous supernatural power is not a game. I felt a rapid flash of intense fear and also a mild disgust. One minute ago Chaiyuth was so alive, so happy, so full of life. And now he had been reduced to a mere shell of himself. All along I had been repressing the possibility that he might be dying before us, but now that thought began to haunt me.

Then as if he had been touched by a magic wand, life suddenly came back into his face. A switch of life turned on, and with it came a moment of exhilaration. He tried to open his eyes, but after a few seconds of struggle he collapsed, and he went limp again.

A sense of controlled panic began to permeate the room. Terry propped him up, began to wipe his face with a wet cloth, and then began to shout for help. Some of the farang helped to put Chaiyuth in a chair, but his muscles seemed nonfunctional. We had to hold his body against the chair to prevent it from falling to the ground. Some of our group members began sobbing, and we still didn't know what to do. We expected that the Thai people would know what to do because it was happening in their homeland, and in accordance with their customs, but they may have assumed that we would take charge of the situation, because we had come to the dance with Chaiyuth.

For the most part, the Thai people remained calm, as if a leaf had just fallen from a tree. They showed no anxiety, panic, fear, or other emotions. And they did nothing to intervene in what was unfolding before us all. Some were watching with looks of concern and curiosity, but they also continued talking, drinking beer, or waiting on the dance floor for the next round of dancing to begin.

Suddenly a Thai woman appeared, a friend of Chaiyuth's whom we had seen at every other dance. She removed the mildly intoxicating leaves that Chaiyuth had been chewing in order to clear his air passage. Others continued to search for a pulse in total silence. Finally somone said there was no pulse. I was sure that one of the Thai people there had already called for an ambulance, but then I realized that no one had done so, and that we were in a small, sleepy village. One of us had a cell phone, and I thrust it in the air shouting, "Please call the doctor. Hospital. Doctor."

At the same time, another woman pointed to the parking area and spoke to the crowd in Thai. It seemed she was saying that we should immediately take Chaiyuth to the hospital. Some of us were already shouting for the driver who had brought us in the white songthaew. Within seconds he appeared, and we picked up Chaiyuth's lifeless body and quickly moved through the long pathway that had been so welcoming only a few hours before.

It seemed to be the farang's responsibility to remove Chaiyuth's body from that place. We reached the parking area and put Chaiyuth's body into the songthaew. Terry asked most of the people in the group to wait there, and she decided that only a few people should accompany the body. The Thai woman who had removed the leaves from Chaiyuth's mouth sat next to the driver. Kaori and I jumped onto her rented motorbike, and I offered to drive, since she felt weakened by the events.

The songthaew began moving, and we followed close behind on the bike. We made our way through the village, and onto the winding roads of the countryside, passing rice fields and small villages in the early afternoon sunshine. I could see in the vehicle ahead of me that they were trying to resuscitate our teacher with artificial respiration and heart pumping.

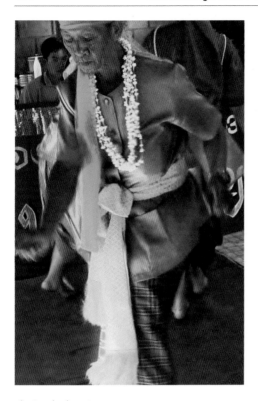

Chaiyuth dancing, moments before entering a trance

We reached the highway, and rather than head toward Chiang Mai, we went in the opposite direction. After a few hundred meters we reached a hospital, directly off the highway. Someone emerged from inside, and brought him in a wheelchair to the emergency room. We could see the doctors attending to him, but after about 15 minutes they looked toward us, shaking their heads. It was over.

One by one, each of us entered the hospital room to say goodbye, and with this act we acknowledged and accepted his death. His skin had already begun to discolor, and small dark specks appeared on the surface of his skin. His body was completely stiff. It was hard to believe that a body as elastic as his had become so stiff in such a short period of time.

The doctors pushed him out to the corridor on a gurney and covered him with a white cloth. They said the cause of death was a heart attack, but most of us who had witnessed his death believed that he had been possessed by a spirit, and that he had died while in a state of trance. It was his time, and Jivaka, his teacher, had come for him.

From the hospital, we walked out into the streets of nowhere. We didn't know what would happen next. Would someone call his family? What would happen to the body? Should we just go home now? After some time, the Thai woman and I got into the songthaew with the driver. We began winding through the countryside, and after a stop at the village of Bo Sang, we returned to Chaiyuth's house in Chiang Mai. No one had returned yet from the dance, nor from the hospital. A young boy came out of the house, and the Thai woman told him what had happened. There was hardly any response, and they both stood there quietly. A girl also appeared, and she didn't react with great emotion, either. I slowly began to understand and internalize that the lack of outward emotion and the stillness I was witnessing is inextricably woven into Thai Buddhist culture, even in times of death.

We politely said goodbye and left that place. I returned there every hour to see if the others had come back, and to hear any news. A large crowd began to assemble in Chaiyuth's garden. Among the crowd were two women who had recently arrived from Europe in order to study with Chaiyuth. They had arrived at Chaiyuth's house expecting to study with him, but instead they were told that the master had just died. We were informed that his body would be transferred the next day to Wat Mahawan, and that it would be there for three days. The cremation would occur on the fourth day. Slowly, the crowd began to dissipate, and we returned to our guest houses and hotels for the evening.

The funeral

The next day I went to Wat Mahawan and saw the coffin in its temporary resting place, along with decorations, burning incense, flowers, and photographs of Chaiyuth spread throughout the room. Each morning and evening for three days, a prayer ceremony was conducted by the resident monks, and each afternoon there was a luncheon for the monks and snacks for the guests who came to pay their respects.

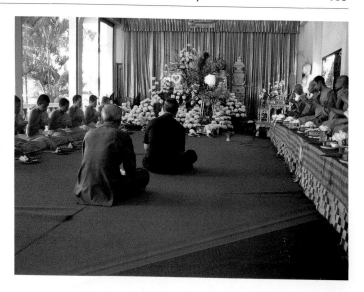

The funeral ceremony at Wat Mahawan in Chiang Mai. Mourners prayed on the floor, friends and guests sat behind in chairs, and monks and novices chanted on the sides

For three days many people came in and out of the temple. Chaiyuth's sister and daughter had arrived from Bangkok, and a large gathering of local Thai people regularly attended the ceremonies, as well as Thai massage teacher Asokananda and several of his students and assistant teachers. I remember thinking that it was good that the coffin would be there for three days, so that friends and mourners could have enough time to let go and become accustomed to the fact that he had left us.

The cremation occurred on the fourth day. The band arrived at the wat very early in the morning, set up a tent, brought in their equipment, and started to play music as if it were a festive occasion. They played for a long time, and guests were offered lunch. A donation box was placed on the side, to help pay for the costs of the funeral. Finally, the coffin was removed from its stand and placed in the hearse. There were three funeral cars. The first carried Chaiyuth's photographic image, the second bore his coffin, and the third transported core members of the band.

One of the organizers asked me to hold Chaiyuth's name on a flag, and to carry incense sticks that were burning inside a coconut shell and contained within a ceramic pot. He asked someone else to carry another flag on the other side of the coffin. A few other farang rode in the first car to display Chaiyuth's photograph. Behind us came the core members of the band in an open car, playing traditional funeral music for the procession.

As we slowly rolled out toward Tha Pae Road, Thai massage teacher Poo told me that the incense ball should be held firmly, because the incense would serve as a guide to allow Chaiyuth's spirit to follow the funeral procession along with the rest of us. We maintained complete silence as the band played music from their car, the sounds echoing off the buildings on the street, bystanders stopping to gaze at the procession.

I saw the whole procession from the vantage point of the hearse carrying the coffin. Chaiyuth was passing through the streets of his hometown for the last time, saying farewell to the city he loved. Slowly we arrived at the place of cremation, and shortly afterward his body and coffin were cremated in a large pyre, accompanied by a display of fireworks.

The chanting monks stood beside the burning coffin and recited over and over again one of the key teachings of the Buddha that is now burned into my memory and consciousness:

> Aniccavata sankhara
> Uppada vaya dhammino
> Uppajjhitva nirujjhanti
> Tesam vupasamo sukho

> All things are impermanent.
> Arising and passing away is their inherent nature.
> When they arise and become extinguished,
> Their eradication brings true happiness.

The Vinaya Pitaka: Stories about Jivaka Kumarabhacca

REDACTION AND NOTES BY BOB HADDAD

The following is a modern redaction of a small portion of the Vinaya Pitaka, one of the three divisions of the Tipitaka (Tripitaka) or Pali Canon. The Tipitaka (literally "three baskets") is the collection of Pali language texts that form the doctrinal foundation of Theravada Buddhism. In a subsection of this sacred text called the Eight Khandaka, circumstances are related surrounding the life of Jivaka Kumarabhacca, the ancestral teacher associated with traditional Thai medicine. The story traces Jivaka's birth and adolescence, his aspiration to the medical field, and momentous events in the professional practice of this famous doctor. At the end of the story, Jivaka converses with the Buddha, and afterward the Buddha decides to allow the *sangha* (spiritual community) to use certain types of robes and garments. With regard to Jivaka's name as it has passed through history, there are several spellings and possible derivations of the name he was given at birth. Early translators imagined that the compound word *Komarabhaccato* was derived from the Sanskrit word for "prince" *(kumara, komara)* and *Abhaya* (the name of the prince who raised Jivaka), so they interpreted Kumarabhacca to mean "raised by Prince Abhaya."

The true meaning of the name may have been different, however, because in Sanskrit, *kumârabhrityâ* and *kaumârabhritya* are technical terms for the division of medicine that deals with the treatment of infants (pediatrics). Therefore, the surname Kumarabhacca could also mean "master of *kaumârabhritya*," or in other words, pediatric specialist. Jivaka's second name is represented with many different spellings, including Kumarbhacca, Kumarabhaccha, and Komarbhacca. His first name is sometimes seen as Givaka, and in Thailand it is known as Shivaga and Shivago. Because of the linguistic confusion in the Thai language of the English consonants r and l, and the similarity between the hard sound of the letter g and the sound of the letter k, Jivaka's last name is sometimes known in Thailand as Gomalapato, Gomalapaj, Gomarapat, or Komarapaj. Several translations of these texts based on various sources have been done over the years, but I couldn't find one that was rendered in easy-to-read language. As I compared the various translations from Pali into English and noted the different interpretations, it occurred to me that it would be an interesting project to prepare and present a new redaction in plain vernacular English for the benefit of students and practitioners of traditional Thai healing arts. As a result, I have updated and edited the text of this interesting document to read in a more contemporary, fluid way. In addition to integrating more modern vocabulary, I've inserted clarifications in italics, and additional notes surrounded by brackets.

There is much talk about the man who is considered the ancestral teacher of Thai medicine and Thai massage, but only a few serious Thai massage practitioners have actually read historical accounts of Jivaka's life and his interactions with the Buddha, the first sangha, and the patients he treated. I hope this contemporary version of ancient stories adds depth to your understanding of this important figure, one whose legacy in India 2,500 years ago is still honored in current-day Thailand.

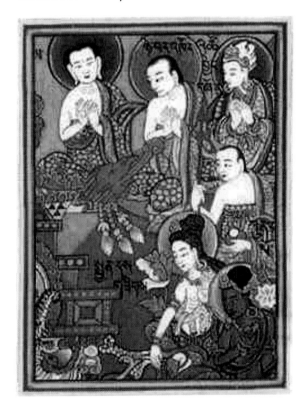

A small section of a 17th-century Tibetan thangka featuring Bodhisattvas and pious attendants of the Buddha. Jivaka Kumarabhacca appears at top right

The story of Jivaka's birth

At that time the blessed Buddha lived in Rajagaha, *[current day Rajgir, Bihar, northern India]* in Venuvana park, near a bamboo grove where many squirrels would gather to eat. In those days Vesali *[current day Vaishali, 150 kilometers to the north]* was an opulent, prosperous town. It was crowded with people and very abundant with food. There were 7,707 storied buildings, 7,707 pinnacled buildings, 7,707 pleasure grounds (*aramas*), and 7,707 lotus ponds.

There was also a courtesan in Vaishali named Ambapali (Ambapalika, Amrapali), who was beautiful, graceful, pleasing, gifted with a wonderful complexion, well versed in dancing, singing, and lute playing, and who was regularly visited by many desirous men. Her fee was 50 *kahapanas* per night. Vaishali was prosperous, but because of the beautiful courtesan Ambapali, the town flourished even more.

One day several merchants who were members of the urban council of Rajgir traveled to Vaishali on business. They noticed how opulent and prosperous Vaishali was, and how populous and abundant with food it was, and they also saw the 7,707 storied buildings. And the courtesan Ambapali was so beautiful! It was clear that Vaishali was a more interesting place because of her.

After finishing their business in Vaishali, the merchants returned to Rajgir and went to the palace of the Magadha king Seniya Bimbisara. Approaching him, they said: "Your Majesty, Vaishali is an opulent, prosperous town, and especially because of the beautiful courtesan Ambapali, it is flourishing more and more these days. Why don't we also install a courtesan in Rajgir?"

The king replied, "Well, then, my good sirs, go ahead and look for a girl that you can install as a courtesan."

Living in Rajgir at that time was a girl by the name of Salavati, who was beautiful, graceful, pleasing, and had an excellent complexion, and she was the one who the merchants chose to be the courtesan. And before long, Salavati became well versed in dancing, singing, and lute playing. She was visited by many desirous men, and she charged 100 kahapanas for one night.

But Salavati soon became pregnant. When this happened, she thought: "Men aren't interested in pregnant courtesans. If anyone finds out that I'm pregnant, I'll lose my job and my entire position. Perhaps I should tell everyone that I am sick."

So she gave orders to her door-keeper saying, "Let no man enter here, my good door-keeper. If anyone calls for me, just tell them that I'm sick." The door-keeper faithfully followed Salavati's orders.

When the child in her womb reached maturity, Salavati gave birth to a baby boy, but afterward she gave orders to her maid-servant saying, "Go, my girl, and put this boy into a winnowing basket. Then take him away, and leave him outside on a trash-heap."

The servant accepted Salavati's order, and she put the baby boy into an old winnowing basket, took him away, and placed him outside, on top of a trash pile.

After some time, a royal prince named Abhaya, while on his way to attend to the king, noticed some crows gathering nearby. When he saw that, he asked the people nearby, "What is over there, my good sirs, where those crows are gathering?"

"It's a baby boy, Your Highness."

"And is he alive?"

"Yes, Your Highness, he is alive."

"Well, then, bring that baby to our palace and give him to the nurses so that they can take care of him."

The people accepted the royal prince's order, and they brought the baby boy to the palace, gave him to the nurses, and told them that the prince wanted him to be nourished.

Now when Prince Abhaya had asked if the baby on the trash heap was alive, the nearby people had responded, *"Jivati,"* which means "He is alive." Because of this, they gave the baby boy the name of Jivaka. And because he had been raised and nourished by the royal prince (Kumarena Posapito), they gave him the name of Kumarabhacca.

Jivaka's training in medicine

Jivaka Kumarabhacca lived a good life throughout his childhood, and eventually he came to his years of discretion. One day, he went to the royal prince's palace, and approaching him, he asked the prince: "Your Highness, please tell me. Who is my mother, and who is my father?"

"I don't know who your mother is, Jivaka, but I am your father, because I've taken care of you for all these years."

Afterward, Jivaka Kumarabhacca thought: "Here in the royal family, it won't be easy to find a livelihood unless I know a craft. I need to learn a craft."

At that time, a well-known physician lived in Takkasila *[now Taxila, in Punjab province of Pakistan]*, and one day Jivaka Kumarabhacca, without even asking Prince Abhaya's permission, set off on a journey to Taxila, *[a distance of approximately 1,900 kilometers, or 1,200 miles]*. After wandering from place to place for a very long time, he finally arrived at the physician's place of practice in Taxila. *[This doctor is known in some texts as Atreya, a world-renowned physician.]*

Jivaka approached him, and he said, "Doctor, I want to learn your craft."

"Well, then, I will teach you," was the answer.

Jivaka Kumarabhacca learned a lot, and he learned very easily, and he understood well, and he didn't forget what he learned. And after a full seven years of study had passed, Jivaka thought: "I've learned a lot. I learn easily, and

I understand well, and I haven't forgotten what I've learned. I've been study-ing medicine now for seven years, but I still can't see an end to all of this. Will there ever be an end to my learning?"

So Jivaka went to the place where his teacher was, and he approached him and said: "I've learned a lot, doctor. I learn easily, I understand well, and I don't forget what I learn. I've studied for seven years now, but I still don't see an end to this art. When will I ever see an end to my learning?"

The doctor replied: "Very well then, Jivaka. Take this spade, and travel far and wide, for a distance of one *yojana* on each side of Taxila. Search all around for as long as necessary, and then bring back to me any plant you can find that has no medicinal value." *[yojana = The exact measurement is unknown, but is believed to be 4–9 miles (6–15 kilometers.]*

So Jivaka took a spade, and he set off to travel all around Taxila for a dis-tance of one yojana on each side. He searched far and wide for a very long time, yet he couldn't find a single plant that was devoid of healing properties.

Finally, Jivaka returned to his teacher, and he approached him and said: "Doctor, I've been searching all around Taxila for a distance of one yojana on each side, but I haven't been able to find anything at all that has no medicinal value."

The doctor replied, "Excellent. You have done your learning well, my dear Jivaka. This knowledge will serve you very well for maintaining your liveli-hood." Then he gave Jivaka some money for his journey home, and he sent him on his way.

Jivaka's first patient

Jivaka gratefully accepted the money given to him by his teacher, and he set out for the long journey back to Rajgir. By the time he reached the town of Saketa, and after the last of the money had been spent, Jivaka thought: "Water and food are very scarce in this wilderness, and it will be very difficult to con-tinue on my journey without more money. I need to earn some money so I can get back to Rajgir." *[Saketa is the ancient Sanskrit name for the current-day city of Ayodhya, which lent its name to the Thai city of Ayutthaya.]*

Now in Saketa at that time, a setthi's wife had been suffering from a head disease for over seven years *[setthi = wealthy merchant]*. Many great and world-renowned physicians had come to attend to her, but none of them could restore her to health. Nevertheless they had received large amounts of gold in payment for their services.

As Jivaka Kumarabhacca entered the town, he asked the people: "Is there anyone sick here, my friends? Is there anyone I can attend to?"

"The setthi's wife, doctor, has been suffering for seven years with a head disease. You can go and try to cure the setthi's wife."

So Jivaka went to that setthi's home, and when he got there, he said to the door-keeper, "Please go and tell the setthi's wife that a physician has arrived who wants to see her."

So the door-keeper went to the setthi's wife. He approached her and said, "A physician has arrived who wants to see you, madam."

"And what kind of man is this physician?"

"He is young, madam."

"How can a young physician help me? Many accomplished and world-renowned doctors have already come here to treat me. We give them our gold in payment, but not a single one of them has been able to cure me."

So the door-keeper went back to Jivaka Kumarabhacca and told him what the setthi's wife had said.

But Jivaka replied: "Please go back and tell her that I don't want any payment beforehand. If I can cure her and restore her to health, then can she pay me whatever she likes."

So the door-keeper went back to the woman and explained what Jivaka had said.

And the woman said, "Well, in that case, let this young physician enter."

Jivaka entered, he approached her, carefully examined her appearance and state, and then he said: "To treat you, madam, I'll need one *pasata* of *ghee* ." [*a measure of clarified butter*] So the setthi's wife ordered one pasata of ghee to be brought to him. Then Jivaka Kumarabhacca boiled that ghee with various drugs. Afterward, he made the woman lie on her back in bed, and he administered the mixture of ghee and herbal medicines to her through the nose. The medicated butter ran through her nose and came out through her mouth. The setthi's wife spat it out into a spittoon, but after she did that, she asked her maid-servant to retrieve the ghee with a piece of cotton, so she could save it for future use.

When Jivaka saw this happen, he thought to himself: "How stingy this woman is! That ghee should be thrown away, yet she's planning to use it again. It makes me wonder what kind of fee she will offer me. I've used many rare and expensive drugs in this treatment."

But the woman noticed Jivaka's change of demeanor, and she said to him: "Don't be concerned, doctor. Householders like us know how to economize. This ghee can be used for the servants and workmen to clean their feet, or it can be poured into a lamp for fuel. Don't be afraid, you won't lose your fee if you cure me."

And as a result of that treatment, with just a single dose of medicine administered through the nose, Jivaka drove away the disease that had plagued the woman for seven years.

The setthi's wife was delighted that she had been completely restored to health, and in payment, she gave Jivaka 4,000 kahapanas. Her son thought,

"My dear mother has finally been cured," and he also gave Jivaka 4,000 kahapanas. Her daughter-in-law thought, "My mother-in-law has finally been cured," and she gave him another 4,000 kahapanas. The setthi himself was so happy that his wife had finally been cured that he gave Jivaka an additional 4,000 kahapanas, plus a pair of servants and a coach with horses.

Jivaka begins practice in Rajgir

So Jivaka Kumarabhacca took those 16,000 kahapanas and the two servants, and he got into the horse-drawn coach, and he set out for Rajgir on the last leg of his long journey home. When he arrived in Rajgir, he went directly to the palace where he was raised, and he approached the royal prince Abhaya, and said to him:

"Your Highness, this is the money I've received for the first work I've done as a doctor. It is 16,000 kahapanas, plus two servants and a coach with horses. Please accept it in payment for all you did to raise me as a child."

"Oh no, my dear Jivaka, please keep it for yourself. Just promise me that now you will build a home for yourself, and that you will live here with us in our compound."

Jivaka Kumarabhacca accepted the prince's order saying, "Yes, Your Highness," and shortly afterward, he had a home built for himself in the compound of the royal prince Abhaya.

Now at that time King Seniya Bimbisara of Magadha had been suffering from an anal fistula, and his garments were constantly becoming stained with blood. Whenever his queens saw the blood stains, they would make fun of the king, saying: "Look, His Majesty is going through his courses, and now he is having a period. Soon our king will be giving birth!"

The king was getting quite annoyed by their comments, and one day he told the prince: "Abhaya, I'm suffering from such a disease that my garments are always stained with blood, and whenever the queens see it, they always ridicule me. Please, my dear Abhaya, find a doctor who can cure me."

"Sire, there is an excellent young physician of ours, Jivaka."

"Very well then, give orders to doctor Jivaka to come and attend to me."

So Abhaya summoned Jivaka and asked him to attend to the king. Jivaka Kumarabhacca gathered some medicine under his fingernail, and he went to the king's residence to see what the problem was. And it is said that Jivaka Kumarabhacca healed King Seniya Bimbisara's fistula with only one treatment.

When the king realized he had been cured, and after he had been fully restored to health, he ordered the women in his household to remove all their jewels and ornaments, and to put them in a big pile. Then the king said: "For your payment, Jivaka, take all these ornaments from my wives."

"No, Sire," said Jivaka. "May Your Majesty simply remember the good work I have done."

"Very well, but from now on, I want you to personally attend to me, and to my family, and also to the entire fraternity of *bhikkus* with the Buddha at its head." [*bhikkus = the monks of the first sangha*]

And so Jivaka accepted his new appointment.

The setthi from Rajgir

Now at that time, a certain setthi from Rajgir had been suffering for seven years from a disease of the head. Many great physicians had come to see him, and not a single one was able to restore him to health. They had all been paid in gold, but before they left, they made some prognoses. Some of the physicians said that the setthi would die on the fifth day, and others said he would die on the seventh day.

Another merchant from Rajgir knew that this particular setthi provided an important service, both to the king and also to the merchants' guild, and he thought: "All the physicians have predicted his imminent death, but now we have Jivaka, the royal physician, who is an excellent young doctor. Maybe I should ask for the king's permission to allow Jivaka to try to cure the setthi."

So this merchant went to King Seniya Bimbisara's palace, and as he approached the king, he said to him; "Sire, the setthi is doing excellent service both to Your Majesty and also to the merchants' guild. All the doctors have predicted his certain death. May it please Your Majesty to order the physician Jivaka to attend to him?"

And so the Magadha king Seniya Bimbisara gave orders to Jivaka Kumarabhacca saying, "Go, my dear Jivaka, and attend to the setthi."

Jivaka Kumarabhacca accepted this order and immediately went to the setthi's house. After examining him, and after carefully observing his condition, he said to him: "If I restore you to health, my good man, what kind of fee will you give me?"

"All that I own will be yours, doctor, and I will become your slave."

"Well then, will you be able to lie down on one side for seven months without moving?"

"Yes, I will lie on my side for seven months, doctor."

"And after that will you be able to lie down on the other side for seven months?"

"Yes, doctor, I will also lie down on the other side for seven months."

"And then, after that, will you be able to lie on your back for another seven months?"

"Yes doctor, I will lie down on my back for seven more months."

So then Jivaka Kumarabhacca ordered the setthi to lie down on his bed. He tied him to the bed, and he began the surgery. He cut through his head, drew apart the flesh on each side of the incision, and he removed two parasitic worms from the afflicted area. He showed them to the people who had gathered nearby and said, "Do you see these two worms, a small one and a bigger one? The doctors who said he would die on the fifth day determined that this big worm would penetrate his brain and that as a result, he would die. They understood the situation quite well. And those doctors who saw the smaller worm realized that it would take seven days to penetrate the setthi's brain, and that he would also die as a result. Those doctors have seen it all quite correctly." After saying that, he closed up the sides of the incision, stitched the skin on his head, and he anointed the area with salve.

After about seven days, the setthi said to Jivaka: "Doctor, I can't stay on my side any longer."

"But didn't you tell me that you'd be able to lie down on your side for seven months?"

"Yes, it's true, I did say that, but if you force me to lie down on one side for seven months, I'm afraid I will die."

"Well, then, just turn over and lie down on your other side for seven months.

And after another seven days, the setthi called for Jivaka, and said to him: "Doctor, I'm not able to lie down on this side for seven months either."

"Well, then, so turn around and lie on your back for seven months."

And after another seven days had elapsed, the setthi once again said to Jivaka Kumarabhacca: "My good doctor, I simply cannot lie down on my back for seven more months."

And then Jivaka said to him: "My friend, if I hadn't told you all of this, you wouldn't have stayed still even for as long as you did. But I knew that after twenty-one days you would probably be restored to health. So stand up, my good man. You are now restored to health. Now please decide how much you will give me in payment."

"I told you that all that I have is yours, doctor, and I will be your slave."

"No, sir, don't give me all that you own, and don't be my slave, either. Give 100,000 kahapanas to the king, and 100,000 kahapanas to me."

So the setthi, having fully regained his health, paid the requested fees to Jivaka and to the King.

The young man from Benares

At that time, the son of a setthi from Benares liked to do *mokkhakika. [tumbling, possibly on a type of trampoline]* One day while doing so, he tangled up his intestines, and as a result, he could no longer digest rice milk or eat any kind of food. He also wasn't able to relieve himself in a normal way. After some time, he began to look disfigured and discolored, his complexion turned yellow, and his veins stood out from his skin.

The setthi thought to himself: "My son is suffering from such a terrible disease. He can't drink rice milk or even eat his food. He has become so sick. I wonder if the king of Rajgir would allow his famous physician Jivaka to cure my son?"

So he went to Rajgir and asked King Bimbisara: "Your Majesty, my son is suffering from such a terrible disease. May it please Your Majesty to order the physician Jivaka to attend to him?"

And so the king gave orders to Jivaka saying, "Go to Benares, and cure the setthi's son."

Jivaka traveled to Benares *[a distance of over 300 kilometers/190 miles]* and finally arrived at the setthi's house. After carefully examining him, he ordered all the people in attendance to leave the room, except for his wife. He closed the curtain, tied the young man to a pillar, and placed his wife in front of him so that he could see her. Then he cut through the skin of his belly, pulled out the twisted intestines, and showed them to his wife saying, "This is what caused your husband's disease. This is why he couldn't drink or eat or relieve himself, and it's also why he has become so thin. This is why he looks disfigured and discolored, and why his complexion is yellow, and why his veins have stood out from his skin." Then he untangled the twisted intestines, put them back into the man's cavity in their correct position, stitched the skin together, and anointed the wound with salve. And before very long the setthi's son regained his health completely.

Happy that his son had been restored to health, the setthi gave Jivaka 16,000 kahapanas as payment. Jivaka Kumarabhacca took that money and he returned to Rajgir.

Jivaka tricks King Paggota and his servant Kaka

Once, king Paggota of Ujjeni was suffering from jaundice, and many doctors had come and gone, receiving plenty of gold in payment, but they were never able to restore him to health. So King Paggota sent a messenger to the Magadha king, Seniya Bimbisara, with a personal note saying that he was suffering from a disease. He asked King Bimbisara to please send his personal physician to attend to him. King Bimbisara then told Jivaka to go there so he could cure King Paggota. *[Ujjeni is current-day Ujjain, in Mahdya Pradesh, 1,000 kilometers away from Rajgir.]*

Jivaka accepted, and he traveled (the long distance) to Ujjain. After a thorough examination of the king, he said to him, "Sire, in order to make the remedy you need I must boil some ghee *[clarified butter]*, which Your Majesty must drink."

"No, my good Jivaka, just do whatever you can to make me better without giving me any ghee. I have a great aversion to ghee, and I simply can't eat it."

So Jivaka thought to himself: "The king's disease is of a type that simply can't be cured without using ghee. Maybe I should boil up my medicines with the ghee so that it takes on the color, the smell, and the taste of an astringent decoction."

So he boiled some ghee with various drugs, but he deliberately gave it the color, smell, and taste of an astringent decoction. But then Jivaka realized that when the king swallowed the butter and digested it, it could make him vomit. This particular king was well known for his cruelty, and he could easily have Jivaka killed as punishment!

After careful thought, Jivaka decided that he would have to leave the palace immediately after administering the drugs. So Jivaka went to King Paggota's residence, and he approached him and said: "Sire, we physicians dig up our roots and collect our medicinal plants and drugs right around this time of day. Could you please send orders to the royal stables and to the guardians of the gates of the town for me? Tell them to allow me to ride out on any animal I wish; let me leave the town by any gate I wish; let me leave at any hour I wish; and let me return again whenever I wish." So King Paggota sent that order to the guardians of the stables and the gates.

Now at that time, King Paggota had a female elephant named Bhaddava-tika, and this famous elephant could travel up to 50 yojanas in just one day. Jivaka gave the medicated ghee to King Paggota and made him drink the decoction. And then, as soon as the king drank the ghee, he went to the elephant stable, and he hurried away from the town on Bhaddavatika.

Sure enough, as soon as King Paggota digested that medicated ghee, it made him vomit, and he said to his attendants: "That wicked Jivaka gave me ghee after all. Go and find him." But the attendants told him that Jivaka had already left town on Bhaddavatika the elephant.

King Paggota had a slave named Kaka who was born of a non-human and who could travel up to 60 yojanas in one day. So King Paggota ordered Kaka to go after Jivaka, and to bring him back, but he also warned Kaka: "Be careful. Physicians are very cunning people, so don't accept anything from him."

Eventually, Kaka overtook Jivaka at the town of Kosambi [current-day Kausambi, Uttar Pradesh] while he was eating breakfast, and he said to him: "Doctor, the king has ordered you to return."

Jivaka replied, "Wait until we've had our breakfast, Kaka. Here, sit down and have some food with me."

And Kaka replied, "No, doctor. The king told me that you physicians are very cunning people, and that I shouldn't accept anything from you."

Now at that time, Jivaka was eating a gooseberry and drinking water. He had properly scraped off the medicinal part of the plant with his nail before he had eaten the fruit. But then he said, "Here, my good Kaka, have some fruit and drink some water."

And the slave Kaka thought: "Well, the doctor is eating this fruit and drinking this water, so there shouldn't be any harm in it." Kaka decided to eat the fruit that Jivaka had offered him, and he drank some of the water, too. And the uncleaned gooseberries that Jivaka gave him opened up his bowels within only a few minutes.

Worried about the serious reaction he was having, Kaka asked Jivaka: "Will I be alright, doctor?"

And Jivaka replied, "Don't be afraid, Kaka. You'll be better in a short time. But you know that your king is very cruel, and if I return he might have me killed, so I won't be going back with you." He handed over the she-elephant Bhaddavatika to Kaka, and he set out on foot for Rajgir.

After some time, he finally arrived in Rajgir, and he went to see King Seniya Bimbisara and told him the whole story of what had happened. After hearing Jivaka's story, Bimbisara said, "You did the right thing, Jivaka. It's good that you didn't return to Ujjain. That king has a reputation for cruelty, and he could have had you killed."

After King Paggota had been fully being restored to health, however, he sent a messenger to Jivaka Kumarabhacca saying, "The king has asked you to visit him, so that he can grant you a boon." *[a special request or favor]*

But Jivaka replied, "No, sir. Tell His Majesty to simply remember my good work."

The suit of precious cloth

Now at that time King Paggota was in possession of a suit made of siveyyaka cloth *[a type of fabric of exceptional quality made in the town of Sivi]*, which was the most excellent and most precious of many suits of cloth. It was better than many hundreds, than many thousands, and even better than many hundreds of thousands of suits of cloth. And King Paggota, in compensation, decided to send this suit of siveyyaka cloth to Jivaka Kumarabhacca for having cured him.

When Jivaka received it, he thought: "This suit of siveyyaka cloth is the best and the most excellent of many hundreds of thousands. No one is worthy to receive it other than the Lord, the blessed one, the perfect Arahat-Buddha, or perhaps King Seniya Bimbisara."

Jivaka purges the Buddha

Now at that time the Lord Buddha, the Truth Seeker, had been suffering from an imbalance of the humors of his body *[humors = bodily fluids]*. And the Lord told the venerable Ananda that he had a disturbance in his body, and that he wished to take a purgative.

So the venerable Ananda went to Jivaka's home, and he approached him and said: "My good Jivaka, the humors of the Lord's body have become disturbed. The Truth Seeker wishes to take a purgative."

Jivaka replied, "Well, my venerable Ananda, in this case you should first rub the Blessed One's body with fat for a few days."

So Ananda attended to the Buddha by rubbing his body with fat for a few days. Afterward he returned to Jivaka to tell him what he had done, and to ask for further advice.

And Jivaka thought: "It's not suitable to give a strong purgative to the Blessed One." So instead, he soaked three handfuls of blue lotuses in mixtures of various medicines, and he personally went to visit the Lord Buddha.

He offered a handful of lotuses to the Buddha saying, "Lord, may the Blessed One inhale the scent of this first handful of lotuses. This will purge the Blessed One ten times." Then he offered the second handful of lotuses to the Blessed One, so he could be purged again ten times, and again he offered the third handful of lotuses so that the Blessed One would be purged another ten times. And after giving the Buddha purgatives for a full thirty times, Jivaka bowed down before him. Then he passed around him with his right side toward him, and he left the room.

When Jivaka exited through the porch, he thought: "I've given the Blessed One a purgative for a full thirty times, but since his humors are imbalanced, the treatment won't actually purge him a full thirty times; it will only purge him twenty-nine times. But if the Blessed One takes a bath, the action of bathing will purge him once more, and then he will be purged a full thirty times."

But the Buddha had already sensed Jivaka's thoughts through the power of his mind, and he said to Ananda: "Ananda, when Jivaka was outside, he thought to himself that I should take a bath in order to be purged a full thirty times, so please get some hot bath water ready for me."

And Ananda began to get the hot water ready for the Buddha's bath.

Jivaka was already in the process of returning to the Blessed One. He approached him, greeted him, he sat down at a respectful distance and asked: "Have you been purged, Blessed One?"

The Buddha replied that, yes, he had been purged.

And then Jivaka explained that once he was outside, he realized that a bath was necessary in order to be purged the full thirty times.

And when Jivaka learned that a bath had already been prepared, he told the Buddha: "Lord, until the Blessed One's body is completely restored, it would be best to abstain from liquid food." And under Jivaka's care, shortly thereafter, the Blessed One's body was completely restored.

Jivaka requests different robes for the monks

After the Buddha was restored to health, Jivaka took the suit of expensive siveyyaka cloth and returned to visit him. He sat down near him, and he said: "Lord, may I ask one boon of the Blessed One?"

The Buddha replied, "Jivaka, the Tathagatas above grant boons before they even know what they are." [*Tathagata = enlightened ones, those who have found the truth*]

But Jivaka said, "Lord, I assure you it is a proper and unobjectionable request."

And the Buddha replied, "Then speak, Jivaka."

"Lord, the Blessed One wears only *pamsukula* robes [*robes made of discarded rags traditionally taken from a trash heap or a cemetery*], and so does the fraternity of bhikkus. Lord, this suit of siveyyaka cloth has been given to me by King Paggota, and it is the most excellent and most noble of many hundreds of thousands of suits of cloth. Lord, may the Blessed One accept this gift from me, and may he also allow the fraternity of bhikkus to wear lay robes."

The Blessed One accepted the suit of siveyyaka cloth. And then he taught Jivaka Kumarabhacca through direct religious discourse [*dhamma*]. Jivaka was so excited and happy that he had been taught directly by the Blessed One, and after receiving this lesson, he rose from his seat, he respectfully saluted the Blessed One, he passed around him with his right side toward him, and he left the room.

And the Blessed One, after delivering this religious discourse in response to Jivaka's visit, addressed the monks by saying: "I allow you, dear bhikkus, to wear lay robes. If you wish, you may wear pamsukula robes, and if you wish, you may wear lay robes. I approve the use of both types of robes."

Soon all those in Rajgir heard that the Blessed One had allowed the monks to wear lay robes, and they were delighted because they thought, "Now we will be able to give more gifts to the monks so that we can acquire more merit through good deeds." And in just one day, many thousands of robes were presented to the monks at Rajgir.

And people throughout the entire region eventually heard that the Blessed One had allowed the monks to wear lay robes, and as a result many more thousands of robes were presented to monks throughout the land.

[*The story continues to describe other types of garments and robes that the Buddha allowed to be used by the order of monks. Jivaka is also mentioned in other texts, including the Jivaka Sutta, a discourse about being a lay follower, the circumstances surrounding the eating of meat, and the merits of maintaining a vegetarian diet.*]

Thai Magic Amulets and Sacred Tattoos

CHRIS JONES

Thai magic amulets

There are four general types of magical amulets in Thai culture. The term to describe these amulets as a whole is *khawng-khlang*, which may be translated as "sacred, potent objects."

The first type is *khruang-rang*, which are material substances sometimes made of stone or copper. These amulets protect people if they are held in the mouth or on the body. They include *khot*, which are objects found in nature, such as stone eggs, meteoric ores, and various types of seeds found in jack-fruit and tamarind pods.

The second type is *phra-khruang*, which are small statues or figurines of the Buddha that protect an individual or, if they are larger, an entire household. These may be cast from a mold or may appear in the form of a votive tablet. They may also be worn as talismans around the neck.

The third type is *khruang-pluk-sek*. These are believed to arouse the potency of a person or an object by means of a spell or incantation. Khruang-pluk-sek are very powerful amulets, and most of the spells used to charge them are incantations based on ancient verses. When magic spells need to be written, the Khmer alphabet is often used since Khmer characters are believed to have runic qualities.

The *takrut* is a long, hollow cylinder made from metal that has passed through many stages of magical arousal. Takrut are worn around the neck, either alone or together, with an odd number of other takrut, perhaps a total of three, five, or seven. A *salika* (mynah bird) is a tiny takrut that can be kept

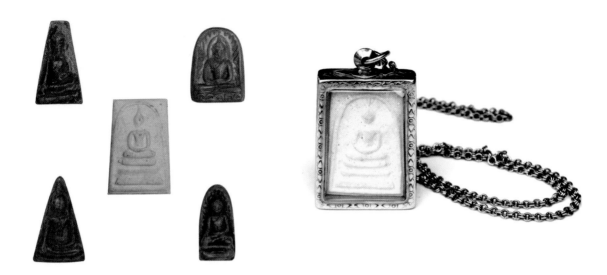

(above) Stylized Buddha amulets in tablet form

(above right) A tablet in a protective silver housing, with silver chain

between the teeth and that allows the user to become a very persuasive talker. Magical items in this class can bestow a variety of benefits on the user, and many have been developed from ancient beliefs and practices.

The fourth type is *wan ya* – plants and roots that combat disease and the actions of *phi,* or spirits. Many people, especially in rural villages, believe that illness and misfortune may be attributed to the actions of malevolent spirits. Fortunately, local shamans are able to combat these spirits with the aid of wan ya, which may be found in surrounding forests and mountains. Every living thing has a spirit, and sometimes even inanimate objects may be brought to life through magic spells.

Sacred tattoos

The art of tattooing has been widely known in Siam for many centuries. Thai tattoos fall into three general categories. Official tattoos are those worn by the military to identify regiments of the royal army, and by prisoners to identify them as having committed serious crimes. These days, art tattoos are very popular, and they are used by the general public, especially young people, for decorative value. We will address the third type, sacred tattoos, in this article.

Sacred tattoos are called *sak yant.* This type of tattooing is popular with Thai men, who wear them as protection from harm caused by weapons. Two types of liquids are used to create sacred tattoos: ink and oil. Ink is used for both art tattoos and sacred tattoos, but ink for sacred tattoos is prepared with extra ingredients, and it sometimes includes extracts of auspicious herbs and sacred plants. Ink formulations have developed and changed over the years, but the traditional preparations are derivatives of a native tree called *ton muek.*

They are also made from soot collected from pots and mixed with buffalo bile, or from a mixture of Chinese ink and sesame oil. Nowadays, commercially available tattoo ink is also used.

Oil tattoos evolved partially as a result of the social stigma that often accompanies a tattooed body. The oil is not visible to the naked eye, but the tattoo provides equal protection. As with sacred ink, the oil is formulated with sacred ingredients and herbs, and sesame oil is often used as the base of the preparation.

A takrut made of a thin sheet of copper engraved by hand with a mantra, and placed in a glass tube

The ink or oil can be applied with a variety of instruments including sharpened sticks, thorns, and needles. Today the most popular method is a sharpened metal stick made from sacred alloys and engraved with magic spells.

Technique

Typically, as with other traditional arts and skills, a serious and respected tattooist spends many years in a master-pupil relationship. In my basic study, I first had to study the characters of the *khom* (ancient Khmer) alphabet, and then learn magical incantations (*katha*) and various types of *na* and *yan* occult writing until I knew them by heart. To steady my hands, my teacher made me practice dry-tattooing on banana trunks for a long time.

Steady hands are needed, since modern electric needles are not favored by Thai tattooists, who instead use a simple pointed steel or brass rod. Holding the needle in one hand and using the fingers of the other hand as a rest and a guide for the pointed end, the tattooist rhythmically jabs at the skin, pricking out the pattern based on his artistic esthetic and his intuition.

Designs

For modern art tattoos, an individual may choose from thousands of art samples, or may even create his own design. But the traditional sacred tattoo is limited to a few basic designs, all of which are based on ancient Buddhist principles, magic, and creatures.

The designs can't be changed significantly, since they have been passed down through generations and any modification may dilute the magic powers. In many circumstances the devotee doesn't choose his own designs, but instead relies on the experience of a revered tattoo artist or a monk or reusi

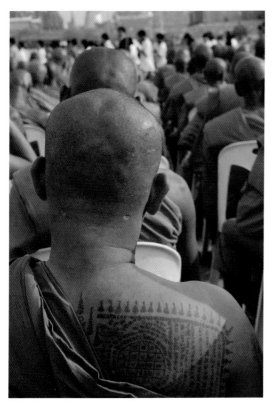

Monks celebrate the Buddha's birthday and the 60th anniversary of the Thai king's accession to the throne, Bangkok

to decide which tattoo is most appropriate.

The precise details of the designs, and especially the complex written spells and magical symbols, are studied and learned by the tattooist. It is said that tattoos can have a greater or lesser effect depending on the extent of the tattooist's knowledge and experience. Designs are respected for their inherent magic power. For example, Hanuman (the monkey god) represents a great and clever fighter; dragons are brave and wise; geckos are loving and compassionate.

The majority of people who get sacred tattoos believe that, in so doing, they acquire two types of strength: *kwam yu yong kong kraphan* and *metta mahaniyom*. As noted earlier, the first is a type of physical protection against weapons, since the tattoos are believed to strengthen the skin against punctures by knives or bullets, while metta mahaniyom is the power to attract admiration and love. This latter type of tattoo is believed to exert positive influence over others.

An important factor in the tattoo tradition of Thailand is the skill and spiritual knowledge possessed by the tattoo artist. These days the art has become flooded with inexperienced practitioners, yet there are still highly respected master tattooists who preserve the tradition based on ancient lore and spiritual beliefs. Some claim to be mediums and execute tattoos while they are possessed by the spirit of a reusi. In this case they may wear a mask and headgear in the likeness of a traditional Thai hermit.

Ceremony for sacred tattoos

Tattooing is usually done in multiple sessions. The entire process can be lengthy, because the receiver must return many times for complex designs to be completed, or to have accompanying tattoos added.

Many worshippers ask that tattoos be placed on parts of the body that are generally covered with clothes. Sacred tattoos are often placed on the upper parts of the body. Aside from choosing the sacred designs, the monk, healer, or spiritual tattoo artist must also organize a sacred ceremony *(wai khru)* to pray to his teachers prior to the actual process of tattooing.

The ritual involved in a tattooing session illustrates the spiritual nature of the practice. The individual brings the tattooist a small offering in addition to the tattoo fee. He makes the traditional *wai* greeting while kneeling reverently in front of the master, and he generally maintains a position of reverence throughout the entire tattooing session.

As the tattoo is being created, the tattoo artist may recite sacred spells in order to transfer magic power into the tattoo. The subject usually doesn't speak during this time since it could interrupt the tattoo artist's concentration and possibly result in a tattoo of diminished power.

The most important stage of the session is at the very end. Tattoos in themselves have no power, and no effectiveness in giving protection, until they are activated by the tattooist. The power is conferred by the tattooist while he recites a sacred incantation and transfers the magic by blowing on the tattoo. A sword or knife may also be ritualistically used to confirm the tattoo's effectiveness. Those who favor sacred tattoos tend to continue adding to their collection until much of the upper body is densely covered. The number of tattoos one receives doesn't necessarily increase one's power or protection. It is believed, for example, that a single dot placed correctly on the face by a true master can provide protection to the entire head.

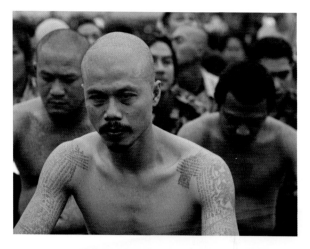

Participants of the Tattoo Festival at Wat Bang Phra, Nakhon Pathom Province

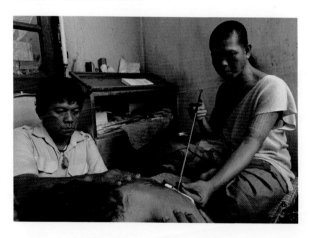

Monk Luang Pi Peaw applying a sak yant

A wealth of tradition

For a variety of reasons, the popularity of sacred tattooing in Thailand has gradually declined in modern times. These days, tattooed individuals are sometimes considered to be of a lower class in Thai society and they may be unfairly stereotyped. Visible tattoos may preclude an individual from being offered gainful employment, for example. However, sacred tattooing is still widely practiced among monks, spiritual devotees, martial arts practitioners, and healers, and this ancient tradition, steeped in magic and Buddhist and animist spirituality, is still alive. If you have an opportunity to closely examine a Thai sacred tattoo, or to hold a protection amulet in your hands, you will behold a wealth of tradition. These traditions have endured for countless generations in Thailand, and are inextricably connected to Thai spirituality and culture.

Introduction to Reusi Dat Ton

ENRICO CORSI

According to Hindu history, the *rishis* (*reusi* or *lersi* in Thai language) were spiritual recluses who lived in isolated places, often in remote Himalayan valleys, in order to dedicate themselves to meditation practices and yoga. In the Ramayana epic, one of the most important texts in Hinduism dating back to approximately 500 BC, rishis are mentioned as engaging in *tapas* (a meditation practice lasting for years under extreme conditions of renunciation) in order to ingratiate themselves with Shiva and absorb supernatural powers.

Reusi dat ton (loosely translated as "ascetic self-stretching") is a Thai physical and spiritual discipline. It is taught to Thai nationals and foreign students within Thailand, and is also becoming more widely known in other countries.

The exercises

Originally there were many different exercises for self-stretching and healing. Several Thai kings, especially Rama I and Rama III, commissioned reproductions in statue form of reusi performing each of the exercises. Artists and writers were also commissioned to create renderings and detailed descriptions of the postures and techniques. There were allegedly 120 original postures, but only 80 of them, based on statues and original drawings, are commonly practiced.

Reusi dat ton is familiar to many Thais, who study it within a historical and religious context, but its practice remains somewhat limited in Thailand. Nevertheless, not long ago, the Thai Ministry of Health decided to standardize a reusi dat ton routine using 15 basic exercises. The routine contained descriptions of the exercises written in metaphorical language, using a style of verse that offers indirect information about the dynamics and execution of the movement. In the image below, for example, text explains that the exercise treats cramps in the hands and feet.

From burning eyes of live flames of the giant mask, assume the dance pose. With outstretched arms, push hands down on hips. This is a remedy for cramping in the hands and feet.

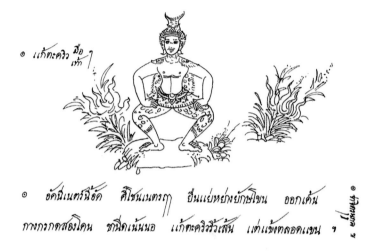

One of the things that distinguishes reusi dat ton from other types of movement therapy is the type of breathing that is used. Unlike other modalities, where breath plays an important part of the movements themselves, the exercises in reusi dat ton are performed in apnea, while holding the breath after an inhalation. It is believed that by performing the exercises while holding the breath, energy may be stored in the body and channeled through one or more *sen* lines in order to affect a particular area.

Reusi dat ton is a self-healing system with dynamic exercises similar to postures and positions used in traditional Thai massage. In some cases, the similarities are apparent since some of the pressure points stimulated in reusi dat ton are also affected in advanced Thai massage techniques.

Many of the statues and drawings of reusi dat ton describe common disorders that are easily understood. Others, however, relate to issues resulting from long periods of immobility, which most likely developed in reusi who engaged in extensive meditation. Regardless of the original therapeutic indications however, reusi dat ton, when practiced regularly, provides substantial benefits to general health and well-being. When an exercise is identified as suitable for treating a particular disorder, it should be practiced daily, or at least as often as possible, in order to achieve optimal results. When the practice is done as a routine exercise, it should be carried out at least once a week. Two or three times a week is an ideal frequency for keeping in shape and maintaining continuous balance to the energy system.

Some of the exercises are easy to perform, even for those who have limited flexibility. A type of "internal stretching" is accomplished as a result of the exercises being performed in apnea. This technique affords a degree of internal elasticity, even when doing movements that are not particularly challenging. At the end of a practice session, the muscles are not only more relaxed but also more toned. A feeling of energetic integration and balance is often felt after a reusi dat ton session.

Some important results of regular practice of reusi dat ton are:

- Treatment of muscle and tendon pain
- Treatment of joint disorders
- Increased muscle tone and flexibility
- Optimization of blood circulation
- Improved breathing
- Alignment of the skeletal system

In traditional Thai massage, problems sometimes manifest that are the topical symptoms of deeper dysfunctions. As in Thai massage, reusi dat ton may also treat a disorder that may have its point of origin elsewhere in the body. Some exercises have therapeutic indications related to body parts that are not directly stimulated by the technique itself. This aspect of the work is often confusing to those who simply follow a sequence without understanding the holistic aspect of traditional Thai healing arts.

Reusi dat ton is an easy discipline to learn and is suitable for almost everyone. Those who are able to practice it regularly will almost certainly reap enormous benefits. Thai massage therapists may find that performing reusi dat ton on a regular basis will complement and help improve their work with clients.

Part of the Thai therapist's job is to help relieve and release stored tension in clients. Reusi dat ton is an excellent tool to support and strengthen the postures and techniques used in Thai massage practice. Over time, a sensitive practitioner may be able to actually feel the sen lines becoming stimulated during the exercises. When this happens, a more complete understanding of the functioning of the human energy system becomes apparent. Additionally, when a Thai therapist learns reusi dat ton techniques, he can, in turn, teach his clients certain exercises so that they can address their individual needs in between Thai sessions, thereby accelerating and supporting the overall healing process.

Sample exercises for the Thai massage therapist

For those who practice the art of traditional Thai massage, here are a few useful exercises that address areas of the body that often become stressed during practice: neck pain, headache, and back/leg pain.

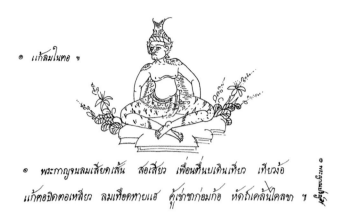

● แก้ลมในคอ ๚

๑ พระกากญจนลมเสียกเส้น สอเสียว เพื่อนที่นบเดินเทียว เทียมอ้อ
แก้คอบิดคอเหลียว ลมเทือดทายแฮ คู่เช่าขาก่อมก้อ หัดถีเคลื่นไคลขา ๚

Neck pain

Sit cross-legged, maintaining a slightly backward balance, and lean backward on your arms. Inhale, and then bend the neck forward as much as possible. Maintain this position for 3–5 seconds while holding your breath, then exhale, and slowly return to the starting position.

Using the same breathing technique, bend the neck backward, hold it, and exhale when returning to the starting position.

Using the same breathing technique, inhale and twist your head to one side, hold it, and return to the center while exhaling. Now twist your head to the other side, and repeat the exercise.

Repeat the entire sequence of movements 3–5 times. Remember to hold your breath for a few seconds, before exhaling and returning to the starting position.

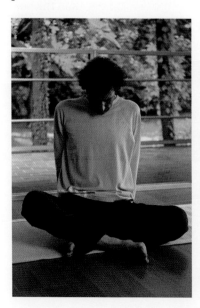 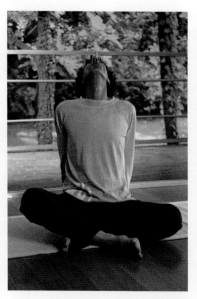 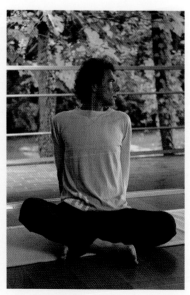

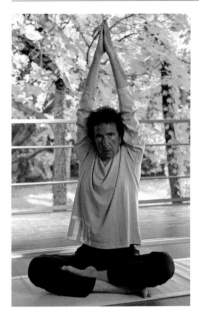

Exercise for headache

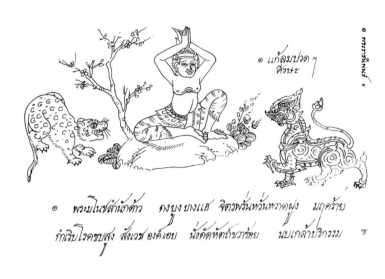

၁ แก้ลมปวด ๆ
ศีวฅ่ะ ๆ

๑   พระมไนยสำนักด๋าว   คงยุง ยงแฮ   จิตรพวั่นหวั่นหวาดผฝง   มฤคร้าย
กำเริบโรคขบูสูง   สังเวช องค์เอย   นั่งดัดหัตถ์บวาซ้าย   นบเกล้าปริกวม   ๚

Headache

Sit in semi-lotus position, with your arms folded in front of you and your hands in prayer position. Inhale, and stretch your arms high above you, while pressing the palms of your hands together. Hold the position in apnea for 3 seconds, and then exhale as you return to the starting position. Repeat the exercise 3–5 times.

Back and leg pain

While balancing on one leg, grasp your foot with your outside hand, and place your other hand on the bent knee.

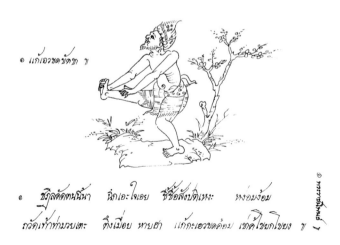

๑ แก้เอวขดขัดขา ๚

๑   ขีลสดัดตนนินา   นึกอะไจเอย   ชี่ชื่อสังปติเหมะ: หง่อมง่อม
ถวัดเท้าทำมวบเตะ   ถึงเมื่อย หาบฮา   แก้กะเอวขดค้อม   เขตค์ไขยกไขยง ๚

Inhale, and extend the leg outward, while bending the knee of your other leg. Hold the position and your breath for at least 3 seconds. Then, as you exhale, slowly return to the starting position.

Repeat the exercise 3–5 times for each leg.

The practice

Reusi dat ton is not intended to be a painful discipline. Some exercises can cause strong reactions and sensations as a result of the stimulation of muscles and organs, but they should not cause acute pain or discomfort. If you experience any pain or cramping while performing an exercise, immediately stop, and don't repeat that exercise until and unless the discomfort passes.

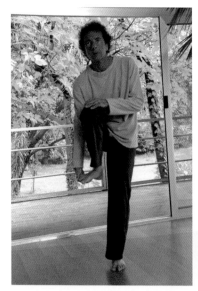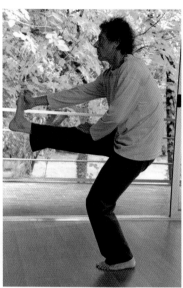

Sequence for back and leg pain

After each exercise, always compose yourself and allow your breath to return to normal before engaging in the next exercise. Always trust your instincts. If you feel light-headed, rest for a few minutes until you are composed. If you experience a headache or any other condition that makes your practice uncomfortable, simply do not engage in exercises that day.

Contraindications for certain reusi dat ton exercises include cardiac problems of any type, hypertension, and a high level of emotional or psychological stress. You should exercise caution with certain exercises if you suffer from osteoporosis, slipped or herniated discs, or unhealed fractures.

Cultivating even a modest practice of reusi dat ton can be beneficial to Thai massage therapists. It is my hope that more professionals in Thai massage will incorporate reusi dat ton into their personal practice and in their preparation for Thai massage sessions. Through the regular practice of reusi dat ton, Thai massage therapists may achieve a greater state of balance and subsequently be better able to treat their patients in accordance with Thai tradition.

The Great Doctor of Northern India: Jivaka Kaumara-Bhrtya

GUNAKAR MULEY

The story is over 2,500 years old. The place is Taxila, a famous center of learning at that time. A young boy of sixteen had come almost 2,000 kilometers from distant Rajgir to study medicine from a world-renowned physician named Atreya. He'd spent seven years studying there, and before declaring that Jivaka's training was complete, his teacher assigned him a practical final examination.

He told him to take a spade and to travel around the area of Taxila, and to bring back any plant that did not possess medicinal properties. The devoted student spent a long period of time examining the plants of the entire region as directed by his teacher, but he couldn't find a single one that was devoid of curative properties and of no use to living beings. When he returned, he reported his findings to his teacher. Satisfied with the answer, the teacher told him that had done his learning well, and that he was ready to begin his professional practice. He gave his student some money for traveling expenses, and sent him on his way.

That young apprentice who studied medicine from the renowned teacher of Taxila was Jivaka, the most famous physician of Gautama Buddha's time (563–483 BC). Much of what we know about him comes from Buddhist canonical texts. His patients included the Buddha; the *bikkhus*, the first order of monks; emperors; rich merchants; and common people.

Jivaka was the son of Salavati, a courtesan of Rajgir, which was the capital of the Magadhan Empire during the reign of King Bimbisara. Soon after birth, the baby Jivaka was thrown on a garbage heap, where prince Abhaya, son of

Bimbisara, noticed that he was still alive *(jivati)*. The prince, therefore, named him Jivaka and had him raised under his own personal care.

Jivaka came to be called Komarabhaccha, meaning "raised by the prince." Interestingly, this name is also derivative of *kaumara bhìtya* (pediatrics), one of the eight branches of Indian Ayurvedic medicine.

Jivaka's notable patients

Jivaka's first patient was a rich merchant's wife who had been suffering from a chronic disease of the head, which many physicians couldn't cure. Because he was young and inexperienced, Jivaka received permission to examine her, on condition that he wouldn't be paid unless she was cured. Jivaka administered the medicine to the patient through her nose and she was completely cured in one treatment.

Jivaka was a contemporary of the Buddha, and was very devoted to him. It is recorded that on one occasion, the Buddha's bodily fluids were imbalanced, and Ananda, the faithful attendant of the Buddha, conveyed this matter to Jivaka. The physician suggested that the Buddha should be massaged with fat for several days. After that, Jivaka selected three lotuses, which he treated with various drugs, and then asked the Buddha to inhale them, thereby ingesting the medicine in a manner appropriate for a holy man.

Jivaka often attended to the holy order of monks. Once, in Vaishali, the monks were offered too much sweet food, and they became very sick. Luckily, Jivaka was in the area at the same time. He treated the sick monks and cured them all.

Jivaka Amravana

Jivaka lived and practiced not far from the center of Rajgir. According to texts, Jivaka one day decided to build a dwelling for the Buddha on his own property. He built ". . . night quarters and day quarters. . . a pavilion . . . and a fragrant hut for the Holy One, surrounded by a mango grove with high walls."

That place, called Jivaka Amravana, was where the Buddha delivered some of his most famous discourses, at least two of them directed to Jivaka. It was also here that on a beautiful moonlit night, the son of King Bimbisara, after having imprisoned and killed his father, came to visit the Buddha to atone for his misdeeds. Here he listened to the Buddha's teaching called Samaññaphala Sutta (the Sutra of the Fruit of Contemplative Life), and became a follower of the Buddha's teachings.

All ancient sources agree that the Jivaka Amravana was located outside the east gate of Rajgir, somewhere between the gate and Gridhakuta hill. The famous Chinese traveler Yuan Chwang (Hiuen Tsiang), who traveled in India during AD 429–45, described his visit to Rajgir in this way:

*North-east from Shrigupta's fire-pit, and in the bend of a mountain wall, was a
tope [stupa] at the spot where Jivaka, the great physician, built a hall for the Buddha. Remains of the walls and of the plants and trees within them still existed.
Tathagata [the Buddha] often stayed here. Beside the tope, the ruins of Jivaka's
private residence still survive.*

Jivaka Amravana, ordered to be built by Jivaka, was discovered and excavated from 1803–1857. Although only the foundations remain, the complex is
interesting in that it includes three long elliptical halls built of stone and bricks.
A visitor to Rajgir must proceed first along the main road to the south, then
take another road that turns to the left. Soon he will arrive at a clearing in the
jungle containing the ruins. From there, about 2.5 kilometers toward the east,
is Gridhakuta Hill, where the Buddha occasionally lived over a period of many
years.

Taxila

After Jivaka Amravana, the second most important place in Jivaka's life was
Taxila, where he completed his medical training. By 500 BC, Taxila was a
renowned education center which attracted students from throughout the
entire region. Many famous doctors, scholars, and scientists, some whose
names are preserved in Indian history, received their higher training at Taxila.
Every medical student of the day underwent extensive study of medical bot-
any. Complicated surgeries were performed there, too, including those on the
skull and the stomach. Aside from the study of medicine, the city was also a
learning center for other disciplines, including the sciences, arts and crafts,
and the humanities.

Although Taxila was a famous center of learning, it was not a university
town with a formal campus, lecture hall, and residential quarters, such as
existed in Nalanda, near Rajgir. References to student life in ancient Buddhist
stories suggest that at Taxila the actual learning took place in teachers' homes.
Students were generally admitted at the age of sixteen. Pupils from rich families boarded with the teachers and paid them handsomely for their studies,
food, and lodging. Pupils from royal families had separate lodgings. Poorer
pupils, not able to pay their own expenses, served as attendants to their teacher
and his family.

Over the course of a thousand years, the city of Taxila was located succes-
sively at three different sites in what is now the Punjab region of Pakistan:
Bhir Mound, Sirkap, and Sirsukh. All three places have been extensively excavated, but archeologists haven't found any site that they believe could have
been the campus of an ancient seat of learning. This supports the theory that
only the teachers' homes were the places of study, at least during Jivaka's time.

Later, a number of Buddhist monasteries were built at Taxila, and they also became seats of learning.

Jivaka's legacy

In ancient times, Buddhist monks often served as doctors among the lay people from whom they obtained food. This Buddhist tradition flourished under the patronage of Emperor Asoka (272–232 BC) who initiated measures for the relief of suffering of both humans and animals. Along with Buddhism, Indian medicine also spread to other Asian countries. For all these endeavors, the inspiration came from the compassionate acts of the Buddha and the wonderful cures of his personal physician Jivaka.

In ancient times, the study of pediatrics was one of the eight components of Ayurveda, and a large body of literature existed on the subject. A twelfth-century commentator on the ancient medical text called the Susruta Samhita says that Jivaka's compendium was regarded as one of the most authoritative texts on the subject. Today, however, no texts by Jivaka are available. The Kashyap Samhita, discovered in Nepal in 1938, is currently the only known text on ancient Indian pediatrics, but it is far too fragmentary to be regarded as a complete volume.

One text that quotes Jivaka's recipes is the *Navanitaka*, a section of the *Bower Manuscript (mss)*, a fourth-century Indian medical manuscript discovered in 1880 in Chinese Turkistan. Based on standard sources, this medical text mentions Jivaka and attributes two pediatric formulas to him, saying, "Iti hovaca Jivakah," *(Thus spoke Jivaka)*. One formula is based on chili pepper and payasya *(coagulated milk)*, mixed with honey, which was used as medical syrup to treat vomiting due to excessive phlegm.

There are several monumental medical texts from ancient India, including the *Caraka Saêhita* and the *Susruta Saêhita,* but almost nothing definite is known about their authors or compilers. Jivaka, on the other hand, is one physician from ancient India who is mentioned in more than only one historical text reference.

Some of the cures brought about by Jivaka as recounted in these ancient texts may indeed be exaggerations, but they certainly indicate the importance attached to astute observation and deduction in the ancient medical sciences of India. For the first time in the history of Indian medicine, these records and accounts tell of a number of patients who were diagnosed and treated by the great physician Jivaka.

The Reusi of Thailand

TEVIJJO YOGI

The Thai word reusi (ruesi) originates from the Sanskrit rishi, meaning "seer." In Thailand, reusi is a blanket term that refers to those who practice the esoteric sciences. In actuality, the practices of individual reusi may be very different from one another. Reusi practice as ascetics or as householders, and they may live in the city or in the wilderness. Some practice mantra, tantra, and yoga, while others practice meditation or medicine. In terms of appearance, some wear robes and some do not. Some dress in animal prints, while others wear robes similar to those of a monk. With so many variations in appearance and practice, we can simply say that reusi are the holders of natural laws and sciences that have been passed down over the millennia.

Bpoo Reusi Sompit invokes deities of the eight directions

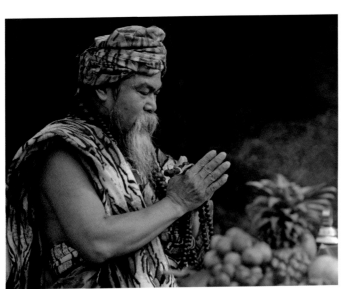

When we speak of sciences, we mean the different types of knowledge on which many ancient cultures and religions have based their practice and theory. These include esoteric sciences such as astrology, alchemy, palmistry, and demonology, as well as mathematics, medicine, and music. In the Thai tradition, reusi are the protectors and holders of all of these sciences.

The reusi tradition

We know from Buddhist texts that reusi lived during the time of the Gautama Buddha. In fact, the Buddha himself practiced as a reusi before attaining enlightenment, and it is believed that he spent numerous past lives as a reusi. Placing a date on the origins of the practice is very difficult. If we look at reusi outside of the Buddhist tradition, we find ascetics as far back as the Indus Valley period (circa 2600–1900 BC). According to tradition, the reusi are those who brought knowledge from the heavens to the human race.

Each culture and religion has its own characteristics, but at heart, all ascetic traditions are similar. The reusi of Thailand are similar to the vijjadharas (weizza) of Burma, the eysey of Cambodia, the yogis of Tibet, the siddhas of India, the immortals of China, the sufis of Islam, the hermits of Europe, the mystics of Christianity, and the shamans of the Americas and Africa. These groups represent the mystical (not the dogmatic or orthodox) traditions within their respective religions. Within Thai Buddhism, for example, monks represent the orthodox path, while reusi adhere to the mystical teachings. Reusi live in accordance with natural law, and they immerse themselves in deep study and contemplation of the basic elements from which all things are composed.

Reusi generally prefer a solitary path, one that keeps them close to nature. They often engage in retreats in isolated areas such as mountains, deserts, caves, and forests, and they take a naturalistic approach to life that deals with the elements, nature, deities, spirits, and ghosts.

The primary goals of a reusi are to understand nature and to aspire to natural law. They learn and practice sciences such as astrology, medicine, and meditation in order to preserve these traditions for future generations. As Buddhists, reusi strive to benefit all sentient beings, while tirelessly promoting and preserving the dharma (spiritual teachings) and maintaining a focused spiritual practice.

Training and daily practice

Technically, anyone can become a reusi, although the training period and the commitment to daily practice is arduous and demanding. It is necessary to have a competent and advanced practitioner as a teacher in order to be initiated into the tradition. Due to the gravity of the commitment to the practice, the teacher puts the disciple through a probationary period in order to test his dedication to the tradition. Many who are initiated as reusi vow to keep their precepts for life. Becoming a reusi is a life decision that should not be made lightly.

The most fundamental guidelines are simple, and they are separated into categories of body, speech, and mind.

Bodily Actions

- To refrain from killing
- To not steal
- To not engage in sexual misconduct

Speech

- To not lie
- To not speak poorly of others in order to create discord
- To not use harsh language
- To not indulge in gossip or idle chatter

Mental Actions

- To not covet others' possessions and to avoid excessive desire
- To avoid thoughts of ill will toward others
- To refrain from false views

The above list of precepts governing body, speech, and mind comes from the Buddha's Eightfold Path, which outlines the proper mode of conduct for any follower of the Buddhist tradition. Though these are the most basic precepts, other guidelines govern things like how and when one eats, proper sleeping periods, and ways in which to interact with others. These disciplines help a reusi to maintain mindfulness throughout the day.

There are precepts about how to relate to the opposite sex, but a reusi's rules of conduct aren't as strict as those that a monk must follow. Some reusi marry or have partners, while others remain celibate for life; regardless, there are rules dealing with when and how sexual relations are permitted. The reusi who give back to the community by teaching or offering their expertise often interact with the opposite sex, and those who practice medicine treat both men and women alike.

Many people are attracted to the reusi path because of a perceived relaxed approach to conduct, but in fact, a reusi's path can be more difficult than that of a monk in many ways. Monks are supported by the community of other monks (sangha), and also by lay people. They are afforded the best conditions, so that they may uphold their precepts and daily practices. Reusi generally don't have these types of support, and instead, they must monitor and care for themselves. New reusi must spend three years in probation, and an additional three years under the direct guidance of a teacher.

Within the reusi tradition, one teaching from the Buddha dharma is applied to govern all actions, whether they relate to body, speech, or mind: This is the observance and cultivation of the brahmavihāras, or the Four Pure Abidings, which are goodwill, compassion, sympathetic joy, and equanimity. This practice is very similar to the cultivation of bodhicitta in the Mahāyāna tradition. The aim of both of these teachings is to develop genuine compassion and unconditional love for all sentient beings, and to apply this love with wisdom.

Daily practice for a reusi consists of meditation, chanting, study, protecting nature and the dharma, and maintaining balance between the unseen world and the seen world. How this is expressed may vary for each individual practitioner, but all reusi aim to study and practice the sciences, to control the mind, to develop goodwill, compassion, sympathetic joy, and equanimity, and most importantly, to help others along their path to enlightenment.

Reusi from different parts of Southeast Asia meet for the blessing of an amulet in Suphanburi, 2012

Clothing and physical appearance

A reusi can wear three types of clothing: white robes, reddish-brown robes, or animal skin. In the past, many reusi lived in the forest and had little or no contact with the outside world. Because of this, they would fashion clothing from things around them, including the skin of dead animals that they would encounter in the forest. The skin of certain animals is believed to prevent a practitioner's negative, downward-flowing energy while in meditation. Use of skin as a meditation seat also symbolically represents mastery over one's "animal mind." In ancient Buddhist texts, including those that recount stories of Jivaka Kumarabhacca, the clothing and robes worn by yogis were white. Although white robes are still worn by reusi in Thailand, animal print cloth has become increasingly popular.

Reusi usually do not cut their hair or beard for the first three years after initiation into the lineage. This is because it is believed that each reusi is empowered with past generations of reusi. Cutting the hair is considered to be a break in the connection to this power, and a break in the commitment to follow the reusi way of life.

Keeping one's word and practicing various types of tapas, or austerities, are major parts of the life of a reusi. Keeping commitments enables a reusi to advance to the next level of training and practice. When performing incantations, one's word is a major source of power. Breaking one's commitment is considered a mental and a spiritual defeat. By keeping commitments, a person develops and evolves spiritually, and accumulates teja, or spiritual power. Teja can be used to help others, and to progress along the true path.

Lineage, status, and preserving the tradition

There are two general lineages of reusi. One has roots in Burma and Tibet, while the other comes from central and eastern Thailand and Cambodia. Though the central teachings of both traditions are very much the same, there are a few differences. The Thai/Cambodian lineage has more influence from Vedic traditions, while the Northern lineage takes more from Burmese and Himalayan practices. The languages used in holy texts and in chanting are also different in the two lineages.

In rural Thailand, especially in the Northeast, reusi still hold a revered place in the community, although monks generally hold a higher status. Typically, monks keep 227 precepts, whereas reusi keep up to 108 precepts.

According to legends and texts, there are 108 important reusi in the Thai tradition. Of these, some are widely acclaimed for specific abilities that set them apart from the others. For example, Reusi Dtah Wua (Reusi with Cow Eyes) was known for his remarkable practice of alchemy and herbal medicine, and Reusi Dtah Fai (Reusi with Eyes of Fire) is remembered for his practice of magic and deep meditation.

Some followers trace their lineage back to these famous reusi, and some mediums channel their spirits in order to work with their direct intercession and guidance. Although these legendary reusi have passed on from the physical realm, they still serve as guides and teachers to help all sentient beings. Powerful deceased reusi, under certain circumstances, may temporarily take on the form of a living human being in order to perform an important act.

In Thailand, the reusi tradition is alive but not thriving. There are few authentic practitioners these days, and increasingly, monks are becoming interested in the esoteric sciences, which is the traditional domain of the reusi. Whether from the Thai tradition or elsewhere, mystics have

Monk and reusi
blessing amulets

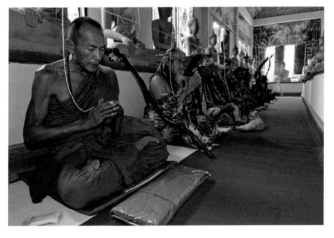

existed for millennia. For the most part, reusi are hermits, and they prefer to keep a low profile. In recent times however, and with issues such as overpopulation, deforestation, and contamination of the planet, reusi have become more public, in order to speak about important issues, and work toward the preservation of nature and a more natural way of life.

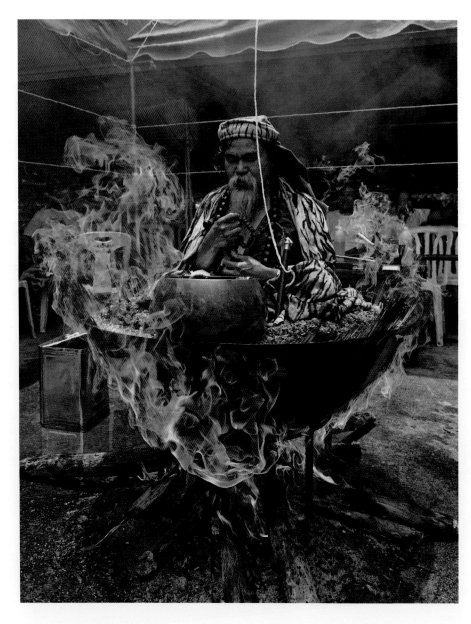

Bpoo Reusi Sompit meditating and blessing herbal medicinal oil in Nakhon Sawan

Traditional Healers of Northern Thailand

GREG LAWRENCE

The traditional medicine of northern Thailand is steeped in a folk tradition with roots stretching back many hundreds of years. Knowledge and learning is based mostly on oral tradition. Training is passed from healer to apprentice, with little or no formal institutionalized training. The current base of traditional medicine is mostly rural and is found in the small villages that make up larger urban areas, such as greater Chiang Mai. Folk medicine differs from the more formalized Thai traditional medicine that is fostered at institutions, and which, in recent years, has gained popularity.

The hill tribes are comprised of different tribal groups that have migrated to various regions of northern Thailand. The traditional folk medicine practices of the Lisu, Lahu, Hmong, Karen, and Akha cultures are also passed down orally from one generation to the next. While each hill tribe group has its own specific perspective on medicine and healing, they all share similarity with each other, and also with the healing traditions of the Lanna Thai of northern Thailand.

Traditional medicine specialists

Mor muang is the general term for "local doctor," and includes several traditional medicine specialties, such as *mor ya* (herbalist), *mor pao* (mantra blower), and *mor song* (spiritual healer). Healers are predominantly male, and outsiders must first be accepted by a master within the tradition, and then pass an initiation ceremony before they can be accepted into a specific discipline of medicine. Although individuals may be skilled in several disciplines, most traditional healers focus on one particular specialty.

The *mor ya* (herbalist) covers the entire spectrum of disease and prepares formulas based on medicinal herbs and other natural substances.

The *mor pao* (mantra blower) specializes in healing through the use of breath and mantras. He often sprays holy water and offers incantations to the affected area by blowing breath or smoke.

The *mor song* (spiritual healer) performs a series of ceremonies and incantations by calling on the spiritual essence of the client and connecting with his spirit guides for assistance. Sometimes the healer may refer the patient to another traditional specialist, or may prescribe specific actions or remedies in order to alleviate the underlying cause of the disorder.

Other Thai healers

Mor nuad carry out traditional massage, an integral part of indigenous Thai medicine. Massage is carried out in the family unit, and many home remedies involve the use of Thai massage techniques. Traditional massage therapists practice in a wide variety of styles and treatments. Mor nuad can be both male and female.

Mor tam yae (midwives) are predominantly female and specialize in childbirth. Their specialized training is generally passed down through several family generations. In areas within easy reach of Western medicine, the traditional practices associated with childbirth are disappearing.

Although names for healing specialists may vary, the northern hill tribe cultures closely parallel the Lanna Thai traditions. In addition, both the village shaman *(mor phi)* and the soul retriever *(mor kwan)* play pivotal roles.

The mor phi (shaman) is the village connection with the spirit world, where ancestors and spirits dwell. The shamans are chosen by the spirits themselves through a near-death experience or through divination by a group of village elders. Trance is the most important vehicle for connecting with the guiding ancestor spirits. Healing treatments are carried out in the spirit world, and/or specific rituals are recommended for the patient to carry out by himself.

The *mor kwan* (soul retriever), is similar to the village shaman, but he specializes in rescuing the spirit of a patient when it has been lost, damaged, or stolen by a vengeful spirit. It is believed that actions caused by a maleficent spirit can result in illness. Specific curative rites and ceremonies are carried out, which sometimes involve a patient's entire family, and even occasionally the participation of an entire village.

Concepts of traditional medicine causality

Traditional healers do not have a tradition of surgery, and their concepts of causality of disease differ strongly from those in the West. Wind and blood are two strong causative factors, and they are often closely connected to each other. Wind *(lom)* surrounds us and is inside us, and it may easily be set out of balance. There may be too much or too little, and lom may even become poisonous. Fainting, uncontrolled movement, and heart pain usually indicate an excess of wind. Certain types of foods and outside odors are believed to contribute to an excess of wind. Lack of wind can affect mobility of the limbs, and in extreme cases may result in paralysis.

Blood *(leuad)* is acknowledged as the basic vital fluid of the body. It may be characterized as normal, hot, or cold, and it may exist in excess or in a diminished state. An imbalance of leuad is said to be the cause of many wind diseases.

Many diseases are brought about by poison *(pid)*. This could be direct poisoning received from a venomous bite or by ingesting contaminated food, but it can also be a result of "poisonous spirits." Healing treatments focus on isolating the poison, restricting its spread, and treating it with herbal medicines in order to expel it from the system. Dietary guidelines and food restrictions are often integral to the healing process.

Hot and cold are important factors in determining illness and in prescribing cures. The patient's perceptions of heat and cold are important diagnostic tools for healers. A fever, for example, may be classified as hot, cold, or neutral, and the healer will prescribe specific treatments based on these classifications. The general rule is that "hot" diseases are treated with "cold" medicines, and vice versa. Left (female) and right (male) energies are also important to bear in mind when making a diagnosis.

In northern Thai traditional medicine, knowledge of disease and corresponding cures has been passed on through the generations, and diagnosis and treatment is derived mainly from the array of symptoms that are displayed by the patient.

Disorders that are commonly diagnosed and treated in northern Thai medicine may be caused by ingestion of (or external contact with) alien materials, bad or inappropriate food, physical or psychological traumas, noxious odors and fumes, insect and animal bites, intestinal worms, diseases caused by spirits, black magic spells, climate conditions, and issues resulting from karma.

The future

Folk medicine in Thailand was outlawed as unscientific many years ago, and this belief was fortified by the advent of Western medicine in the region during the first quarter of the 20th century. As a result, ancient folk healing practices were often cast aside because practitioners were afraid of being arrested as charlatans. Only recently has the ban been lifted, and since then, what had once been pushed underground has begun to be practiced openly once again.

Knowledge is still passed on by word of mouth, with no centralized teaching. Herbal remedies are often held in secret, and even when recipes are written down, some of the most potent ingredients are deliberately omitted. Students often learn from one master, usually a specialist, and then they widen their studies and perspectives by working with other teachers.

Although it is struggling, northern Thai traditional medicine still has a chance to survive. A determining factor in its success depends on the healers themselves, and on whether they can abandon their secretive practices in order to create a centralized base of knowledge. From the patient's point of view, more choices in health care are always better. The West has gone through a similar process, and now alternative healing and herbal medicine are gaining more popularity and credibility each year. There is every reason to hope for a similar process in northern Thailand.

In the words of Phra Khru Uppakara Pattanakij, healer and abbot of Nong Yah Nang Temple: "We want to offer ordinary people more choices in health care. And we can do this by respecting the wisdom of our ancestors, and by keeping it alive through practice."

Om Namo ... What ?
The Thai Massage Wai Khru

BOB HADDAD

Every serious practitioner of traditional Thai massage is familiar with the *wai khru* – the famous prayer that begins "Om namo Shivago," and which invokes Jivaka (Shivago), the Ayurvedic doctor who is revered in Thailand as an ancestral teacher. Thai massage practitioners may recite it silently or chant it aloud in a group before beginning their lessons, but what does this prayer really mean?

Pali is an ancient language from India, and although many Thai people recite or chant in Pali within the context of Theravada Buddhist ceremonies, they often don't know the meaning of the prayers, much like Christians who routinely memorized and recited prayers in Latin years ago. Adaptation to Thai language over the years makes it more difficult to decipher the original Pali words. For Thai massage, the situation becomes even more complicated because the translations offered by those who composed, modified, or promoted the prayers have been spread all over the world in English, mostly by foreign students who have studied Thai massage. From these English translations, additional translations have been made by practitioners whose first language is not English. In addition, the common translations of several versions of the Thai massage wai khru are simply not correct.

For these and many more reasons, the Thai massage wai khru is often misrepresented, misinterpreted, and misunderstood. The purpose of this article is to address the wai khru ceremony, to shed light on the Pali words, and to discuss the common translations and true meanings of the words in this prayer.

The wai khru ceremony

The wai khru is not unique to practitioners of traditional Thai massage. Throughout Thailand, people perform wai khru ceremonies that are specific to individual jobs and ways of life. Schoolchildren gather in schoolyards and classrooms to recite a wai khru to thank the Buddha, their parents, and their school teachers. Graduation celebrations for any type of study or discipline always include a wai khru. Muay Thai kick boxers perform ceremonies that feature a dance to honor their teachers and the ancestral teacher and founder of this martial art. Musicians, performers, doctors, and soldiers all perform wai khru ceremonies. Although each of these may involve the recitation or chanting of different prayers, all pay homage to the Buddha, all include offerings of flowers, incense, and candles, and all invoke the intercession of a higher power in order to carry out a specific deed or action with respect, clarity, and integrity.

The Thai word *wai* means "respect"; it is also the name for the common gesture of bringing two hands together in prayer position while slightly bowing with deference toward the receiver of the action. The word *khru* is a Thai language adaptation of the Pali/Sanskrit word *guru*. So wai khru literally means "respect teacher."

Buddhist veneration

In the Theravada tradition, it is customary to pay homage to the Buddha, to recite a prayer called the Three Refuges (the Triple Gem), and to observe the *Pancha Sila* (The Five Disciplines) upon visiting a place of worship, or at the start of a Buddhist ceremony. One may recite the stanzas alone, or they may be led by a Buddhist monk. The prayer is in the Pali language.

In addition to the two main versions of the Thai massage wai khru known today, other variations may also be found throughout Thailand. These may include the Triple Gem, chants that pay homage to one's parents and teachers, and even prayers directed toward reusi, who are credited with transmission of *reusi dat ton,* Thai massage, incantations, traditional medicine, and other sciences.

In some places in Thailand, it's customary to recite prayers immediately preceding the main wai khru to Jivaka. Reproduced below are the Vandana (the homage to the Buddha that is recited three times) and the Tisarana (also known as The Three Refuges, the Triple Gem, and the Three Jewels):

Namo tassa bhagavato arahato samma sambhuddhassa.	Honor to the blessed one, the exalted one, the fully enlightened one.
Buddham saranam gacchami	I go to the Buddha for my refuge.
Dhammam saranam gacchami	I go to the dhamma for my refuge.
Sangham saranam gacchami	I go to the sangha for my refuge.
Dutiyampi Buddham saranam gacchami	For the second time I go to the Buddha for my refuge.
Dutiyampi Dhammam saranam gacchami	For the second time I go to the dhamma for my refuge.
Dutiyampi Sangham saranam gacchami	For the second time I go to the sangha for my refuge.
Tatiyampi Buddham saranam gacchami	For the third time I go to the Buddha for my refuge.
Tatiyampi Dhammam saranam gacchami	For the third time I go to the dhamma for my refuge.
Tatiyampi Sangham saranam gacchami	For the third time I go to the sangha for my refuge.

The Thai massage wai khru

Most students who arrive in Chiang Mai to study Thai massage will encounter the northern-style wai khru, the one that was spread largely through the Old Medicine Hospital and ITM Massage School. This wai khru reads as follows, with slight variations in spelling from place to place:

Om Namo Shivago Silasa Ahang

Karuniko Sapasatanang Osata Tipa Mantang

Papaso Suriya Jantang Gomalapato Paka Sesi

Wantami Bantito Sumetaso

Aroha Sumana Homi *(recite 3 times)*

Piyo Tewa Manussanang Piyo Proma Namutamo

Piyo Nakha Supananang

Pininsiang Nama Mihang Namo Puttaya

Navon Navien Nasatit Nasatien

Ehi Mama Navien Nawe

Napai Tangvien Navien Mahaku

Ehi Mama Piyong Mama Namo Puttaya *(recite one time)*

Na-a Na-wa Roh-kha Payati Vinasanti *(recite three times)*

And this is the common translation that has been offered to Thai massage students in recent years:

> We pray to you, Shivago, you who led a saintly life.
>
> We pray that you bring us knowledge, and that you allow our prayers
>
> to bring us the true medicine of the Universe.
>
> We pray that you will bring us health and all good things.
>
> The God of healing lives in the heavens, and we live in the world below.
>
> We pray to you so that heaven may be reflected
>
> in the world below, and that healing medicine
>
> may encircle the world.
>
> We pray for the one we touch, that he will be happy,
>
> and that all illness will be released from him.

According to several trust-worthy sources, however, this translation is not accurate. In addition, the Thai massage wai khru mentioned above is not as old as is commonly believed. The English translation of the northern-style wai khru was probably done in the 1980s, and the prayer itself was put together only a short time before that.

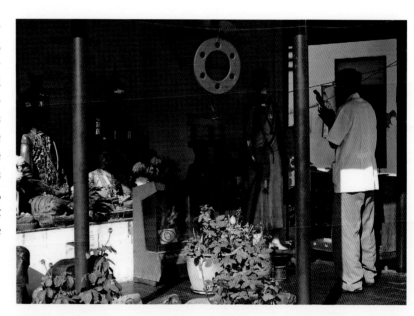

The Wat Po wai khru

The wai khru used at the Wat Po massage school in Bangkok is quite different from the Old Medicine Hospital version. The first verse is the same as its northern counterpart, but it is preceded by the standard Buddhist veneration that begins with "Namo tassa," which was described previously in this essay. In addition, the consonants of several words of the first section are pronounced differently. The northern spelling "*silasa*" is pronounced "*sirasa*." The letter r reflects the original Pali pronunciation and is not necessarily the result of the common linguistic confusion of the letters l and r. Finally, the word "*aroha*," as in "*aroha sumana homi*," is absent.

Ajahn Sintorn prays at the Old Medicine Hospital's altar, 2003

The Wat Po wai khru contains three main sections, and each section is preceded by the familiar *Namo Tassa* ("Homage to the Buddha"). Here is the Wat Po version of the Thai massage wai khru. Note in the first section the variations in spelling and pronunciation from the northern version:

Namo tassa prakawatoe arahatoe samma samphudtasa (3x)

Ohm namo Chevago sirasa arhang   Karuniko Shapphasattanang

Osata Tipphamantang   Praphaso suriyajantang

Komarawattoe Pakasaysi   Wontami Phantitoe

Sumaythatoe Sumanahomi

Namo Tassa Prakawatoe Arahatoe Samma Samphudtasa (3x)

Sahamuti Sumuhakatoe Saymatang Phatasaymayang

Sahanitampho Aewang Aehe Nathod Mothon Phudkhon Takhueain

Yaluelain Ludloihai Sawaha Sawahai

Namo Tassa Prakawatoe Arahatoe Samma Samphudtasa (3x)

Phuttang Pajakame Thammang Pajakame Sankhang Pajakame

The truth about the Thai massage wai khru

As may be seen above, the Wat Po wai khru doesn't contain the second and third sections of the northern version. Instead, two other sections are found, described as "spell before massage" and "spell for protection against bad incantations." The presence of these two sections in the Wat Po version, and the way they are described, reflect the fact that the second and third sections of the northern-style mantra also have their roots in magical incantations.

When Ajahn Sinthorn Chaichakan moved to Chiang Mai and founded what would become known as the Old Medicine Hospital (Thai Massage School Shivagakomarapaj), he developed a new style and sequence of Thai massage techniques based, in part, on what he'd learned when he studied at Wat Po. Around that same time, he put together a new wai khru to use in his business endeavors in Chiang Mai. This new northern-style wai khru was based on the older first verse from Wat Po, plus two additional sections based on incantations and magic spells. This has been confirmed to me personally by Ajahn Preeda Tangtrongchitr, the founder and long-time director of the Wat Po massage school, and also by Sintorn's son, Wasan Chaichakan, the current director of the Old Medicine Hospital.

In addition to its use at Old Medicine Hospital, this version of the wai khru was used by Chongkol Setthakorn, who had spent several years working at the Old Medicine Hospital in the 1980s, when he opened his Chiang Mai school, ITM.

As a result of the commercial success of these two schools among Western students, the northern-style wai khru (and its incomplete and misleading English translation) began to be spread all over the world, and was even translated into other languages. All of the teachers mentioned above have acknowledged to me that magic spells are contained in the wai khrus, and that they have deliberately not been translated, in keeping with Thai traditions regarding *khathas* and magic incantations.

Meanings of individual words

Here is a list of many of the individual words used in the commonly known Thai massage wai khru, along with reasonable translations. The majority of them come from Pali, though there is also some intermixing of Thai words. This information was supplied to me by one of my teachers, and many of these words are available through research:

ahang	I, me, my
arahato	an arhat, a worthy one
aroga (aroha)	to be free from disease
chandang (jantan, candam)	moon
dewa	see *tewa*, below
dibba (tipa)	divine
dibbamantang (tipa mantang)	divine mantra
Jivako	one who has life, Jivaka
bhagavato (bhagawato)	blessed one
homi	to me, for me
jantang (jantam)	moon
karuniko	compassion, one who has compassion
Komarabhacco (Gomalapato)	Jivaka's second name
kru (khru)	(Thai) teacher, guru
mantam (mantang)	mantra
manusanang	the human race
naa (nakha)	naga, a deity that takes the shape of a great serpent
namo	homage
vien (wien)	(Thai) spin, spinning
osadha (osatha)	medicine
pabhaso (pabaso, papaso)	luminous, to give light

pakasesi	to shine, to declare
pandito (bantito)	pandit, or wise man
piyinsiang (pininsiang)	one who has clarity of the senses and control of their faculties
piyo	beloved, revered
proma	Thai pronunciation for Brahma, of the Indian pantheon
Putaya	Thai pronunciation of *Buddhaya* or *Buddhaaya*, which means Buddha
pujaya	(Thai) worship, from *puja*
samma	perfectly, fully, or in a correct way
sapasatanang (sabbasattanam)	all sentient beings
sirasa (silasa)	The correct meaning of sirasa is "head."
sumana	healthy, happy
sumedhaso (sumetasso)	intelligent, wise, accomplished
supananang	heavenly beings
suriya	sun
tewa	*deva*, celestial being
vandami (wantami)	to pay respect
wai	to respect

Prayer to Jivaka, first section

Om namo Shivago sirasa ahang	I pay homage to Jivaka with my head
karuniko sapasatanan	with compassion for all sentient beings
osatha (osadha) tipa mantang	He who gave divine medicine
papaso suriya jantang	Kumarabhaccha glows as
Gomalapato paka sesi	brightly as the sun and the moon
wandhami (wantami) bantito	We pay obeisance to the pandit, the
sumethaso arokha	wise one, to be healthy
sumana homi	and at peace

Second section, first part

Some words in the first part of the second section are taken from the Buddhist *ratanamala*, which is well known in Thailand, Burma, and throughout Southeast Asia, and which is used primarily to pay homage to the Buddha. In this context, however, it does not appear to be specific to the Buddha. It is generally used as an incantation (a magic spell) to attract beneficial people and things to oneself, and to become more beloved by those beings. It prays that actions may have a beneficial outcome:

Piyo dewa (tewa) manussanang piyo proma namutamo

I revere the one who is beloved by devas, by Brahma, and by mankind

piyo nakha supananang pininsiang

beloved by nagas, cherubs, and those with pure senses

nama mihang

I pay homage

Second section, second part

The rest of the second section is a magical incantation used for disorienting and overpowering people. After confusing them and spinning them around, it then reestablishes them and attracts them closer to the one who is casting the spell. It is generally forbidden to literally translate magic incantations, and in keeping with Thai tradition I will not offer a complete translation of this section of the wai khru. It's important to keep in mind that this portion has never been accurately represented in commonly available explanations of the prayer. In fact, in a way, it has been deliberately misrepresented. It represents a magic spell that should be respected and held secret:

namo Puttaya

Nawon (navon) nawien (navien) nasatit nasatien

Ehi mama navien (nawien) nawe napai tangvien navien (nawien) mahaku (makaku)

Ehi mama piyong mama namo Puttaya

Last section

The last section of the wai khru is a mantra in and of itself, though not all words are translatable:

Na-a Na-wa

These are known as "heart syllables" in Thai, and "seed syllables" in Sanskrit. They don't have a direct translation and have no meaning in and of themselves. They are short mantras that are generally attached to a longer text.

Roga (rokha) payati (vyadhi) vinasanti

May all illness and disease be healed

A new, more accurate translation

Keeping all of the above information in mind, and without translating the magic incantations, I offer to the international Thai massage community a new, accurate, and vernacular translation of the commonly known northern style wai khru:

> I pay homage with my head to Jivaka.
>
> With compassion for all beings, he has brought us divine medicine.
>
> Kumarabhacca shines as brightly as the sun and the moon.
>
> I pay respect to the great pandit, to the wise one.
>
> May there be happiness and freedom from illness.
>
> I revere the one who is adored by deities, by humans, and by Brahma;
>
> the one who is adored by nagas and by heavenly beings;
>
> the one who is of pure faculties.
>
> May all illness and disease be healed.

The practice

For students, practitioners, and teachers of Thai healing arts, performing a wai khru is an integral part of practice. It helps calm the body and mind; it establishes a respectful, humble atmosphere within which to live and work; and it reinforces the practice of Thai massage through prayer, reflection, and gratitude.

The wai khru may be carried out on a daily basis, and can be added to a regimen of meditation, yoga, or other spiritual and physical practices, whether in the morning or in the evening. It is considered most important in the morning, before the start of a day's work. It is performed before an altar containing images or statues of the Buddha, Jivaka, and sometimes other deities or respected ones such as a reusi, a monk, or a revered person. Photos or mementos of deceased parents and teachers are also customary to include on an altar, as well as candles, incense, and other offerings, such as old coins and fruit. Traditionally, offerings that represent the elements are routinely placed and changed on an altar. Incense represents wind *(lom)*, candles represent fire *(fai)*, water represents water *(naam)*, food represents earth *(din)*, and flowers represent space *(aagaasathaat)*.

The Wai Khru is performed kneeling, with the feet behind the body. In Thailand, men curl their feet under their toes, rather than laying the top of the foot flat on the ground. The practitioner bows three times before beginning the recitation of prayers, and three times afterward. If candles are lit during the ceremony, they may be extinguished with the fingers or with a candle snuffer, but not with the breath. Blowing out a candle is believed to disperse the offerings.

Although the wai khru ceremony is inextricably connected to Buddhism, Thai massage practitioners who follow other faiths and religious beliefs can adapt their altars and prayers accordingly. Prayers for guidance and intercession in your work may be offered to other gods and deities, but you should still give thanks to your teachers of Thai massage, your life teachers, and to Jivaka, if possible.

However you structure your wai khru, it is important to recognize and respect that traditional Thai healing arts are inextricably connected to the life concepts and teachings of the Buddha, and that to practice Thai healing without embracing these basic concepts is not in keeping with tradition. Fortunately, the teachings of the Buddha are such that it would be difficult to find a person, whatever religion they may follow, who disagrees with the basic underlying truths embodied in Buddhist philosophy.

I hope this essay has provided Thai massage practitioners around the world with a deeper understanding of the wai khru and its history, meaning, and translation. Maintaining an attitude filled with respect, reverence, compassion, and loving-kindness is essential to a deep and effective practice in traditional Thai healing arts. Regular practice of the wai khru can help to promote and prolong these spiritual elements, and can strengthen our abilities to help others through our work. Remember to practice safely, and with great respect for your teachers, for your lineage of instruction, and for Thai spiritual traditions.

The Thai Massage Wai Khru

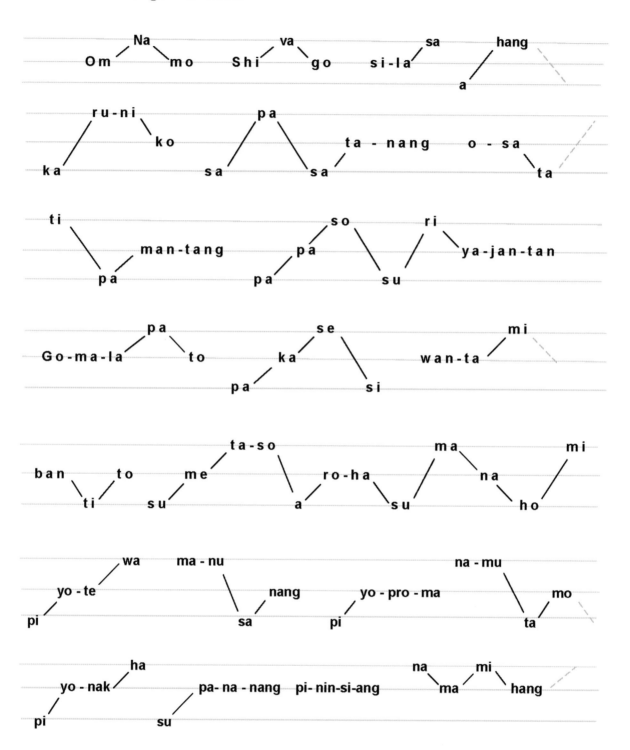

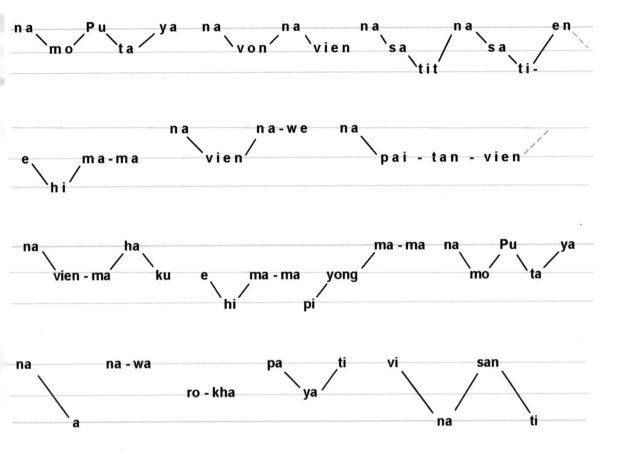

Chanting the Thai Massage Wai Khru (Om Namo Shivago)

In some lineages, this mantra is chanted, not simply recited. This is a transcription of the three-note melody, annotated in an easy-to-use format. The solid lines between syllables guide the singer from one note to the next, and the dashed lines indicate when there is a different tone at the beginning of a new line.

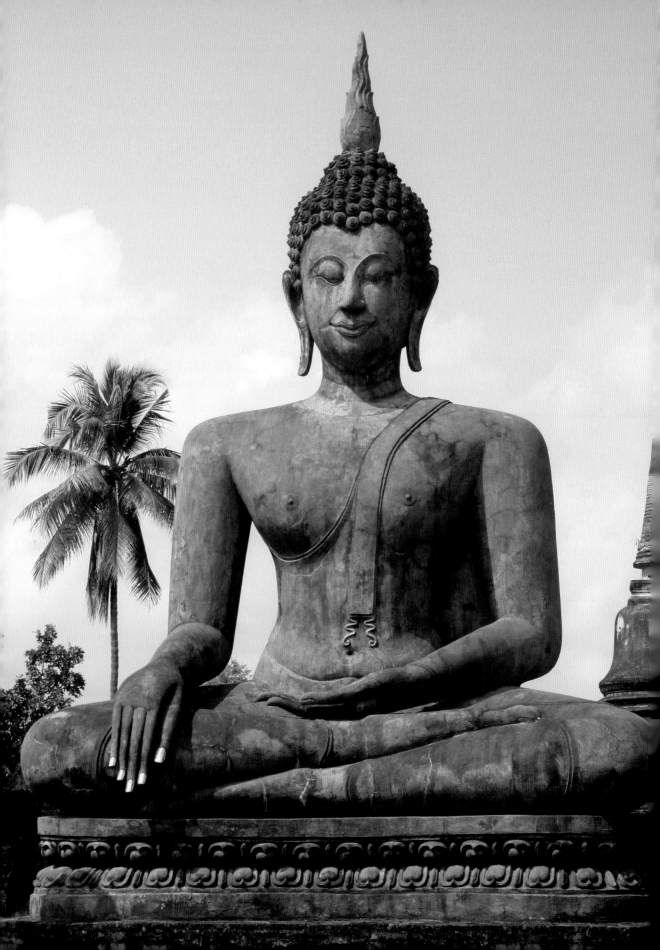

Section 4

Thai Therapists Speak

Diabetes and Thai Massage – No Contraindication

KAREN UFER

The story I'd like to share is about a strong experience I had in the treatment room. It's a story about the impact of conditions that are beyond our control, which nevertheless influence the outcome of a Thai therapy session. It's also a story about recognizing that the people we touch are our teachers.

What happened?

I was giving a Thai bodywork session to a client of mine who had come to my treatment room for his second Thai session. It was a Tuesday afternoon, and no one else was present in the house. Toward the end of the 90-minute session, it looked like my client Jeff had relaxed completely and had fallen asleep. He was even snoring lightly. I left the room, went to the restroom, washed my hands, drank some water, and changed my shirt. When I returned to the room and asked if he was alright, Jeff didn't answer. His eyes were wide open, but he had lost consciousness. He was bathed in sweat, and his shirt was wet. He was breathing and had a pulse, but it seemed like his physical body was shutting down.

"Jeff, what are you doing? What's going on?" I shouted. I grabbed the phone and called 911.

"Do you want to report an emergency?"

"Yes!"

I stayed next to Jeff, holding his left hand. Both of his arms and hands began to spasm. A tsunami of fear flooded the treatment room. After a few minutes, family members arrived, and we waited for the ambulance. The paramedics realized very quickly that we were dealing with diabetic shock. His blood sugar was down to 19 – the threshold is 40, and anything below that is life threatening. They managed to bring Jeff back, they stabilized him, and by the time they left for the hospital, he had regained consciousness. The next day, Jeff and his wife came back to pick up his car and some personal belongings. He had completely recovered.

Background information

The first time I met Jeff, he had come to try Thai bodywork because of chronic pain in the area around his left hip. After he completed the intake form, we spent a considerable amount of time discussing all the health issues he'd reported.

Jeff is a 73-year-old man with long-term type 2 diabetes, high blood pressure, triple bypass heart surgery, three spinal surgeries (including fusion of several lumbar vertebrae), one surgery on the cervical spine, two surgeries on the right rotator cuff, one surgery on the left shoulder, and one surgery on the piriformis muscle near his hip, which was done in order to relieve his sciatica pain. He was hoping to address this hip pain in his sessions with me.

After the session that had ended in diabetic shock, I realized that the complexity of his health issues had distracted me from asking more about the stability of his diabetic condition. I was much more concerned about the implications of his vascular and spinal conditions, and how that would affect my work.

This was the first time in my practice that I had had to deal with such a complexity of disorders in a single client. Did I feel comfortable about it? Not exactly, and I doubted that I could find a way to give him what he needed. I had thought that his body could introduce me to a new level of sensitivity, sensing, and feeling, but I could have never imagined what would happen on my mat that day.

Because of his delicate health history, my repertoire of Thai techniques was very limited. My focus was on intensive foot reflexology, careful line work along the legs, no deep compressions, no double leg work, no arterial compressions, and no twisting. I tried to guide him to breathe deeply in order to facilitate deep relaxation.

The boomerang area around the left hip joint seemed to be inflamed, and I felt an unusual heat there. This meant that I could only approach this area indirectly. So I worked around the hip, not on the inflamed area, using line work. I also gently laid my hand on the inflamed area, intending to send it healing energy. Instead, I received a transfer of heat into my hands, and from there my whole body became warm, and I began to sweat.

Despite the diabetic shock and the emergency medical situation that occurred in the second session, that first session went well from a therapeutic perspective. Jeff said he felt great, and he even reported some pain relief. I was exhausted, and although I generally don't like cold showers, I needed one after that session.

While speaking to Jeff's family after the incident, I learned that a similar event had happened before his diabetic shock on my Thai mat that day. He had suffered a sudden and dramatic decrease in his blood sugar because of a change of medication a few weeks before. This resulted in a dangerous instability that he hadn't mentioned in the pre-session consultation for his first appointment. He couldn't feel that his blood sugar was falling, so he couldn't warn others about it and take action. He had eaten lunch that day, but our session began at 4 p.m., so by the time it was over, too much time had elapsed since his last food intake.

Conclusions

We know that traditional Thai bodywork is not contraindicated for diabetes. I searched the Internet for information, and I spoke to experienced Thai teachers and shiatsu practitioners to see if they had any advice. I found only one incident of a diabetic crisis at the end of a *reiki* session on an older woman, and that was mostly related to nutritional factors. Interestingly, there were many reports about successful management of diabetic disorders with Thai massage, shiatsu, acupuncture, even yoga. As a result of this experience, I've learned to take into account two very important conditions, especially in older clients: stability of medication and nutrition status. In the future, if a client circles "diabetes" on my intake form, I will insist on more detailed information about the current condition of the person, including, for example:

- How stable is your medication?
- When was your last incident of a sudden drop of blood sugar, and what happened as a result?
- Have you ever suffered from diabetic shock?
- When did you last eat food?
- Do you carry anything with you that I should know about in case of an emergency?

Only when I know this information will I feel comfortable enough to give a Thai bodywork session to another client with diabetes.

Revelations

We connect to the healing energy of the universe through our prayers and through right action, but risk is present anywhere (even on your mat), at any time (even during your Thai sessions), and with anyone (either you or your client). My experience with Jeff allowed me to surrender to this truth. I experienced an energy flow in the physical body that I'd never felt before, and the vital energies with which we are so familiar in our work had completely drained from my client's body. Realizing I had no control, my mind bombarded me with my worst fears: my client was having a stroke, going into a coma, probably dying. If I'd done something wrong, if I'd harmed a human being on my mat, I would never be able to treat another person again. I felt completely helpless as I waited for the ambulance to arrive. And Jeff was in a raging river, holding on to a weak branch of a tree, resisting a powerful current. All I could do was to hold on to his hand and tell him repeatedly, "Please, Jeff, stay with me." That was my mantra for an endless moment.

When the paramedics arrived, I wanted to move aside and make room for them, but Jeff's grip was so tight, it was difficult to remove my hand. In our training we learn that we are one with the body that we touch; now I truly know what that means.

I am grateful that my client's soul didn't depart from my mat, and that he remained unharmed. I am even grateful that his attack occurred on my mat and not on his way home, alone, in his car. I am also grateful that the universal plan allows me to continue to touch others, and to maintain the awareness that we are all constantly dying.

Om namo Shivago.

Acupuncture and Thai Massage: Same-Same, but Different

ERIC SPIVACK

Thai massage and acupuncture are ancient healing arts that have existed for thousands of years. Thai massage is rooted in Ayurvedic medicine, Buddhist spiritual practice, and yoga. Acupuncture and Chinese medicine have their origins in China.

While both acupuncture and Thai massage are distinct modalities, they share some similarities, and could perhaps be described with the popular Thai expression "Same-same, but different."

Acupuncture and Thai massage are individual elements of more complex systems of medicine. Both Chinese medicine and traditional Thai medicine utilize herbal medicine, nutritional and food cures, spiritual practice, and physical medicine.

Neither acupuncture nor Thai massage is based on the Western system of anatomy. In many places in the East, dissection was forbidden until the introduction of Western medicine, so the earliest references to the human body were based on external observations. As a result, both modalities are complete energy-based healing systems. In Thai massage, we use the term *sen* to describe the pathways along which energy travels, and that energy is referred to as *lom*. In acupuncture, the pathways are called meridians or channels, and the energy that moves throughout the body is called *qi* (pronounced "chee"). Other Eastern names for this energy force are *ki* (Japanese), and *prana* (Indian Ayurvedic medicine).

This energy powers all our physical, mental, and emotional processes. In both acupuncture and Thai massage, the practitioner's intent is to harmonize and clear energetic imbalances. Such imbalances may present themselves physically in a number of ways, such as body pain, muscle cramping, stiffness, insomnia, irritability, anxiety, constipation, or disease.

When the system is working well, a person feels happy, relaxed, and free from pain, though according to Chinese medicine, being symptom-free does not necessarily mean a person is in complete balance. Whereas an acupuncturist inserts sterile, hair-thin pins at various points on the body, the Thai massage practitioner uses his fingers, palms, elbows, knees, and feet to adjust for energetic blockages.

The Ayurvedic tradition speaks of untold thousands of *nadis* (channels), which run through the human body. Of these channels, ten major sen lines are the focus for Thai massage practitioners. Acupuncturists address twelve major meridians and eight additional pathways called "extraordinary vessels." While there is some overlap of Thai sen and Chinese meridians, they are not the same. For example, in Thai medicine, the ten sen begin and end at or near the navel, and energy travels in both directions along each sen. In acupuncture, the meridians either begin or end at the finger tips or toes, and when energy is flowing properly, it travels in only one direction.

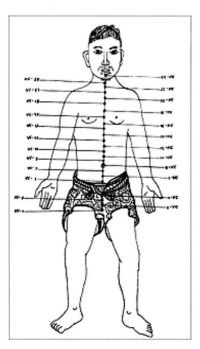

Ren Mai

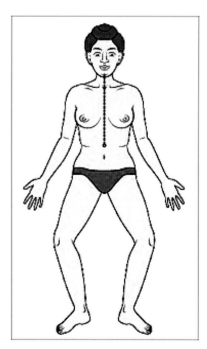

Sen Sumana

As the energy pathways are different, so are the treatment points along them. For example, in Chinese medicine, the *ren* meridian originates in the uterus in women and in the lower abdomen in men. It emerges at the perineum, travels up the anterior midline of the body, and ends just below the lower lip, where it curves around the lips and terminates below the eyes, where it then meets the stomach meridian.

In Thai massage, this pathway may be similarly comprised of several lines:

1   *Sen Sumana*, which originates at the navel and travels to the tip of the tongue;

2   *Sen Nanthakrawat*, which subdivides into two lines: *Sen Sukhumang*, which travels from the navel to the anus, and *Sen Sikhin*, which travels from the navel to the urethra;

3   *Sen Khitchana*, which also subdivides into two lines: *Sen Pitakun*, running from the navel to the penis in men, and *Sen Kitcha*, running from the navel to the vagina in women.

Though strong differences exist between traditional Chinese medicine and traditional Thai medicine, there are enough similarities for these two systems to complement one another. In my experience, I have found that combining acupuncture and Thai massage in a single session can be extremely beneficial. I have noticed that my patients respond best when they are able to receive 30 minutes of acupuncture followed by one or two hours of Thai massage. Acupuncture helps clear energetic blockages and enables patients to benefit more from the Thai massage work. People feel more relaxed. They breathe more deeply, they experience deeper stretches, and they feel like they've received a truly holistic treatment.

One Week with Pichest Boonthumme

MICHELLE TUPKO

Ajahn Pichest is always smiling . . . except when he pretends to hit you on the head with his Buddhist cane as he says "pok pok!" Well, even then, he's smiling. Though I've studied with Pichest over a period of several years, this is a story that I wrote during my first week of study with him.

Pichest's classroom is in the middle of a suburb called Hang Dong that was once a village of its own. Even now, it feels like the countryside compared to Chiang Mai, and there are still a few cultivated fields alongside his family home. The practice room has a very large shrine area, occupying nearly one-third of the total area of the space. There are three sections: one part for teachers and family, one part for the Buddha and the *dhamma*, and one part that contains a free-standing white spirit house. Near this house is a large sculpture – a boat covered in gold leaf.

Each day is structured in basically the same way, with some variations and improvisations. In general, Pichest speaks about keeping the Five Precepts of Buddhism, honoring one's mother and father, not thinking too much, not thinking at all, the illusion of the body, and the certainty of death.

He often refers to the many 7-11 convenience stores throughout Thailand as a metaphor for all that's gone wrong in contemporary society. He once explained that if trying to be a Thai massage therapist makes you too worried, or makes you think too much, you should become someone who sells boxes, because that is a job without stress, and anyway, everyone always needs boxes, all kinds of boxes, including the one you that you find yourself in when you "stop life."

Every day we pray a formal set of Buddhist prayers, including a recitation of a vow to observe the Five Precepts. We recite some of these prayers together, and Pichest offers a series of prayers by himself as we listen and sit in meditation. We pray to all three areas of the shrine. We chant the *wai khru* to Jivaka and then more prayers follow. After prayers, Pichest usually gives a dharma talk. He elaborates on the same subjects mentioned above, and sometimes directs much of his speaking to a particular student. When he does this, I believe it's an example of what is called "transmission" in Buddhism – the teaching he gives is heard by all, but the inner energy of the teaching is directed to someone in particular. I believe, in fact, that this direct transmission is a very important part of his bodywork, and it is also one of the ways he works as a teacher.

Somehow arising from the dharma talk, he chooses someone and makes comments about what's going on in their body. He may suddenly go over to someone and say, "See, block here," and point to a particular area. He elaborates, and sometimes does some work on that person's afflicted area. Oftentimes, he'll say to the students, "Feel, sense. Where is the block?" He will have that person lie down and the other students will gather around to explore and work on that person's body. This all happens in a very organic and fluid way. Sometimes students ask questions, but if they ask a very "thinking" type of question, they'll get threatened with a hit on the head in a playful way. In response to questions, he may demonstrate something extremely interesting, and sometimes he may not respond at all.

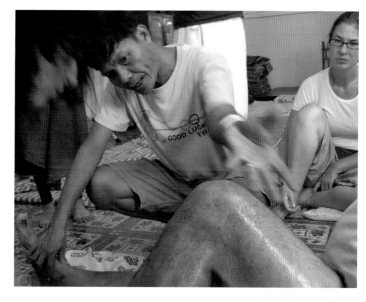

Ajahn Pichest with students

Ajahn Pichest teaches entirely in the moment. He works only with what is there, and he rejects conceptualization and abstraction. This can be utterly maddening for students, but it also forces us to look very closely at who is actually lying on the mat in front of us, and to surrender the belief that we can work from our own ideas about what someone else needs.

After the morning session we have lunch. Sometimes, Pichest's wife kindly cooks vegetarian food. Other times, we go to the food stand down the road. There, we drink *cha nom* (Thai iced tea with condensed milk) or *cha manao* (Thai iced tea with lime). It is served in plastic bags, and that is just delightful. It's also funny, because when you need to put aside your tea, you can't, because it's in a plastic bag! Maybe you should hang it on a hook, as we once saw Pichest do.

After lunch, we return to the classroom and begin to work with someone. This, like the rest of the day, happens very organically. At times, Pichest may receive work from one of the students, or he will show the class new techniques by working on someone. Other times, he will circulate around the room, making adjustments and offering advice. Sometimes, Pichest may even close his eyes and rest.

In class, one finds oneself looking to the other students as well as to Pichest for answers, for ways to work, and for guidance. This is one of my favorite aspects of his way of teaching. The room is a mix of beginner, intermediate, and advanced students, so a lot of knowledge is exchanged among the students.

If you can't understand something, like how to use your knee pressure in the right way, Pichest will place your hand under his knee so you can feel how the pressure should be transmitted to the receiver. This "feeling" way of learning is very direct, and like so much that Pichest does, it avoids over-conceptualizing. At around 4 p.m., we pray again, this time with a short invocation to the Buddha, and then we again chant the wai khru. After that, we are free to go home. After class, Pichest sometimes sits outside the classroom and talks with students. This is the daily rhythm of study.

One day, an American man who lives in Chiang Mai, and who suffers from Parkinson's, came to receive a treatment from Pichest. The session was carried out in the main room, with the students watching, some even taking photos. Pichest had one of his students open the man's wind gate in side-lying position, but other than that, he did all of the work himself.

I was glad to have this chance to watch him work. He didn't talk or explain much while he worked, but watching him and following the thread of his thought – that is, his nonthinking – was an amazing learning experience. Pichest is truly a master of finding the simplest, most direct, and most effective way to work at any given moment in any position, and he works with astounding fluidity.

On another day, a Thai woman arrived with an older Indian man who had polio as a child. He had recently undergone surgery to have his Achilles tendon lengthened, and his leg was still stiff and swollen, and was causing him a lot of pain. Pichest examined the man and gave him the exact same diagnosis as the doctor had given. The most surprising thing that Pichest said was that he should definitely not receive Thai massage, because the pressure could worsen his condition.

Instead, he recommended oil massage. He went to the back of the room, where there was a big tub of dark, herbed sesame oil. One of his students brought him a variety of containers, bowls, and cups to put the oil in, but none of them were appropriate. Pichest apparently wanted an earthenware container for the oil. Finally, after ten minutes of searching for the right container, he began to give a type of slapping massage to the man's leg, a technique meant to stimulate blood flow.

One week with Pichest is both a long time and a short time to be in his presence. He always works based on the bodies and the energies of the students in his room each day. The usual classroom structure that is typical of most Thai massage courses is totally absent from his way of teaching. He teaches from each situation as it is, in the present moment. I am realizing more and more that this is the essence of meditation. I once mentioned to Pichest that it would be good if he taught meditation in class, but now I realize that he is already doing this.

At the end of class one day, just before closing prayers, he suddenly stood up, went to the window, and called for us to come and look at the light. As we crowded around him, he opened a bottle of water and poured a few drops into a cavity made by the veins of a large leaf outside. Then he held that beautiful and simple water droplet up to the light, so that the light could shine through it. "Like that," he said. "Just like that."

Integrating General Acupressure into Traditional Thai Massage

MICHAEL REED GACH

Traditional Thai massage techniques stimulate various acupressure points using the fingers, palms, forearms, elbows, knees, feet, and toes in order to trigger the body's natural self-curative abilities. Thai stretches, similar to assisted yoga postures, also stimulate the healing energy pathways known as *sen*, whose Chinese counterparts are known as meridians. Each of these energy lines reinforces all the functions of the body, and the acupressure points are often where this healing energy gets blocked.

This essay attempts to highlight common acupressure points that may be stimulated while performing a traditional Thai massage. A wide variety of wonderful Thai massage stretching techniques focus only on the stretches themselves. Why not incorporate acupressure as we engage our clients in assisted stretching? If we are holding our client's feet and pulling them toward us to bring about a lower back opening, can we lodge our fingers and thumbs into strong acupressure points nearby as we execute the stretch? In many instances the answer is yes. When I perform a Thai massage, I integrate my knowledge of Chinese acupressure into my traditional Thai massage routines and stretches. In most cases, these two ancient healing systems work very well together.

The origins and history of acupressure

The origins of acupressure are based upon instinct. For example, it is instinctive to hold your forehead or your temples when you have a headache. Everyone at one time or another has spontaneously held painful or tight areas on the body. Ancient civilizations around the world have independently developed hands-on folk remedies within their own cultures. Acupressure and massage methods that were found to be effective were handed down from generation to generation.

Acupressure therapy developed in cultures that honored healing arts. In the early dynasties, when stones and arrows were the implements of war, soldiers on the battlefield reported that symptoms of disease that had bothered them for years suddenly vanished after they had been wounded. Naturally, such strange occurrences baffled physicians who could find no logical relationship between the trauma points and the ensuing recovery of health. After years of conscientious observation, ancient Chinese physicians developed ways of curing certain illnesses by piercing specific points on the surface of the body. They also discovered that pressing certain points relieved pain where it was felt, and also benefitted other parts of the body, far away from the point itself. Other cultures made similar discoveries, and developed ways of working specific pressure points along energy lines in order to relieve pain.

How acupressure works

Muscular pain and tension tend to concentrate around acupressure points, and this tension, in turn, affects other areas of the body. Acupressure relaxes muscular tension and balances the vital life forces of the body that run through energy channels. The points have a high electrical conductivity on the surface of the skin, and by gradually increasing the pressure, energy may be manipulated and balanced. Thai sen lines, Indian nadis, and Chinese meridians are pathways that carry the body's healing energy as it flows from point to point. The stimulation of specific acupressure points helps to charge the body's homeostatic process by directly reducing tension and stress, restoring calm, and allowing the body to heal itself more effectively.

Healing energy (known as *chi* or *qi* in Chinese medicine, *prana* in Indian Ayurvedic medicine, and *lom* in traditional Thai medicine) is the source of life, and its flow is the key to radiant health. It functions to regulate all human body systems, and also balances our emotional and mental states. Acupressure works to effectively create a feeling of balance and well-being. When our energy is flowing properly, we feel alive, happy, peaceful, and in harmony with others and with ourselves.

Acupressure for pain relief

Traditional Thai massage stimulates sen lines and acupressure points that are associated with specific health benefits, so understanding how acupressure works can further clarify how Thai massage activates healing and relieves pain. Pain perception is closely related to the amount of bodily stress, tension, and emotional anxiety that is present in the client. Acupressure increases circulation, which decreases lactic acid, carbon dioxide, histamines, bradykinins (mediators for pain reception), and a variety of toxins. Enhanced blood flow brings oxygen and other nutrients to the affected areas.

The client's focus on pain is often distracted by touching and stimulating the corresponding acupressure points, which in turn decreases tension. In these ways, acupressure therapy provides a natural way for the client to cope with pain and stress.

One explanation of this pain relief phenomenon is the "pain-gateway" theory. This theory postulates that the transmission of pain impulses can be modulated by a gating mechanism in the pain signaling system. An open gate results in pain; a partially open gate, less intense pain; and a closed gate, no pain. This "gating" is affected in part by the activity of sensory nerves. Stimulation of these large cutaneous fibers tends to close the gate, inhibiting the transmission of pain impulses from the spinal cord to the brain. Acupressure produces a mild, fairly painless stimulation, which causes the gates to close, so painful sensations can't pass through.

Another theory is that prolonged pressure on the acupressure points releases endorphins, which have a natural analgesic effect on the body. Endorphins are neurotransmitters that appear to be produced by the pituitary gland. Acupressure and acupuncture stimulate the pituitary gland to release endorphins. Endorphins don't entirely block the sensation of pain, but they do alter a person's perception of the sensation, similar to the effect of narcotics. This might explain why traditional Thai massage often brings about a "natural high" after the bodywork session.

Acupressure for emotional healing

Acupressure and Thai massage relax tight muscles resulting from emotional stress and trauma. A hurtful emotional incident can cause the body to contract its muscles, like protective armor, in order to shield the inner self. When something frightens you or someone treats you abrasively, your neck and shoulders may tighten in response, and this reaction prevents energy from circulating throughout your body. Consequently, your body may overreact and lock up, causing a mixture of physical ailments and emotional imbalances.

Spiritual aspects of our lives may also shut down, causing depression, apathy, and diminished self-awareness. Many therapies deal with the cognitive and emotional characteristics of trauma, but do not deal with the physiological component. Thai massage and acupressure have a distinct advantage over other therapies since they work directly with the energetic core, which is affected by the trauma.

Tension and emotional pain accumulate at acupressure points. As an acupressure point or a Thai stretch is held, tension yields to the finger pressure or elongation, enabling muscle fibers to relax, blood to circulate freely, and toxins to be released and eliminated. Acupressure and Thai bodywork reach to the core of many emotional disorders and stress-related problems. By freeing unresolved emotional experiences stored in the body, acupressure and traditional Thai massage can alleviate many everyday complaints such as headaches, insomnia, sluggishness, and depression. When healing energy flows, anxiety turns to calm, encouraging physical health and overall wellness.

Acupressure in Thai massage

Yoga postures stimulate specific acupressure points, and Thai massage naturally stimulates many of these same healing points during a session. When I work in Thai massage, I try to constantly stay aware of the points that my hands can hold as well as other points that are being released in each Thai technique or stretch. Knowledge of point therapeutics in Thai techniques can intensify the benefits of individual Thai postures. The goal of this essay is to raise awareness of the many ways to further enhance a traditional Thai session by integrating more acupressure. This can be done while staying true to traditional Thai techniques and postures. A client of mine who also practices Thai massage once described one of my Thai sessions in this way: "As you engaged me in a standard Thai massage posture and slowly brought me into a full body stretch, you began to gradually apply firm pressure on acupressure points that were totally unknown to me. I could tell you knew exactly what you were working on, and although I was enjoying the Thai stretch, it was the combination of the stretch plus the strong acupressure that brought about the entire healing effect".

Both Thai massage and general acupressure relax muscle tension and balance vital life forces of the body. Acupressure does this by manipulating body energy through a system of points and meridians. The energy flows through the meridians, and the points are precise areas that can be manipulated for specific healing purposes. Tension collects around these acupressure points, and working with them creatively and sensitively is important in order to effectively relieve tension. In Thai massage, we compress and stretch areas of the body that may be blocked, and individual acupressure points along the energy lines that correspond to these areas are usually worked independently of stretches. Even if you were taught to execute a certain Thai yoga stretch without applying simultaneous acupressure, however, it can be helpful to hold specific points within your reach as you execute the stretch. Once your body positioning is comfortable, take a moment to become still, take a breath, and then begin to apply point pressure.

A Thai massage practitioner's ability to facilitate healing can be further enhanced by knowing basic acupressure points, whether the source is Thai, Chinese, Indian, or from other traditions. If your Thai massage training didn't incorporate extensive knowledge of individual acupressure points from within the body of Thai medicine, you may research some of the points referenced by Wat Po, Asokananda, and Noam Tyroler, or search out Northern Thai (Lanna) points from other sources. Fortunately these days, more acupressure is being integrated into current-day Thai massage teaching, so if you wish to stay true to the Thai system, you can certainly do it. However, you may also integrate Chinese point pressure into your Thai treatments, if you already have knowledge of traditional Chinese medicine, or if you want to study it in more depth. Chinese acupressure is the most widely known acupressure system, and it is easy to find programs of study and reference books around the world.

Applying the pressure

Use gradual, steady, firm pressure. Each point feels different when you press it; some points feel tense, while others may be sore or numb. The pressure should be firm enough to bring the client almost to the edge of his threshold of pain. Generally, the more developed your client's muscles are, the more pressure you should apply. If your touch brings about pain, gradually decrease the pressure until you find a balance between pain and pleasure. If a point is sore or painful, hold it lightly for a few minutes using the middle finger with your index and ring fingers on either side for support. The pain will usually diminish. Sometimes when you hold a point, the receiver will feel a pain or sensation in another part of their body. This indicates that those areas may be blocked, and working points there can often release the referred pain.

The middle finger is well suited for emotional healing because it is the longest and strongest finger, and because a major healing energy channel travels through it. The thumb is better suited for areas of large muscle mass, but avoid using your thumb excessively or in an area that requires more sensitivity. If more pressure is needed and your hand hurts when you apply finger pressure, you can use other parts of your hand or your body.

Acupressure is most effective when you hold points steadily with direct finger pressure at a 90-degree angle from the surface of the skin. If you pull or stretch the skin, the angle of pressure is incorrect. Gradually direct your pressure into the center of the area of the body that is receiving your touch. Release the pressure gradually to allow time for the tissues to respond naturally, and in order to effectuate deeper healing.

When you hold points for at least three minutes with great awareness, and while breathing slowly and deeply, you may feel a pulse at the point. This pulsation is a good sign – it means circulation has increased. Pay attention to the type of pulse you feel. If it throbs or is very faint, hold the point gently until the rhythm becomes more balanced and smooth. If you don't feel a pulse, you may sense other signs of release, such as temperature variation, a change in texture, or an inner feeling of deep relaxation.

If your hands get tired, slowly withdraw pressure from the point, rotate your wrists, gently shake your hand out, and take a few deep breaths. When you're ready, return to the point, and gradually apply incremental pressure until you reach a depth that feels comfortable. Again, press directly on the sensitive area. It will often move, so follow it and stay with it until you feel a regular pulse or until you sense that the pain has diminished. Then slowly decrease your finger pressure, and end with a few seconds of light touch for a softer finish.

When you've located a good point and your fingers are comfortably positioned right on the spot, gradually lean your bodyweight toward the point to apply your pressure. If you're pressing a point on the foot, for example, you may bend or move the leg first and apply pressure by slowly leaning forward. By using the weight of your upper body, not only your hands, you can apply firm pressure without straining.

Every individual body and each area of the body requires a different amount of pressure. If your client shows signs of pain or discomfort when you apply pressure on a particular point, then use a lighter touch, or use palming instead of thumb pressure. The calves, face, and inguinal and abdominal areas are generally more sensitive to pressure. The back, buttocks, and shoulders, especially if the musculature is developed, usually need deeper, firmer pressure. Traditional Thai massage postures provide an excellent platform for applying deeper pressure to these areas by using your whole body to lean in, while allowing the receiver to stretch and breathe deeply.

Acupressure points for enhancing Thai massage techniques

Stimulating acupressure points while engaging a client in Thai massage stretches can bring positive results. Although the Chinese and Thai medicine systems vary greatly, many of the points illustrated in the following postures are known to both healing systems. The intention is not to dilute or modify the original Thai postures and traditions, but rather to bring about a more effective Thai massage session for your clients.

Thai acupressure is not usually done while clients are simultaneously engaged in yoga stretches, suspensions, inversions, and other Thai bodywork applications, but I suggest that you consider doing so. As clients surrender to powerful Thai stretches, working acupressure points within your reach can heighten their experience and bring enhanced results. Enhanced awareness is a major result of receiving a well-balanced Thai massage session. This awareness fosters peace of mind and calmness, and by extension, it positively affects other pursuits in life. By developing an awareness of the body's acupressure points and energy channels, an individual's healing paths can unfold to their fullest potential.

The following examples are only a few of the many traditional Thai massage postures that allow for simultaneous stimulation of acupressure points. While the Thai postures themselves have specific therapeutic values, acupressure points may be integrated into each technique, further benefitting the body by activating endocrine glands, trigger nerves, muscles, and corresponding energy lines. The points mentioned here are described in accordance with traditional Chinese medicine, which is my base of knowledge for acupressure. Try them, and get feedback from your clients.

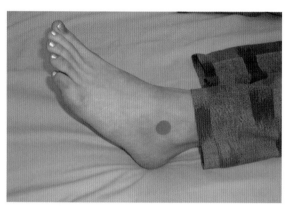

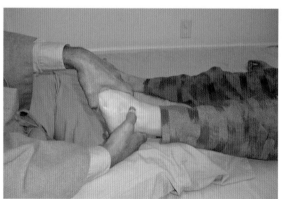

Leg twist and pull

Description: This basic Thai technique involves grasping the foot, twisting it medially, and pulling backward. In this version, as you grasp the top of the foot with one hand, place your thumb on the large indentation in front of the ankle bone. Twist the foot inward, and gradually apply firm pressure into this hollow as you lean back slowly to stretch. Every time you lean back, engage the acupressure point.

Acupressure benefits: This point balances the gall bladder and is an excellent point for strengthening the ankle joint to prevent ankle sprains, toe cramps, and sciatic pain, which travel into the side of the foot. This point balances a generally tight and stiff body, and relieves aches and pains along the side of the body, including headaches. Adding this point to this traditional Thai leg stretch may also decrease a client's frustration and irritability. Be aware that many lateral ankle points should be avoided for pregnant women.

Twisting feet inward

Description: There are many variations of twisting the feet inward in Thai massage. To engage this point, use your thumbs to press between the bones attached to the big toe and second toe, in a natural indentation. Apply firm pressure downward and inward, and support the rest of the foot with your other fingers as you press the feet toward the mat.

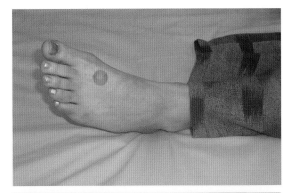

Acupressure benefits: This point is the source or balancing point for the liver meridian, known for its ability to balance the body's energy system. This healing point benefits the eyes and the nervous system, and it relieves general stiffness, headaches, hangovers, and congestion.

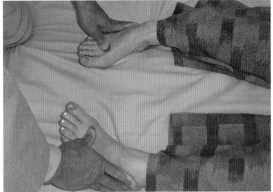

Stretching feet downward and inward

Description: Here's another variation of a traditional Thai foot press. Place your thumbs in the indentation on top of the foot, in between the fourth and fifth toes. Press downward toward the mat and then twist inward. Hold for a few seconds, and repeat if desired.

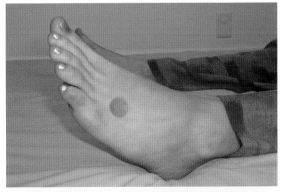

Acupressure benefits: This point balances the gall bladder, regulates body pain, and relieves headaches and stiffness. It eases frustration and irritability, and relieves pain along the sides of the body and the sides of the head.

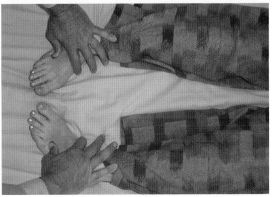

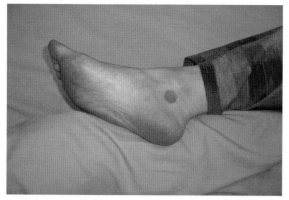

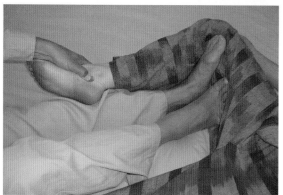

Foot walking on thighs

Description: Instead of just gripping the foot as you do this traditional Thai foot walk, thumb-press the indentation that lies midway between the protrusion of the inside anklebone and the Achilles tendon. Once you are on that point, you can foot-press or foot-walk according to Thai tradition.

Acupressure benefits: This ankle point relieves swollen feet, fatigue, fears, phobias, and bedwetting. It also treats sexual problems such as premature ejaculation, semen leakage, genital pain, vaginal discharge, and menstrual irregularity. This point must be avoided for pregnant women.

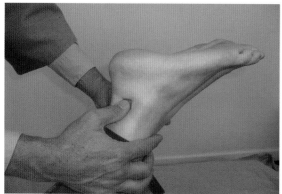

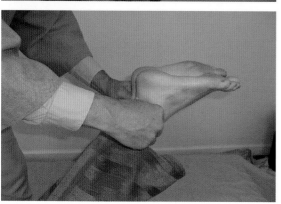

Half plow

Description: With the client in supine position, bring the legs up over your client's head. This is a traditional Thai half plow, but instead of merely holding the ankles as you lunge forward, press into the point between the outer ankle bone and the Achilles tendon. This can be done as the client rests her arms on the mat, or as she braces her hands against her knees with locked elbows.

Acupressure benefits: This point, on the outside of the ankles, relieves rheumatism and lumbago, and it's an excellent point for lower-back pain.

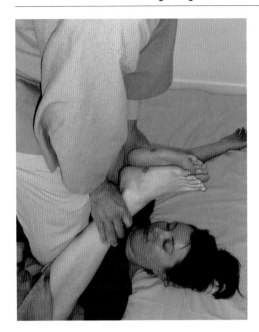 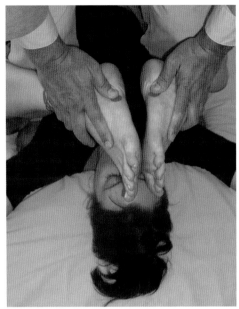

Frog stretch

Description: This is based on the traditional Thai stretch where you step inside your partner's legs with your toes near her armpits. Then, with the bottoms of her feet together, you stretch the legs three times forward over the head, then three times downward toward the nose. Rather than merely grasping the ankles, thumb-press into the acupressure points on the sides of the feet as you execute this technique.

Acupressure benefits: This point, on the sides of the feet, is the source point for balancing energy in the bladder meridian, which travels through the neck and the back.

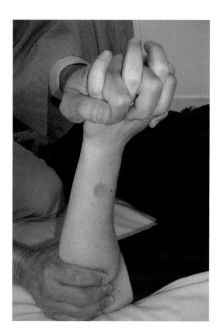 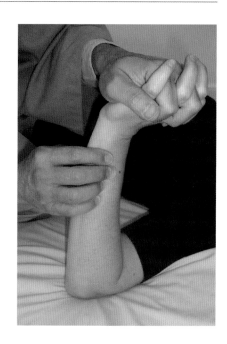

Wrist rotation

Description: The Thai technique involves interlacing fingers and slowly rotating the wrist several times in one direction, then in the other direction. In this variation, as you rotate, press your second and third finger into this point, which is three finger widths below the outer wrist crease.

Acupressure benefits: This point, called the *Outer Gate* in Chinese medicine, relieves allergic reactions, rheumatism, carpal tunnel pain, and wrist tendonitis. The point also boosts the immune system and relaxes the entire body.

Incorporate more acupressure

Thai sen lines, Indian nadis, and Chinese meridians are all healing pathways that carry the body's vital life force from one point to another. The stimulation of acupressure points in traditional Thai massage opens the body's natural homeostatic (balancing) mechanisms by reducing tension so that the body may heal itself more effectively. During the course of a Thai massage session, acupressure points along sen lines are stimulated naturally, but many postures and stretches provide additional opportunities to simultaneously apply deep finger pressure into specific acupressure points. Acupressure therapy and Thai massage are complementary modalities, and increased benefits and pain relief can result by simultaneously combining these two systems of healing. I encourage you to integrate more acupressure, regardless of the source, into your traditional Thai massage practice.

"Stop the Blood" or "Open the Gates"?

TIM HOLT

Most experienced therapists and instructors of traditional Thai massage include inguinal and axillary circulatory restrictions in their treatments. This clears stagnation of energy (*lom*) in the large gates of the pelvis and in the small gates of the shoulder/neck area. From a Western perspective, it helps the body clear toxins and bring nutrient-rich blood to areas that are receiving bodywork. It is presented in Thailand as "stop the blood" or "blood stop."

This use of the English phrase "stop the blood," however, is a negative and inaccurate term for such a positively healing treatment. I have no historical data on when this English phrase was first employed, but I originally learned this term at the Old Medicine Hospital in 1988. Many other teachers in the Chiang Mai area also use this phrase, and it has now spread worldwide.

I believe this technique would be better served by using a more positive name. We are temporarily restricting the flow of blood to the extremities, but the intention and effect is to open the gates, to move energy, to flush tissues, and to distribute nutrients and oxygen. In essence, we are *increasing* the blood flow to those areas; we are not really *stopping* blood flow. We are encouraging it to go deeper and to find new pathways. We are also slowing the heart rate and providing deep relaxation for the client.

It is analogous to the use of ice on injuries in Western sports massage. Ice creates retrostasis, and blood retreats from the cold stimulus. Once the cold stimulus is removed, there is a surge of circulation back into the affected area, which flushes metabolic debris and brings nutrients to the area. Blood flow is temporarily restricted, but healing occurs when the tissues are engorged by fresh blood.

When I present the "stop the blood" technique in my classes, I normally get a few raised eyebrows and some mild fear about this treatment. I sense that the fear is a reaction to the words themselves, and not the technique. If you stop the blood flow to healthy tissue, it will die! This is the mental image students often have when this technique is initially presented, so because of this, I no longer use the phrase. I teach the Old Medicine style as well as Pichest's techniques, but I introduce them as opening the energetic large gates of the pelvis and the small gates of the shoulders. I present this from a Western perspective as a circulatory flush. We are opening the gates, not stopping the blood.

This is an open request to the international community of Thai therapists and instructors to reframe these valuable traditional techniques with a more positive and accurate introduction and name.

Om namo Shivago.

Exploring Energy in Thai Massage

ROBERT HENDERSON

Much is written in Thai massage literature about the use of Thai massage as a means to release energy blocks or to restore harmony and balance to the energy system of a client. Most Thai massage schools or teachers refer to energy or energy blocks in their teachings, but unfortunately these phenomena are usually left unexplored.

Through the use of applied acupressure on energy lines, Thai massage is probably the most energy-intensive of all massage and healing modalities. In addition to stimulating the ten major *sen* lines *(sip sen),* Thai massage also activates energy centers on the front and the back of the body. In short, a basic two-hour Thai routine activates an enormous part of a person's energy system, a fact rarely addressed in beginner's Thai massage classes.

All of this activation of energy can trigger a wide range of unexpected feelings, thoughts, or emotions during a treatment, which may be experienced by both the receiver and the giver. The purpose of this essay is to look at some of the more common manifestations of energy in traditional Thai massage, and to explain ways in which both the client and the therapist may experience and react to these energies. The goal is to help practitioners guide themselves and their clients with more awareness during a Thai session.

My awakening of energy in Thai massage

In November 2002, I received my first treatment from Chaiyuth Priyasith on the veranda of his massage room on Tha Pae Road in Chiang Mai. At the time,

Chaiyuth's reputation as a magical healer was well known. His treatments lasted 3–7 hours in length, and he was said to be able to revitalize an entire energy system in a single treatment. He also had treated a member of the Thai royal family, an honor that is rarely bestowed on a lay person in Thailand. The prospect of receiving from Master Chaiyuth was very exciting, and I eagerly anticipated what was in store for me. It was a warm and sunny day, and Chaiyuth worked with his eyes closed, seemingly in a trance. And then things started happening.

Halfway through the treatment I began to feel cold – not cold from the outside, but cold from the inside. I began to shake and shiver. I developed goose bumps, and the hairs on my body stood on end. I remember thinking it was very strange for me to be feeling so cold when it was sunny and warm outside. I began to lose control of my breathing, and I soon became very uncomfortable. This was not the type of Thai massage I was expecting. By the end of the treatment I was soaking wet, and I was cold and exhausted. I also felt like I weighed twice my normal weight. It took me about 15 minutes to get up from the mat. I said nothing. I couldn't say anything. I didn't have enough energy.

After a while, I quietly made my way outside. I began to stumble home to my guest house. The short walk took over an hour because I had to sit down and compose myself every 20–30 steps. The treatment was late on a Tuesday afternoon, and I spent most of Wednesday and Thursday shaking, sweating, and unable to eat anything. On Friday morning I finally vomited, after which everything magically settled, and I felt my normal self again.

I returned to Chaiyuth and asked him what had happened. In his usual cryptic and playful manner, he replied: "You closed; now you open." I knew right away that he was referring to energy, but it wasn't until much later that I fully understood what had happened during that treatment, and how common strong reactions can be in a serious Thai healing session. Chaiyuth had touched my energy, and the entire massage he gave me was nothing more than a dance, a movement, a flow of this energy.

This was my first real experience of energy work in Thai massage. Since then I have learned that you first have to experience energy and energy release before you can understand how to work with it. During a session, signs of energy release may include internal coldness, shivering, heaviness, sleepiness, irregular breathing, sweatiness, anxiety, and changes in complexion. After a deep session, symptoms can sometimes manifest as loss of energy, loss of appetite, speech and vision impairment, dehydration, and even vomiting. It was only by experiencing these things personally that I was able to understand how energy can be released through traditional Thai massage.

The activation of certain types of energy during a Thai massage treatment can sometimes continue long after the treatment is over. This is why clients and receivers can sometimes feel unsettled for a few days after a treatment, particularly if they experienced a deep and transformative session. The intensity diminishes as the movement of energy subsides, and things eventually return to a state of calm and internal harmony.

The cycle of energy release

Whether in our home regions or in Thailand, our most important lessons about energy healing are the experiences that we have with our own energy. As we become aware of different forms of energy arising in our bodies, we can learn to identify a particular energy by how it feels, what it's connected to, and where it is stored in the body. The final part of the learning comes from understanding the origin of the energy and why it is being held in the body. When it is fully acknowledged, the energy can release itself from you, as you no longer have any need of it, and it no longer has any need of you. This is the cycle of energetic release, and the way it works for you is the exact same way it works for your client during a Thai massage treatment.

I believe that without an awareness of our clients' energy, standard Thai massage treatment for lower-back weakness, for example, may have only limited success. The physical condition of the lower back may be connected to an underlying energy imbalance. If it does not reference the underlying energy, isolated treatment of the physical condition treats only part of the condition, and therefore may have only partial success.

We each have our own natural energy – energy that is transmitted to our clients through our touch. The type of energy we ourselves have determines where we enter our client's cycle of energy, and how deeply we can guide and support our client in the process of release during a Thai massage treatment. I believe our experiences of energy in Thai massage depend on three factors: our own natural energy levels, our natural abilities to sense energy in others, and our experiences of energy as it unfolds in Thai massage.

Your natural energy level

Each of us has a natural energy level. Some people are natural athletes, others are naturally good with finances, and others make excellent parents. Sports, money, and parenting each require very different types of energy.

In Thai massage, it is helpful to know something about your own natural energy level, since this knowledge can guide you in a direction that is best suited for your practice. Thai massage is a physical therapy, a dance of movement and flow, a medical treatment, an expression of compassion, and a medium for spiritual healing. It's important to know how well suited we are to serve one or more of these treats from the cosmic menu of Thai massage.

Natural sensitivity and developing sensitivity to energy

Some people have a natural sensitivity to energy. They see color, they can read auras, and they may receive intuitive messages. When they touch you, they can somehow be intuitively drawn to the parts of your body that need healing or treatment. You could say they are naturally gifted healers. I'm not one of those people.

When I studied Thai massage with my first teachers, I had very little sensitivity. But now, many years later, things have changed. I developed my sensitivity to energy through years of practice, and also through the work I've done with my teachers. I found that by developing sensitivity to my own energy, I could also become sensitive to the energies of my clients.

Over the years, I explored energies held in different parts of my body, and as I did so, I became more aware of the energies held in the same body parts of my clients. As a result, I was better able to understand the nature of the energy and energy blocks in my clients. Because of this, I have become more able to help my clients to process, understand, and release these energies.

Our sensitivities to energy can be enhanced and improved by examining our own energy system, by studying with an energy teacher or a spiritual teacher, and by maintaining awareness during our regular massage practice.

Primary and secondary manifestations of energy

For many of us, the heat of our client's body is an expression of energy we can easily relate to. Because of this, it can serve as a good entry point to begin to experience and understand energy. A good way to tune in to energy in Thai massage work is to check how hot or cold certain parts of a client's body feel. This may be considered a primary manifestation of energy.

Hold one hand about an inch over your client's skin, and slowly scan her body to see if you can sense areas that feel hotter or colder. You may find that one of your hands is better at sensing energy than the other. After some practice, you may begin to experience body temperature that feels normal, as well as body temperature that feels hotter or colder than normal.

While scanning a body, let's say that you sense that your client's feet seem cold. Perhaps your visual analysis also confirms this, because they seem pale in color. Now touch them. Do they feel hard or soft, dry or wet? These can be considered as secondary expressions of your client's energy, and by understanding these expressions, you may slowly begin to develop an energetic diagnosis of your client. Regardless of color or temperature, feet that feel dry, soft, and yielding generally don't require specific massage treatment. In fact, any body area that is generally warm, dry to the touch, and soft and yielding generally doesn't require deep, intensive work. On the other hand, feet that are hard, spongy, wet, or sticky often reveal an imbalance in energy.

Tension

Tension is another manifestation of energy that is evident in traditional Thai massage. The release of energy sometimes creates temporary tension, and that is one of the reasons why a client can sometimes feel stiff or sore the morning after a session. The stiffness indicates an ongoing release of energy, and when the release of energy subsides, so does the feeling of stiffness. It is a natural process.

Tension can also indicate the presence of an acute or chronic energy blockage. A client may come to you during a stressful or volatile period in her life, and you can often sense the energy of tension when you touch her. You may also have a client with a long-term chronic health condition, or someone who is on heavy medication. These conditions can result in certain types of tension that are held deeper in the body, and that are often beyond the reach of treatment with Thai massage.

There is no single approach to treating tension with Thai massage. There may be two equally tense clients in one day who require different treatments – one vigorous and one gentle. Tension should be dealt with on a case-by-case basis; we locate effective approaches to treatment only through experimentation and practice. Some people respond best to gentle touch, while others need more vigorous work. If you have a client with tightness in the lower back, for example, see if the area responds better to a slow, gentle, and warming touch, or to a more structured and vigorous approach. Be guided by what you feel. After the session, take notes, get your client's feedback, and continue to refine your work with that person based on what you've learned from him in previous sessions.

Pain

Pain is another indicator of energy blockage. If a client tells you she has a pain, ask her to show you where it is with her index finger. Physiological pains, such as bruises, torn or ruptured muscles or ligaments, or inflammations and swellings, will be sore to the touch. Energy block pain is harder to locate, however. It's something beyond topical touch and needs to be addressed differently. It is pain that a Western doctor can't diagnose, yet to your clients it is very real. The pain can last days, weeks, months, or years and then mysteriously vanish, leaving no physical damage. It is a pain without rules: sometimes it's sudden and sharp, and sometimes dull and long-lasting. If you have a client with this type of pain, you may very likely be dealing with an energy block.

Energy block pain can also play a little trick on you. Clients may complain of a pain in the lower back, for instance, yet when you touch them there, they don't feel any pain. This doesn't mean the pain has gone away. It may simply lie outside the realm of topical treatment. Treating the area in question, however, even if your client feels nothing, may still address the block that is causing the pain. As our experience and understanding of energy grows, so does our ability to help clients who suffer from energy block pain.

Energy blocks

In basic terms, an energy block is an area of unprocessed and unbalanced energy that has gotten stuck somewhere. It is something that an experienced therapist is able to feel and sense. In some cases, energy blocks need to be released in order for a person to move forward in good health, but sometimes energy blocks serve as coping devices for things that may otherwise cause harm. The following are a few examples of the way emotions may manifest as energy.

Let's say you win the lottery and become overcome with joy. The unexpected energy of joy that is released into your body is too sudden and too intense for you to process and release. As a result, you faint and fall to the ground. You were unable to process the jolt of energy quickly enough, so as a result, your body shut down. Other people who experience joy may scream and jump up and down, and this is their body's way of processing energy through physical release. Joy is fire energy. It can be fast and strong, but it can also burn out quickly. Whatever the reaction, people usually recover and restabilize themselves quickly after a sudden outburst of joy.

You may lose a loved one, someone who has been close to you for many years. You become devastated with grief. Your body is unable to process and release the burst of emotion that was suddenly released into your system. The lack of physical activity that often accompanies grief means the energy can more easily remain unprocessed and unreleased in your system, and this can lead to a blockage. Short-term blockages are usually found in the upper chest, close to the heart, in the soft area between the breast and the clavicle. The area may feel cold if you scan it with your hand, and it also may be spongy to the touch. If an energy blockage is large, its presence can fill the entire upper chest cavity; it can also be felt behind the upper chest, in the soft area near the posterior shoulder.

Thai massage is a very effective treatment in the release of grief, especially in the hands of a compassionate therapist, but one needs to work slowly and with great sensitivity. Place a warm hand directly on the sternum just below the clavicle, and let the heat of your hand do the work. If after a minute or so they are not responsive, this may not be the right time to release grief, so simply move on. Alternately, you may see a slight trembling in your client's face, and some emotion may begin to surface. Ask your client if she will allow you to continue to rest your hand where it is. You may need to remove your hand, re-warm it, and re-place it from time to time, but always make sure your client is comfortable enough to continue. Never force a release on a client by using trigger points or strong pressure in an unannounced or unexpected way. This would be insensitive, and it would be an invasion of your client's privacy. The body area between the breasts and the clavicle can be very sensitive since it holds energies of despair, loneliness, and sadness. Be sensitive, and allow your client to express what they are feeling, if they wish to do so.

Chronic energy blocks

The older the blockage is, the deeper it is believed to be. Grief from the loss of a loved one ten years ago may be buried under layers of other, more recent events and energies. Layers of unprocessed energy can build on top of each other, and this is why dealing with energy blocks can be so difficult. To work with the deepest block, we sometimes have to slowly release the blocks that are layered on top of it.

Stress

The unreleased energy of stress accounts for many energy blockages in our modern society. These blockages often start on the anterior of the body, at the solar plexus, then work through the back of the body. From there, stress may travel upward along sens *ittha* and *pingkala* to the base of the skull, and from there, it can move to the shoulder area. This is why stress is one of the main causes of shoulder tightness. If the energy block is severe, the energy may work through the base of the skull into the back of the head, resulting in a headache or a migraine.

In my opinion, *nuad boran* is the best treatment for stress, but all body areas need to be addressed, not only where the client feels discomfort. Dissipating stress energy can also release emotions commonly associated with stress, such as anger and frustration. If you, as a therapist, begin to feel frustrated or upset during a treatment, stop your work for a few moments, re-center yourself, and then continue. The feelings should pass as the energies dissipate.

Stress may surface when a client wants to be in control, or if he or she is unable to relax. Clients sometimes raise a leg for you when you begin a single leg routine, or lift themselves up during a cobra. This is not intentional, and they are probably unaware that they are doing it. Some clients may also engage you in conversation throughout a treatment, or keep their eyes open. To work with these behavior patterns, consistent rhythm and pressure can be helpful. After the feet, work the leg lines with a constant rhythm and uniform pressure. This can help to create a safe space into which your client can relax. Work slowly, and take your time. Stressed clients need time to unwind. Work the leg lines several times – palming, rocking, thumbing, and rocking. Once a client relaxes more fully, your work as a therapist will be more effective.

Practice with awareness and compassion

In this essay I have tried to describe some concepts, sources, and manifestations of energy in ourselves and in our clients, and I've discussed ideas for treatment of several types of energy blockages. As Thai massage therapists, we learn more about energy and energy transference as we progress in our study, experience, and practice. Awareness, knowledge, intuition, and ability to sense energy come from constant practice, and from careful listening to the body.

It is always best to work with the body and not "on" the body. When we come up against resistance, we must be patient and compassionate, and we must never force anything on our clients. If the person before you on the mat is not ready or willing to surrender, don't force yourself or your techniques or your ego onto him. Remember that we are merely witnesses to our clients as they unfold into the process of self-healing.

I respect clients who block my work because they are not ready or willing to release or surrender. They are the ones who must carry their energies, their emotions, their memories, and their life experiences. Whatever they do to help themselves at any given time is their rightful decision. As therapists, we must respect whatever coping mechanism they may choose to use, even if doing so results in an energy block. Remember that energy blocks shouldn't be prematurely pushed to resolution. The client must be ready and willing to let go, and to surrender to the origins of the block, and the therapist must be patient, loving, supportive, and consoling. Practice sensitively, with awareness and compassion, and always create a safe place for your client to surrender to the process of healing.

Thai Massage for Multiple Sclerosis Patients

GORAN MILOVANOV

Multiple sclerosis (or MS) is a chronic, often disabling disease that attacks the central nervous system, which is made up of the brain, spinal cord, and optic nerves. Symptoms may be mild, such as numbness in the limbs, or severe, such as paralysis or loss of vision. The progress, severity, and specific symptoms of MS are unpredictable and vary from one person to another.

The exact cause of the condition is unknown, and the disease is still incurable. In some cases, the disease is progressive and chronic, with slow, continual degradation. In other cases, it is acute and traumatic, resulting in severe disability within a few years.

Symptoms include:

- Numbness and tingling sensations in different regions;
- Double vision, blurred vision, general weakness, muscle paralysis that affects one or more limbs, tremors, gait problems, and exaggerated reflexes;
- Mood swings, irritability, and depression;
- For some, there may be difficulty with speaking and swallowing.

I have worked in Thai massage with MS patients over a period of several years, and so far I have learned that each patient has an individual situation worthy of individual attention. Even though the symptoms of the disease are consistent, each patient suffers physical damage and consequences of varying intensity and progression. In addition, the physical and emotional states of each person vary widely, and this is important to take into consideration when working on the mat. The experience of working with an individual patient is valuable, but it is not necessarily transferrable to your work with other patients. Each new treatment with an MS client requires your maximum attention, as if it were your very first session with that person.

At the beginning of a long-term course of treatment, it may be helpful, if you are qualified, to administer one or more relaxing Western-style massage treatments, in order to understand the physical conditions of the patient and the level of mobility of his body.

When you begin your first Thai massage treatment, be aware that you won't be able to perform stretches and point pressure routines with the intensity that you would normally use for other people. Go easy at first, and incorporate plenty of constant, gentle rocking. As you begin working on the sen lines, you'll be able to gain better insight into the patient's condition, and you'll have a better understanding of an appropriate level of stretching.

One of the possible physical consequences of MS is decreased topical sensitivity, so because of this, the patient may occasionally ask you what you are doing. You may explain in a few words the goal of the move or the technique that you are executing at that time. Unnecessary talking during the treatment is not encouraged, but you should be understanding, and you should always make sure your client feels assured and supported. Thai massage is a unique experience, and when you show compassion and patience, you will earn your clients' confidence in no time. Once they trust you, they may be able to escape their harsh reality and become more open to your work.

When you work with the sen lines, pay special attention to sens *kalathari*, *sahatsarangsi,* and *thawari*. Kalatahari has a very strong healing quality. It is a conduit of emotional and psychic energy, and it affects emotions, hidden memories, and fears. Sahatsarangsi and thawari are detoxification lines, and working on them can help to circulate energy, especially for patients with restricted mobility.

Stiffness in the extremities (especially the legs) is a common condition for MS patients, so when you do leg stretches you may sense a natural resistance. At the subconscious level, your client may have a need to control your every move. Be tolerant and patient, because much of this reflex may be a result of the disease itself. Multiple sclerosis patients often find that they're not able to control their extremities, so they subconsciously struggle to gain control over them, even when they are supposed to be at rest. They want to relax, but they are not able to do so very easily. Because of this, be prepared to suggest to them over and over again how good it feels to completely relax, and gently encourage them to let go as much as possible. Sometimes, just a tender touch on a stiff area is enough to bring about relaxation.

I have also seen MS patients whose legs are extremely elastic, but don't be deceived: you must not treat them like a healthy, flexible person's. When this is the case, take extreme care around the tendons and joints, especially at the hips and knees. Whenever you transition from one move to another, always hold and support the knee as you work the leg. Your client may have good flexibility in his hip, but at the same time, his posterior thigh may be compressed and stiff. Perform palming, thumbing, and acupressure on the stiffest part of the back of the leg, and don't insist on doing stretches. You can add light stretching techniques only if you feel the other work is bringing about positive results.

Whether the hips are stiff or hyper-elastic, never attempt to perform lifting poses, inversions, or complicated stretches. These postures will almost always be too intense for their condition, and you could easily hurt them.

While working on the leg lines, sudden uncontrolled jerks and tremors may occur due to direct stimulation of the nerves near the lines. The tremors are not necessarily painful, so don't stop your palming or thumbing – just do it with less intensity. Also, when you are working the sen lines of one leg, you may encounter a reflex reaction on the other leg. This is normal, and it generally indicates a release of energy from the body.

Working the spine and the muscles around it can be very beneficial if it's done carefully and with sensitivity. Every form of acupressure is allowed, but don't expect your clients to withstand pain for too long while you treat a stiff or blocked area.

A good strategy for blocked areas is to work for longer periods, but with less intensity, and with occasional pauses in between. Always keep in mind that their life is one of suffering, so don't add to their pain in any way with your work. Stretching the spine can be pleasant for them, and you can perform light torsions in supine position, as well as torsions and side stretches in sitting position.

Once you reach their first point of resistance, don't hold the patient for too long in that position. Release and gently return to the starting point in a supportive manner. Don't push your MS clients to their limit each and every time, as you might do with more healthy clients. The first point of resistance for MS patients may differ from one day to another. Don't work routinely through a fixed sequence. Instead, work with extreme care, as if each treatment were their very first treatment with you.

Keep these things in mind as you work:

- Each patient's experience of the disease is unique, and their physical and emotional states can change continuously.
- It's important to understand and respect their limited ability to relax, and their often subconcious response to help you as you work.
- When executing stretches, maintain communication with your client as you move them into position. Never bring about pain or stretch them beyond their level of comfort.

In closing, I'd like to say that the suggestions I offer here are based only on my personal experiences with my clients and are not necessarily applicable to all clients with multiple sclerosis. However I do believe that my work has helped my clients to maintain mobility and has afforded them a greater sense of ease. My clients have confirmed this to me, and their comments have supported me and have validated my efforts.

If you ever have a chance to work with a multiple sclerosis patient in Thai massage, you will surely establish your own guidelines and inspirations for practice. Never forget, however, that your work should always be done in accordance with the manifestations of the disease, and with great respect for the psycho-physical state of each individual at each moment in time.

Notes from the Mat

ACCOUNTS OF THAI MASSAGE SESSIONS WRITTEN BY THERAPISTS AND CLIENTS

Body memory

I recently had an interesting experience while working with a client whom I've seen on a weekly basis for the past year. He's a large, muscular guy, and I tend to work on him with my knees and my feet, since he requires fairly deep pressure. During one particular session, I placed him in prone position, with his left knee bent to the side. I was working with my knee in his hip and buttock, to address his piriformis muscle, which was particularly tight that day.

As I moved medially, I was drawn to one spot, and I immediately sensed that I needed to stay there and work for a while. After about a minute of relaxing myself into his body, he told me he was beginning to feel nauseous. I released the pressure, and he lay there feeling sick for a few minutes. I suggested that he may have been having an emotional reaction. Sometimes early trauma is stored in the tissues of our bodies, and when they are touched deeply, the trauma is brought up again through memory and physical reaction. He looked at me with surprise, and he said that as I was working there, he suddenly remembered being attacked and bitten by a large dog when he was eight years old. It was strange to him that this thought would suddenly come to his mind, because he hadn't thought about it in over twenty years. He looked at me and said, "I guess there's more to this than meets the eye, isn't there?" I smiled, and I secretly thanked Jivaka.

Paul Fowler

Sympathetic pain

Recently, I had a session with a regular client of mine whom I've seen every month for the past few years. She usually holds tension in her hips, stomach, and shoulders, but that day, in addition to her usual stress areas, she mentioned that her right side seemed blocked. Sure enough, we found some pockets of tension in her upper right torso. I continued to work in supine, and then I worked a bit in side position, so that I could follow the flow of energy upward. It was a fairly normal session, and she had some nice releases during the first 90 minutes. Little did I know what was about to happen in the last few minutes of final supine position.

As I continued to work on the blockage that I sensed in her right lower neck, I suddenly began to feel a sharp pain at the end of my jaw bone, directly below the medial end of my ear lobe. Almost immediately I sensed that this was sympathetic pain – that what I was feeling in my jaw was a signal that I should go there for my client. So I slowly released my pressure on her upper neck and positioned my third and fourth fingers directly on the spot on her jaw where I was feeling my own sudden and sharp pain. Immediately, my client began to cough intensely. The pain in my jaw grew sharper, but as she continued to cough violently for about 15 seconds, I felt the pain ease in my jaw. She returned to stillness, and I finished the session, gazing occasionally at my Jivaka altar.

After the session she felt light and relaxed, and in an e-mail follow-up, she wrote that she believed the release in her jaw had its roots deep inside her belly. She said she was feeling open and spiritually grounded after that experience. My own jaw pain gradually disappeared after about two days.

Bob Haddad

I need 3 inches

Once, when I was working at a health club, a young man came in, inquired about a session, and then said, "I need 3 more inches!" I cleared my throat and asked him jokingly what type of massage he was expecting. He laughed and explained that he was applying to be a police officer, and that he had passed every section of the very rigorous physical exam except for one: the sit-and-reach flexibility test. "When I'm sitting on the floor with my legs in front of me," he said, "I must be able to reach my fingers past my feet, but my hamstrings are just too tight. Can you help me?"

After a session of Thai stretches aimed at the legs and hips, he left to take his examination, and he passed it.

Kay Rynerson

Ancient wisdom

A friend of mine was scheduled to undergo oral surgery to remove his wisdom teeth. He is a student of natural therapy and follows a natural lifestyle. Much to the dismay of his friends and family, he decided to not take antibiotics or painkillers, and he approached me to find an alternative therapy. Using Thai medicine theory, I was able to prescribe to him an oral rinse, along with an antiseptic/anti-inflammatory herbal formula.

When he returned to his dentist a week later, the dentist remarked on how well his wounds were healing and told him that his recovery process had been much shorter than with most people. My friend didn't tell the dentist he had never taken the antibiotics or painkillers, or what had happened in our treatment sessions. At the end of his checkup visit, the dentist reminded him to finish all of his antibiotics.

David Bliss

Don't tell my wife

A married couple has regularly come to me for table massage every two weeks, one after the other, on the same day. The wife always arrives first, then she returns home to the children and then her husband comes for his massage. One day, the husband said to me, "Let's do one of those Thai massages you've been talking about. I am very curious." We proceeded with a full body Thai treatment.

Two weeks later, his wife came for her session and asked, "What did you do to my husband?" At first I thought to myself, "Oh no, I must have pulled a muscle somewhere. I was afraid that adductor stretch was too deep." But then she elaborated: "Usually when he comes home from his massage, he takes off his shoes, opens a beer, puts his feet up, and he relaxes for the rest of the day. But after your Thai massage, he came home, cleaned the garage, trimmed the rose bushes and then he mowed the lawn! From now on, don't ask him what kind of massage he wants – just give him Thai."

Kay Rynerson

Deep rivers

My first experience with Thai massage was profound. Before the session began, the therapist knelt and offered a prayer for my welfare and asked to be guided. At that moment, I felt the amazing effect of that small act of loving-kindness, and the room became filled with peace. I felt weightless as he moved my body into various positions. He coached me to be aware of my breath and to be open. As he pressed energy points with his hands, feet, and elbows, I sensed deep rivers stirring inside me. Fingertips and toes became alive, and breath flowed through my body and mind.

Now, years later, with each new session I discover new truths about myself. Thai massage not only awakens the deep physical body, it releases the spirit and enlivens the mind.

Della French

Shared moments of release

Every few weeks, my first client of the day is an older man who has been coming to see me for several years. He doesn't always appreciate the meditative aspect of *nuad boran*. He often talks during a session, he keeps me updated on his wife's health, and he arrives and departs quickly.

One day he told me his wife's health was deteriorating, and that the only touch he ever receives is my massage because his wife is in so much pain, that all they can do is hold hands. As I worked on his left hip/adductor area, which is chronically tight, a thought drifted through me, "feminine side," and as I moved deeper I realized that my client was beginning to cry.

I continued to work with deep gentle movements and rocking postures, and he continued to move in and out of emotions. Before he left my office I offered a parting hug – the first time I had ever done this to him. He accepted it with enthusiasm, and I was privileged to be able to offer my support, to receive his acceptance, and to sense a release of tension in him. Shared moments of release, relief of pain, joy in our bodies, and supporting healing relationships – these are the reasons why I love my practice.

Kath Rutland

Clear lungs and relief of soreness

My mother, a registered nurse, was recently taking a second round of antibiotics in order to cure pneumonia. Her progress had slowed, and her mucus stopped moving. A few hours after her Thai massage, she released more mucus than had come out of her in many days. Her lungs felt clearer after each Thai massage session, until she was restored to health. In another case, a serious weight-training client had been feeling sore about two days after her workouts. But when she received a Thai massage session the day after her workout, her body felt absolutely no soreness afterward, and she said she felt increased mobility.

Jill Roberts

Connections previously thought unimaginable

When I received my first Thai massage, the experience and the effect were unlike anything I had ever known. During the session itself, it felt as if things were moving around inside my body, not only on the surface where I was being touched and compressed. There were clear connections between different parts of my body that I would have previously thought unimaginable. Following the therapist's advice, I gave more awareness to my breath, and to the effect my breath had on my state, which was one of continual release and relaxation. After the therapist left the room, I opened my eyes and immediately noticed that my senses had been enhanced. My vision, smell, and awareness had dramatically improved.

Dwight Parrodin

No interpretation needed

Reading over the intake form of a new client, I didn't notice anything unusual, and I wondered why she had come for a treatment that day. As she lay down on the mat, she said, as if as an afterthought, "Oh, I have a pain in the left side of my back. Maybe it is my heart chakra."

At one point, moving with thoughtless awareness, I found myself at her left shoulder, and instead of leaning firmly into it, I placed one hand under her shoulder and my other hand on top of it. I have no idea why I did that, but as my touch firmly held this position, she began to sob. I reached for some tissues to put at her side, and I told her that if she wanted me to stop working that she should just raise her hand. Then I continued my work, palming and brushing the energy across her pectorals, down her arms, and out through her hands.

She muttered that she felt the weight of the world's sorrow in her heart and that she needed to forgive her parents. She was crying so intensely that she began to hyperventilate. I stopped my work, sat near her head, and while touching her forehead, I asked her to inhale and exhale deeply and completely. I suggested that old, stored energy was being released, and that it didn't need to be judged as good or bad; it just needed to be released.

As she inhaled and exhaled deeply, her crying began to subside, and I continued my work for almost another hour. Afterward, she asked me to sit with her, and she thanked me. I felt grateful, because this beautiful person was able to trust me and to release all her emotional pain through my lightest touch. Truly our clients are our greatest teachers.

Later, as a follow up to the session, she wrote to me: "You were right. The mind habitually wants to interpret everything, but that is missing the point entirely. Some things need no interpretation."

Jaci Daly Fraser

Pure light energy

I once gave a nuad boran session to my yoga teacher. At first he wanted to pay me for the session, but I would have paid *him* for the opportunity to work with such an open yoga body. The session lasted over 2 ½ hours, and it moved into total darkness as the sun set outside our palm-roofed pavilion. The last 30 minutes or so, I worked by intuition, and I ended with a comprehensive head massage. When I brought my thumbs to his third-eye point, I felt an intense rush of pure energy pass through my hands and up through my body. It was so strong that I had to make a determined effort to ground myself and to keep my own energy centered. The sense of euphoria and completeness at the end of the session was overwhelming for both of us.

That experience has brought about an awareness that I now aspire to in my work with all my clients. I have felt a greater awareness and sensitivity. I am more physically aware of alignment, tension, and contact. I have always explained to people that nuad boran is meditation for me. Now it becomes more and more profound the more I practice.

Kath Rutland

Pilgrimage to Rajgir

BOB HADDAD

I'd had a strong desire for such a long time, and now was my chance. Many years before my visit, I'd learned that an archeological site excavated in the mid-1800s in Rajgir, Bihar, northern India was believed to be Jivaka's famous mango garden, residence, and dispensary. I knew I would go there one day.

Jivaka's presence in my practice became very strong a few years after my first instruction in Thai massage, and over the years I've witnessed and sensed many things that have led me to fully believe in the power of ancestral transmission. The circumstances surrounding Chaiyuth's death, other teachers' beliefs in Jivaka's intercession, and my own personal interests encouraged me to delve deeper into the spiritual healing aspect of *nuad boran*. Along the way, there were other unusual experiences, some too personal or strange to mention here, that sparked my desire to learn more about this person named Jivaka Kumarabhacca.

I remember when I commissioned bronze statues of Jivaka to be made in a Bangkok foundry for distribution to colleagues, teachers, and students around the world. The sculptor patiently and skillfully refined the details of the mold over a period of several weeks, constantly adjusting the hair, facial features, muscles, garments, and other aspects of the prototype, until we were happy with the results. When they were finally issued, I felt as if I had done something, some small thing, to help dignify Jivaka's presence in the world of Thai healing arts.

My ongoing study helped me to understand that many of the stories surrounding Jivaka and traditional Thai massage were illogical distortions of the truth, and not based on historical facts. Later, the development, translations, and true meanings of the Thai massage *wai khru* became known to me through research and discussion with colleagues and teachers.

For those readers who still may not know, the plain and simple truth is that Jivaka Kumarabhacca had little or no influence at all on the direct development of traditional Thai massage. He probably never practiced massage, there is no proof that he ever taught monks how to practice massage or Ayurvedic medicine, and he certainly never traveled to Thailand! Yet although these and other myths continue to be spread into the twenty-first century, they do not invalidate or weaken the widespread belief in, and devotion to this legendary doctor from ancient India. What is most important is that a cult following of Jivaka evolved in Thailand, based in a sociocultural and spiritual need to revere him as the ancestral teacher of Thai medicine, so that prayers could be directed to him and through him in order to bring about healing.

Jivaka's presence and intercession in my practice and life had been so apparent in recent years that I felt a strong desire to visit him in his home town. In order to complete the circuit from my first lessons in Thai massage to the present time, I wanted to pay my respects, to pray and give thanks, and to spend some time alone, in communion with spirits of the ancestral past.

Preparations

I planned the trip so that it coincided with a long-term stay in Thailand, and I bought an airline ticket from Bangkok to India for a reasonable price on a discount air carrier. I had the idea to bring back a small amount of earth from the site of Jivaka Amravana, so that I could place it on my altar and also share it with those of my teachers and colleagues who truly believe in his powers of intercession.

Some months before my departure, I spoke to a long-time Thai massage friend who indirectly became one of my teachers, about my upcoming trip to Rajgir. I told him that I wanted to pay my respects to Jivaka by personally bringing an offering of some type, and I asked for his advice. We decided to prepare a special offering that I would deliver to Jivaka's apothecary. My hope was to carry out a *puja*, and to leave the offering there on that sacred land. I was excited about the prospect of bringing a spiritual gift from Thailand to Jivaka, and also bringing samples of soil from Jivaka Amravana back to Thailand, where he was more revered than in India.

A few weeks before my flight, my friend called and asked if I'd like to visit with his teacher, a Thai *reusi,* before I left for India. I jumped at the opportunity to meet a reusi, and to ask for his blessings for my pilgrimage. We traveled about one hour from Bangkok to a suburban neighborhood where the reusi lives and practices. During the several hours I and others spent in his presence, he performed various types of ceremonies and blessings for people in the area, and he recommended a specific type of *sak yant* tattoo for a devotee, which was carried out in an adjoining room. After learning that I was going to visit Jivaka's home and mango garden, he agreed to give me a blessing of protection for my journey. The blessing was long, and it involved a protection amulet, reciting prayers, blowing with breath, sprinkling of holy water with a bamboo whisk, and the use of a sword.

I felt myself changing from the inside as the ceremony unfolded. Afterward, he told me how I should make my offering to Jivaka when I arrived at the site. I was to light sixteen sticks of incense; to pray to the Buddha, the dhamma, the sangha, my parents and my teachers, and then to ask permission from the local spirits that govern that place before I left my offering and removed some soil.

The next day I flew to Kolkata and spent a few days with friends before heading out on my pilgrimage. From Kolkata I flew to Patna, the capital of Bihar, and I spent the night there. Early the next morning, the car and driver I had hired took me on a bumpy road for about 3 hours, until we finally arrived in the town of Rajgir, about 100 kilometers away. The last leg of the journey, to Jivaka Amravana, was by *tanga*, a horse-drawn cart.

A visit with Jivaka and the Buddha

The tanga driver wanted to wait for me, but I let him know that I would be there for a long time. I paid him, and he left me alone with Jivaka. No one was there except for me, and I felt a stillness there that I have experienced only in a few other places on Earth. I could hardly believe my eyes. The elliptical gardens and the foundations of the structures were where Jivaka had grown his medicinal herbs, and where he had lived and practiced medicine! According to Pali scriptures, the Buddha had been treated at least once by Jivaka at this very spot, and lived here for some time.

After about ten minutes of being still, and looking and listening and sensing and feeling, I walked near the road to a blue sign on a rusty metal frame that marked the spot in Hindi and English. The sign read:

JIVAKA AMRAVANA VIHARA
Jivaka was a renowned physician in the royal court of Bimbisara and Ajatshatru during sixth–fifth century BC. He presented his extensive mango grove to Lord Buddha and constructed a monastery for the community. These elliptical structures have been identified as Jivaka Amravana Vihara.

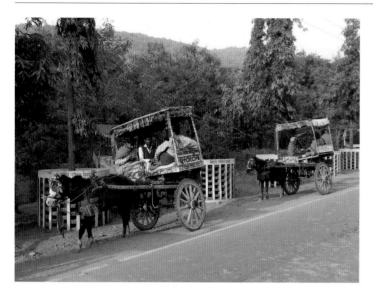

Tangas are an important means of local transport in Rajgir

I heard some sounds, and I turned my head to notice that a troop of monkeys was clambering down from the trees and noisily scavenging through paper and plastic containers for bits of food that were left in a pile of garbage near the eastern fence. Upon seeing this, I remembered that it was on top of a garbage heap where baby Jivaka was found in a basket by Prince Abhaya, son of King Bimbisara.

Then I began a very slow circumambulation of the entire area. I walked slowly, taking it all in, and trying to imagine what it might have looked like over 2,500 years ago. At one point, a few tourists came to visit, stopping no longer than a few minutes before moving on. It occurred to me that for most people, this place was probably an uninteresting pile of rocks. That thought, how our perceptions are shaped by our personal experiences and beliefs, made me feel simultaneously connected to those tourists and also very separate from them.

Once again, I walked around slowly, but this time I was looking for a place to leave the offering, and after a few minutes I found the perfect place. The tourists had gone, and I was alone again. I dug a small hole in the ground to support the sixteen incense sticks. I lit them and then began what for me was a deeply meaningful personal ceremony – one of the highest points in the chronology of my work as a student, therapist, and teacher of traditional Thai massage.

As I finished my puja, a group of about twenty local people arrived, with many children and even a cow, and they proceeded to have a picnic right there on the grounds of Jivaka Amravana. The kids began to play and run and jump all over the ruins, and the women laid out blankets and baskets of food. I smiled and thought to myself that Jivaka would have approved.

It was mid-afternoon, and I decided to continue on to Gridhakuta Hill, or Vulture Peak, as it is sometimes called, because of a rock formation that resembles a vulture's beak. This was the second most important place I wanted to visit in the area, since it is believed to be the Buddha's favorite meditation spot, and a place where he lived in caves and preached over a period of many years. It was here that he delivered the Lotus Sutra, which speaks of the concept and use of skillful means, and of salvation for all beings. The Prajnaparamitra Sutra (Perfection of Wisdom) was also sermonized here, suggesting that all things, including ourselves, appear as thought-forms and conceptual constructs.

From Jivaka Amravana, I walked on a road lined with trees and flowering shrubs for about 3 kilometers, until I reached the base of Ratanagiri Hill. From there I took a rickety chairlift to the top, and stopped at a modern *stupa* called Vishwa Shanti before hiking to the Buddha's meditation place.

The approach to Gridhakuta Hill, from an adjoining mountain, provided fabulous views of the surrounding hills, the valley below, and the meandering Banganga River. It was foggy, and sunset was approaching. I reached the final ascent to the actual altar, and by this time, all the monks and tourists were gone. The security policeman and the maintenance person allowed me to enter, and again I was alone at a sacred site, this time at the top of Gridhakuta Hill. I felt so grateful to be there, especially as the last visitor of the day, in silence, at sunset. I said a prayer as the earth continued its slow rotation, bringing with it the illusion that the sun was sinking. After a while, I began the slow descent all the way down to the base of the hill.

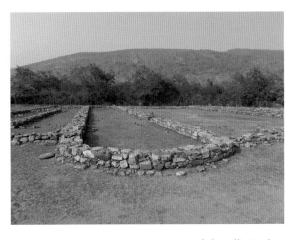

One of the elliptical foundations or garden walls on the site of Jivaka Amravana

Suggestions for travel to the area

Although Jivaka Amravana and Gridhakuta Hill were the highlights of my days in Rajgir, other places are also worth visiting. Venuvana is the pleasure garden of King Bimbisara, which was bestowed to the Buddha and the first sangha. It is the site of the famous bamboo grove mentioned in Buddhist scriptures. There are numerous Jain and Hindu temples in the area, and several sets of ancient walls surround Rajgir, which provided fortification and

(below left) Gridhakuta Hill (Vulture Peak) from a distance

(below right) The altar at the top of Gridhakuta Hill

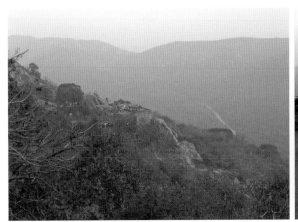

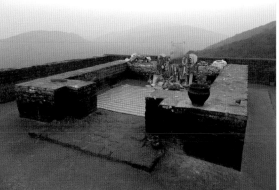

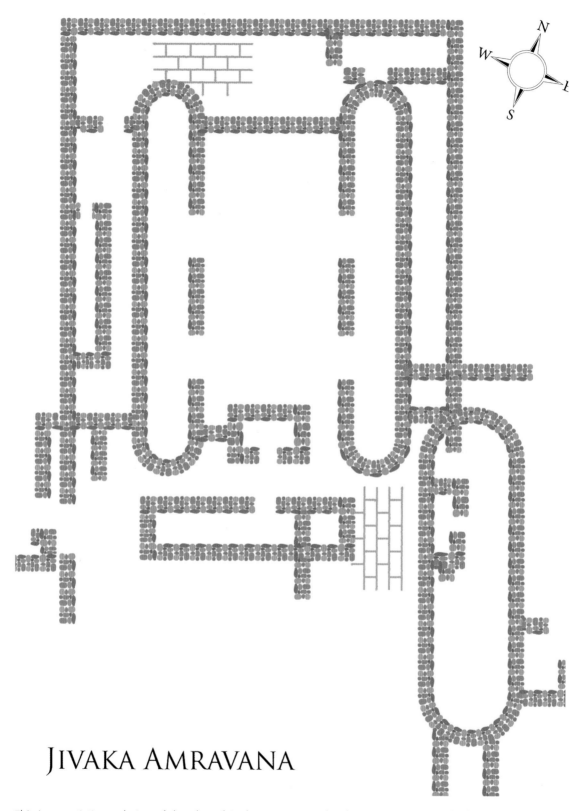

JIVAKA AMRAVANA

This is an artistic rendering of the plan of Jivaka Amravana. The drawing is not to scale, but the actual site is about 100 meters wide. There are remains of paving stones on the ground in several areas, which may indicate that there were pathways within and around the walls. There also appears to be a courtyard in the center of the two upper elliptical enclosures.

protection in ancient times. The Topada hot springs, mentioned as far back as the epic Mahabharata, are part of the Lakshminarayan temple complex. The impressive ruins of Nalanda, around 12 kilometers away, date from the fifth century AD, and mark the site of an ancient seat of learning in the sciences and arts. Finally, Bodhgaya, the most well-known Buddhist pilgrimage site, and where the Buddha is believed to have attained enlightenment under a bodhi tree, is about 3 hours away by bus or car.

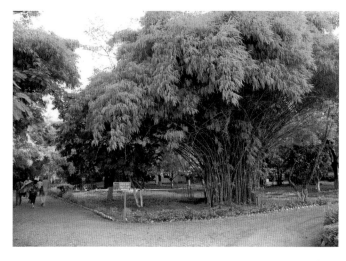

An outcropping of bamboo at Venuvana gardens, once a residence of the Buddha

Professionals in the field of traditional Thai massage, and those who are interested in Jivaka and the Buddha, will enjoy a trip to Rajgir and adjoining areas. There are numerous Buddhist pilgrimage tours you might join, but if you do the trip on your own, it can be rewarding because it allows more time to explore the area and you can decide on your own itinerary. There are airports in Patna and in Gaya, and from either place you can find transportation to Rajgir and to other areas on the Buddhist pilgrimage circuit.

My time in Rajgir helped me to complete a circuit in my professional practice and spiritual growth. I encourage all Thai massage practitioners who believe in the intercession and guidance of Jivaka Kumarabhacca to travel to Rajgir someday, and to pay respects to Jivaka at his home.

Compassion and Ethics in Thai Massage

EMILY CANIBANO

According to Thai healing traditions, the Thai massage *wai khru* shows respect for Jivaka and the Buddha and helps us connect with the long lineage of practitioners of traditional Thai massage. It is a request for guidance to help alleviate suffering, unhappiness, and disease in our clients. These rituals don't specifically mention compassion by name, but the Buddha teaches that compassion is what "makes the heart of the good move at the pain of others."

The word compassion means literally "to suffer together with." It is a human emotion that is triggered by the pain of others. When we suffer together with another person, we distance ourselves from the solitary ego. We get closer to the concept of interconnectedness among all living beings, and we share in the universal spirit. As we begin to see ourselves as less separate from other people, it becomes more difficult to cause suffering to others because we realize that this will also cause suffering to ourselves. The desire to alleviate pain in others becomes almost innate, because in doing so we also lessen our own pain.

Major religions, spiritual philosophies, and professions laud compassion as one of the highest virtues. Clients seek out Thai practitioners to help remove physical manifestations of suffering, such as pain and tension. It is the therapist's desire and intention to meet this suffering with compassion, and to help lessen the client's pain. Although the practice of Thai massage may sometimes cause discomfort similar to that of other physical exertions, such as yoga or strenuous exercise, the goal of the Thai practitioner should be to lessen pain and suffering compassionately – not create more of it. Because of Thai massage's connection to Theravada Buddhism, one of its most essential elements is compassion.

Pain and suffering come in many forms, and it's important for Thai massage professionals to understand what lies within the scope of practice of our work. As practitioners, we must act ethically and responsibly, and we must also be compassionate. In order to alleviate the pain of others and embrace the distressed, we must be aware of our own limitations and act and speak accordingly. Often, there can be more compassion in silence than in words.

Nuad boran is a powerful healing practice, but it has limitations, and so do its practitioners. Practitioners may gain insights into a client's state during an intake discussion prior to beginning a treatment, but it's unlikely they will get to know the deeper inner workings of a client's psyche, or the abstract concepts that cause this person's emotional and psychological pain. In some cases a practitioner may have the training and credentials to deal with a client's psychological state, but even if this is the case, this is not the role of a Thai therapist. Physical pain can manifest from emotional and psychological pain, and vice versa, and it can be hard to determine which comes first, and harder still to address these types of traumas.

For example, on a physical level, when we view a client with lopsided shoulders and pain in the upper back it may suggest to us that tight pectoral muscles may be involved, and we might confirm this by palpating the area. Asking the client about his shoulder pain might prompt a discussion about this physical asymmetry, leading to further insight into the condition. The practitioner may then suggest to the client that stretching exercises, being mindful of overstraining, or using the opposite side of the body more frequently, could help improve the condition. These words and actions are within the scope of our practice: they are not based in judgment, and they make no diagnosis of the situation, except to offer suggestions that may help the condition.

If, on the other hand, this same client offers information about the physical asymmetry of his shoulders, and how it relates to working at a job that requires him to carry a heavy load, or that he is depressed, or has family problems, at that point it is not within our scope of practice to counsel him on how to quit his job, relieve his depression, or address his family situation. This type of advice should be left to licensed specialists who are trained to handle such issues. Although a Thai massage therapist may want to personally help the client in some way, taking on such a task would be unethical, illegal, irresponsible, and could even bring about more pain and suffering for the client. Wanting to help is a positive attribute in a Thai massage practitioner, as it demonstrates compassion for our clients; however, we must always act within the scope of our practice.

The practice of compassion touches our work on three separate levels: mental, physical, and verbal. On the mental level, a Thai massage therapist should have a clear mind when working with a client, and be free of conflicting thoughts and actions. On the verbal level, we should refrain from offering advice, and never discuss subjects that are questionable, uncomfortable, or that may cause emotional or psychological pain. As practitioners, we must be responsible for what we do and say, and we should act and speak exclusively within our scope of knowledge and practice.

Eastern medicine is based on a holistic model of health that emphasizes spiritual and energy healing. On the surface, it may seem to have less regard for ethics; however, that is not the case. One of the earliest representations of medical ethics in history is attributed to Sun Ssu-Miao (AD 581–682), a traditional Chinese doctor who emphasized the need for education, conscientiousness, self-discipline, and compassion. His written works, and those of others, led to what is known as ancient Chinese medical ethics. Interestingly, concepts of respect for autonomy, non-maleficence, beneficence, and justice were clearly identified in these ancient documents, along with the key principle of compassion.

Traditional Thai massage, with its mix of assisted yoga, acupressure, energy work, spirituality, and herbal medicine, falls outside clear lines of definition and regulation. This, however, cannot be an excuse for Thai practitioners to forgo ethics, responsibility, and compassion. Thai massage therapists may have the ability to help clients heal, but we must always keep these things as the cornerstones of our practice.

Interview with Asokananda

BOB HADDAD

The following are excerpts from an interview with Asokananda by Bob Haddad which took place on Feb 12, 2004, at Asokananda's home in Chiang Mai, Thailand.

What was your first experience with Thai yoga massage?
My first experience with Thai yoga massage was watching my two teachers practice at the Old Medicine Hospital [in Chiang Mai, Thailand]. I had no previous experience with Thai massage before that, but I'd been studying a type of massage as part of my yoga training. My introduction to Thai massage was quite interesting. I was teaching yoga to a friend on the beach at Ko Samet, and two Dutch people came over and asked if they could join our morning yoga session. They were the ones who first told me about Thai massage. That was in 1986.

Were you already living in Thailand at that time?
No, I was primarily doing meditation in Burma, and I'd spent quite a bit of time in Sri Lanka and India, and I would occasionally visit Thailand. I had met up with one of my students at my teacher's monastery in Burma, and he was with me when I was doing that yoga session on the beach. I had absolutely no idea that serious yoga therapy existed in Thailand. It was virtually unknown back in the eighties. Even in Thailand, only a few people knew about it, and there were practically no formalized schools where you could learn it. The Dutch people told me that there were two places where one could learn Thai

massage – at Wat Pho in Bangkok and at the Old Medicine Hospital in Chiang Mai. I didn't really want to spend much time in Bangkok, so on my next trip to Chiang Mai, I went to have a look at what they were doing at the Old Medicine Hospital. Back then, there were no regularly structured classes – it was simply based on ongoing study. For the first half-year I spent there, I think there were only two or three students in the school. Anyway, I watched two teachers working there, and what they were doing amazed me. I knew immediately that I wanted to learn it, so I asked them if I could learn from them, and they said I could start right away. That was my introduction to Thai massage.

How was Thai massage thought of at that time in Thailand?
Thai massage was virtually unknown at that time. Very few people were interested in learning the art, but shortly afterward, about three years later, Thai massage began to establish a name for itself, and more and more people arrived in Thailand hoping to study. Attendance at the massage hospital grew from the handful of people I began with to a group of 40–50 students by 1989, when I left. Interest in Thai massage had exploded.

Do you owe that to any particular phenomenon?
Well I think it was a combination of things. On the one hand, this was a time when alternative medical practices had begun to gain popularity and acceptance all over the world, and consequently people began to be interested in traditional Thai massage. Also, within Thailand, this was a time when a group of Thai intellectuals began to question their country's complete dependence on Western medicine. Traditional Thai medicine and Thai massage had been pretty much pushed aside since the 1930s, when Western medicine began to gain prominence. Also, in the mid-eighties, the Thai Massage Revival project was implemented by the government, and more emphasis was placed on reviving what was still left of traditional Thai massage. It was a time of change, and within four or five years, the whole situation with Thai massage had become completely transformed. When I first started, no one was interested in Thai massage, neither Thai nationals nor foreigners; yet four or five years later, there was considerable interest within Thai society, as well as from the outside world.

What do you know about the Thai Massage Revival Project? Was it an effort to bring about standardization in the teaching and practice of Thai massage?
Initially it was a project to simply revive Thai massage. People had begun to realize that Thailand had a serious tradition of profound, therapeutic massage and of traditional medicine, whose revival was running parallel to that of Thai massage. So it was an attempt to bring back the knowledge and to spread it further, and at the same time to make sure that it was somehow maintained at a certain standard of practice.

Do you think it was successful in achieving its goals?
It certainly did raise awareness of Thai massage within Thai society, and by now, Thai massage has regained a certain level of status within Thai society that was lacking at that time. A few years ago, there was a government attempt to get every Thai massage teacher registered in Bangkok, and teachers were supposed to have done some training there in order to get officially registered. One of my teachers sent in some materials at one point, but he never received an answer. I remember when I asked my other teacher about it – he just looked at me, smiling, and said, "Do you really think I need that?" So the people I was working with were not very concerned about any sort of government affiliation.

Can you tell me about your teachers?
My teachers were Pichest Boonthumme and Chaiyuth Priyasith.

Were they both teaching simultaneously at Old Medicine Hospital?
Well nobody was really teaching there, actually; they were both working there, practicing as therapists. The teaching consisted of being around them, observing them, working with them, and getting feedback from them.

So the Old Medicine Hospital was functioning as a therapeutic center where people in the area would be attended to, as it was in the Buddhist wat tradition?
Yes, it was a place where people with health issues would go and receive serious treatments, and the main therapists there at that time were Chaiyuth and Pichest. They both started there in the mid-eighties and worked together for a period of two or three years. Chaiyuth left sometime in '87, as far as I remember, and Pichest stayed on until the early nineties.

Could you say something about the presence of Ayurveda in the practice of Thai massage?
Thai massage is a part of Thai medicine, and anyone here in Thailand who is engaged in serious Thai massage sees it that way, because that's the history of its development. Medical knowledge from India probably began to arrive in the Mon kingdoms of what is now northern Thailand as early as 200 or 300 BC. As Mon rulers developed contact with India, Theravada Buddhist monks and Ayurvedic medicine practitioners began traveling to Southeast Asia. Eventually a system of healing now known as Thai

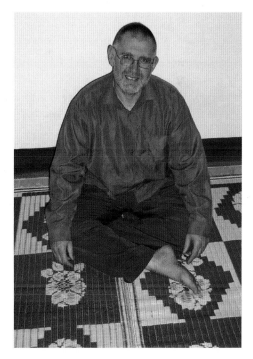

Asokananda at his home in Chiang Mai, 2004

Ayurveda developed in Thailand, which is quite different in theory and practice from Indian Ayurveda, and earlier yoga and massage elements developed into what is now known as Thai massage.

To what extent have the original elements of Indian Ayurveda been lost or changed in current-day Thai practice?
Well for example, in the actual practice of Thai Ayurveda, the *doshas* [bodily humors used in diagnosis] do not play a significant role. The major source of diagnosis and of treatment protocol in Thai Ayurveda is based on tastes, which is not the case in Indian Ayurveda. In Indian Ayurvedic medicine there are eight tastes, but in Thai Ayurveda there can be up to ten. It can be difficult for an outside observer to understand Thai Ayurveda, because it's based on a theoretical background containing ancient Indian principles which are rarely used in actual practice. Thais are not particularly concerned with those elements. They pay respect to the source, but they work within their own tradition.

Does Thai massage reflect any indigenous Southeast Asian healing practices?
No one has any idea about this. There must have been some native healing traditions in Thailand, but there are no known sources of information about this.

To what extent does Thai massage reflect ancient Chinese healing practices?
I think Chinese influence in Thai yoga massage is completely overrated in much of the current literature on Thai medicine and in Thai massage. I often smile when I read articles on Thai massage where the Thai energy system is compared to the Chinese meridian system, arguing that it is more or less the same thing. There are even books that claim that the Thai massage *sen* system is the same as the Chinese meridian system, and they then conclude that practitioners should utilize Chinese meridians when engaging in Thai massage.

I believe this is not a good way to look at the Thai healing tradition because upon serious investigation, one will see that the Thai tradition is clearly derived from the Indian *prana nadi* system and from Ayurvedic medicine. Chinese medicine and the Chinese meridian system had little influence on the actual practice of Thai Ayurveda and traditional Thai massage. It's historically easy to understand this, because the first Thais were refugees driven out of China by the Han Dynasty. So the idea that these people would happily embrace the Chinese system and incorporate it into their own practice is somewhat unlikely. Only recently have an increasing number of Chinese traders brought Chinese medical knowledge and herbal products to Thailand. Currently in Thailand, Chinese medical treatment has become popular, but I still think there is very little mixing of the two healing arts. Chinese practitioners in Thailand are still quite separate from Thai Ayurvedic practitioners, and there is a clear distinction between traditional Thai medicine doctors and Chinese doctors in Thailand who practice Chinese medicine.

So how do traditional Thai medicine practitioners work with their patients?
They will often perform a taste analysis on their patients, and prescribe medicinal herbs and sometimes minerals. They would possibly perform Thai massage, apply hot herbal compresses, and prescribe herbal remedies. There is a wide range of practices that form the basis of traditional Thai medicine. To qualify as a Thai medicine practitioner you first have to undergo rigorous training these days. One can study to become either a Thai Ayurvedic doctor or a Thai Ayurvedic pharmacist.

How do you feel about the commercialization of Thai massage by relatively unqualified practitioners?
Well, I'm sure sad about it, but I also don't think there's much we can do. One of the side effects of the increasing popularity of Thai massage is that there are also quacks who try to ride the wave and then wind up teaching things that are incorrect or nontraditional. But as with most fads, I'm confident that those who wish to practice seriously will eventually prevail, and that the quality teachers will eventually have the strongest impact. Even the substandard schools in Thailand and in the West are raising interest in Thai massage, and anyone who gets started and can see the great potential of Thai massage will ultimately look for a serious teacher.

How important is Thai yoga massage to one's spirituality?
I don't think they can be separated, because Thai massage evolved in Thailand in conjunction with Buddhism. Historically, Thai massage was taught alongside the teachings of the Buddha, and it remained closely connected to Buddhist tradition and also to meditation. The approach was that massage was an act of loving-kindness and mindfulness applied to another person. The spirit of Thai massage is essentially a Buddhist spirit, and to take it out of that context is to remove the heart of the process. If a massage is not practiced with loving-kindness and mindfulness, a certain quality can be missing from the end result. For me it's essential that the teachings of Thai massage also incorporate the teachings of meditation and yoga.

To make one point clear that often appears as somewhat of a misunderstanding – Buddhist monks were not the ones responsible for teaching massage in Thailand; it was the Ayurvedic doctors who arrived with the monks and who, in the same Buddhist spirit, worked in the region to spread medical knowledge. Buddhist monasteries were the first places where massage was carried out in Thailand, so there was a very close link between traditional Thai massage and Buddhist spirituality and principles. As far as is known, the first emigrations of Indian Ayurvedic practitioners and Buddhist monks began a few hundred years after the Buddha's death, around 300 BC.

And what about Jivaka Komarabhacca?

Jivaka Komarabhacca is a mythological figurehead. He never set foot on Thai soil, because he lived a few hundred years before the first Buddhist travelers came to the region. Those who began to spread knowledge of Thai massage, however, practiced in his spirit. He is specifically revered because he is the famous doctor mentioned in ancient Buddhist scriptures. He was the Buddha's doctor, the physician of the Buddha's *sangha*, so anything medical that was associated with Buddhism automatically became associated with him. When Ayurvedic medicine was brought to this region, it was brought and transmitted in Jivaka's spirit and tradition.

So the elements of mindfulness, metta, and loving-kindness inherent in Thai massage have been transmitted over the years largely as a result of Jivaka's personal relationship and interaction with the Buddha.

Yes, exactly.

Tell me a little bit about sen line blockages. How does energy healing take place?

Any kind of influence that we go through in our lives, whether emotional or physical, leaves an imprint on all the levels of energy manifestation that make up a human being. We most directly relate to the physical body, but there is also an energy body, a memory or subconscious body, an intuitive body, and our link to cosmic energy flow. Each of these are different manifestations that are so closely linked to each other that any disturbance on one level can become apparent on another level.

If, for example, we go through emotional turmoil, we may end up with physical problems. Or if we are involved in a car crash and we break a leg, then this may have effects on our emotional or energetic levels. In Thai massage, our main tool is the individual's energy body that we follow with the *sen* lines. We try to balance disturbances that exist on the energetic level, and in doing so, we influence other levels, too. If a physical problem is causing a disturbance in the energy flow, our work can have a balancing effect on both physical and energetic levels, or on another combination of levels, or on all the levels combined.

Can intuitive sensitivity be taught?

Only to a certain extent. You can teach people how to develop their sensitivity, but intuition has to come by playing with the energy lines and feeling the

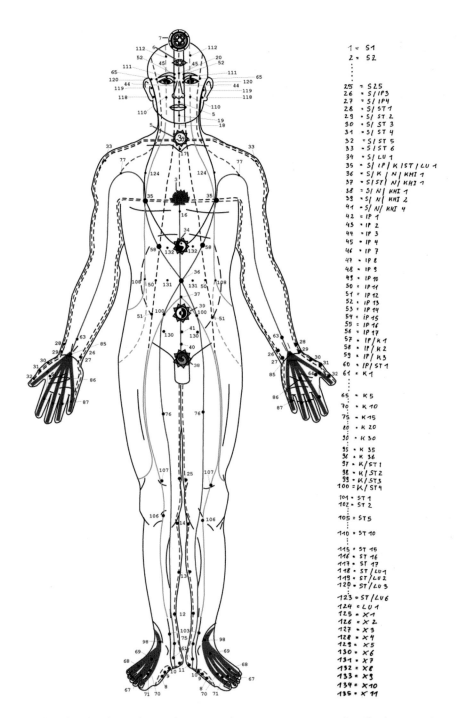

Before his death, Asokananda was working on a system to identify therapeutic points in the northern Thai system. The goal was to systematically plot and number each point with letters and numbers for each main sen line, much the way acupuncture points are documented in traditional Chinese medicine. His work was never completed or made available on a wide scale. This is the last anterior point chart that he completed, along with a hand-written key to pressure points and intersecting lines.

energy. Ultimately, it comes from one's intuition, and most people have the ability to tap into it. Some people are naturals; they're right there from the first moment, and they can hone into energy flow. Others may look on in confusion and not understand what the heck we're talking about.

How do you guide your students in this regard?
I try to give very precise feedback on whether they are actually on the energy lines or not, and I ask them to feel the difference. It's important to try to develop a sense for how differently it feels to actually be working on a line. After some time, the sensing ability usually develops quite well.

Traditionally, we begin and end a session in supine position. Others some-times deviate from this structure. What's your opinion on this?
My preference is to begin and end lying on the back. The final touch in Thai massage is to bring major energy streams together at the forehead and at the top of the head and then to balance the energy from there. This can also be done in sitting position, and I'm not dogmatic about people having to lie down at the end. But the final work on the head is an important aspect of Thai massage, and my preference is to do it while the patient is in supine position.

Is there a major release at the top of the head?
Yes, but this is actually happening throughout the whole workout, not just at the end. We release tension through the whole body during the entire massage. There's an energy exchange happening between the therapist and the patient all the time. Whenever we touch, we tap into the patient's energy. That's why it's also very important that the therapist take care of himself, making sure he protects himself properly before the session, and cleans his energy system afterward.

In addition to meditation and yoga, what can practitioners do to prepare for and to unwind from a session?
I usually recommend an exercise to create an energy shield to protect yourself before you work, such as *prana eggs,* and then to do an exercise after the session like *kaya kriya,* where you release tension very strongly from the body. Especially when we know that we have a patient under duress, I'd recommend doing prana eggs before you start, and then take a shower or do a salt-water cleanse, and perform kaya kriya after the patient has left.

Understanding Clients in Nuad Boran

DANKO LARA RADIC

Unlike in the recent past, when *nuad boran* was shrouded in a veil of mystery, it's much easier to find information about traditional Thai massage these days. Much has already been said about the nature, techniques, and benefits of nuad boran, but there is little information available about the internal process of clients during treatment. What are our clients' understandings and perceptions of this therapy? How does their awareness of Thai massage influence the overall effectiveness of treatment? These and other questions are the focus of this article.

A new client's perception of nuad boran

Partly as a result of a global interest in health and wellness, nuad boran is sometimes perceived by newcomers as a spa product, or even, in some cases of gross misperception, as an erotic service. In wellness centers around the world, and even in Thailand, treatments are carried out in routine fashion in order to bring about relaxation, but without careful assessment or attention to the client's individual needs. Therefore, to help educate clients and to dispel incorrect perceptions about this healing art, therapists should take time to explain to new clients that Thai massage is an ancient and spiritual healing practice, and that it is a component of the traditional Thai medicine system.

Many people are unaware of their overall health until painful symptoms occur. Some disorders develop over an extended period of time, starting as a subtle imbalance on the energy level and ending up as a manifestation on a physical level. This process can sometimes go on for years. Since painful symptoms appear only in the terminal stage, people often react too late, but this doesn't prevent them from expecting instant healing. New clients may have such expectations, so they should be informed that disorders that have accumulated over years cannot usually be remedied with one or two treatments.

Some clients have little awareness of the responsibility they can take for their own well-being. Many illnesses and disorders are caused by deeper psychological patterns, and unless the individual assumes an active role in maintaining his own health, a Thai therapist is restricted in the ways he is able to help.

Excessive talking

Some people find it hard to be quiet, and they come to the mat with excessive wordiness. This may be due to nervousness, insecurity, stress, or anxiety, or a conditioning that prevents the person from fully relaxing and being present. Some clients continue talking, even when the treatment begins, and they won't stop unless you ask them to do so. Unlike other modalities, nuad boran does not require constant verbal communication between the giver and receiver. Conversation can take place before and after the session, but to bring about the best effect, talking should be kept to an absolute minimum during treatment. Nuad boran is a meditative style of bodywork, and it requires the therapist and the receiver to maintain full awareness, and to focus on breath. Words should be exchanged only when processing certain sensations, when providing or offering feedback or assistance, or when making a brief observation.

Understanding pain

During Thai massage therapy, a client may experience various types of pain in differing intensity. Pain can be of a physical or psychological nature, and it usually serves as a signal that something is wrong. Aside from the pain that results from poor execution of a technique by a therapist who lacks skill, many forms of pain may be considered "beneficial pain." In modern times, people undergo stressful situations daily, and negative emotions and patterns that are repressed or unexpressed may remain etched in the body as information. During therapy, these memories can be stimulated, emotions can be revived, and the client may feel them as pain. It is important for the client to understand this phenomenon in order to be able to process painful sensations, because sometimes it may be the only way that pain can be reduced. Many people understand this process intuitively, but nevertheless it may be important to communicate this to new or unaware clients.

Clients who want to help

Unlike other therapies, in Thai massage the client's body is in movement most of the time. While moving or stretching, some clients often want to "help" by moving a certain part of their body by themselves, rather than relaxing completely. This can be due to certain factors. Sometimes, if clients feel that the movement you are about to execute may go beyond their comfort zone, they'll become afraid and will subconsciously engage their muscles and execute the movement by themselves. Other clients may do this because they want to stay in control or because they are unable to surrender completely. Clients who need to be in control are a great challenge for every therapist.

Another way a client may want to help is if he is larger or heavier than the therapist and thinks it is difficult for the therapist to physically manipulate his body. This shows that the client is not familiar with the techniques used in nuad boran, which are not based on brute strength but rather physics and proper body mechanics. It can be helpful for the therapist to determine why the client wants to help, and to gently explain that it is not necessary to do so.

Unpleasant positions for the client

Sometimes, a client finds herself in a position that is not painful, yet it still arouses an unpleasant sensation. This may happen because as the body is worked, information is released in the form of emotion. This phenomenon can also have psychological underpinnings, if a position or a technique reminds the client's body of a time when it suffered a traumatic experience. A skilled Thai massage therapist should learn to recognize when a client experiences pain or discomfort, and to either ease up on the pressure, or change the technique and move on with the session. Reassuring, verbal recognition of a client's discomfort, and of the therapist's adjustments, can be given when necessary.

Inability to relax

When therapists encounter resistance, they may ask a client to relax a certain part of their body, yet when the movement is repeated, there is still resistance. This tension exists largely on an unconscious level, so it's good to be aware that the client cannot control it easily. Sometimes this can be overcome by introducing gentle and smooth repetitive movements, such as rotations, which may make it easier for the client to relax.

Some people find it hard to keep their eyes closed during an entire treatment. These people may be seeking external stimulation or reassurance, or they may have a subconscious desire to remove themselves from the context of the massage treatment. Other times, a client may just be gazing into nothingness, but in a relaxed state. A therapist should take note when a client's eyes are open, but it's best to not interfere with the client's natural process by asking him to close his eyes.

Breathing patterns

Many people have shallow breathing and don't understand the importance of breathing deeply during treatments. Some react to pain by contorting their body and holding their breath. Breath is the carrier of vital energy – we bring it into our body and then let it go. Sometimes it can be helpful to softly remind clients to deeply inhale and exhale, and to guide them through the process of breath awareness during critical points in a session.

Stoicism and lack of communication

Some people go through an entire Thai massage treatment without displaying any type of emotion or sensation on their face, either physically or vocally. This doesn't mean they are not having a good experience. Therapists may feel tension, trembling, or uneasiness in a client, but sometimes a client may keep it hidden and not let it out in any way. A compassionate therapist may gently encourage the client to explore his emotions and sensations, to feel comfortable enough to let go, to breathe deeply, and to relax.

Emotional reactions

Sometimes, Thai massage treatments trigger trauma in our clients, during which they experience strong emotions, such as intense sorrow, anger, guilt, and many other emotions. Again, use gentle reassurance, patience, and working within each person's limits to handle this type of situation in a professional manner.

Sexual energy

Thai massage is an intimate healing modality, and if the work is not channeled properly, it can lead to misunderstandings. During the course of a nuad boran treatment sexual energy can arise, due to the actions of the client, the therapist, or both of them simultaneously. Sexual energy can be triggered consciously or unconsciously, but whatever the case, the responsibility lies with the therapist to diffuse it. Thai massage therapists are the bearers of a spiritual healing art that in no way should be confused with sexuality. If the therapist feels sexual energy in the air, he should remove himself from the situation, attempt to dissipate the energy, and carry on in a professional manner. If the energy cannot be dispelled, the session should be brought to a close.

Relapsing symptoms

After a Thai massage session, a client may report that she temporarily felt better, but that the same symptoms returned shortly after the session. This happens because the problem itself is not fully resolved. Some people suffer from chronic pathologies, which take a long time to develop, and correspondingly, a long time to heal. Often, without the client committing to a serious change in lifestyle, the root of the problem can't be resolved, regardless of how many Thai massage treatments he receives. In addition, many conditions cannot be treated by Thai massage, and may require medicine or other therapies. Ultimately, clients must understand that the responsibility lies with them to make life-changing decisions that will affect their well-being. The therapist's role is to provide support and encouragement.

Guidance and change

When we are children, we develop specific patterns of behavior in order to adapt to our immediate environment and survive physically, mentally, and emotionally. These patterns remain deeply rooted in our subconscious, and also continue through adulthood, even though our environments may change. Many people don't recognize their patterns, because they have lost touch with their inner selves.

Nuad boran is a complex, spiritual healing art, and when it's performed skillfully and sensitively, it can permeate our very essence. Accomplished Thai massage therapists may help clients through techniques and concepts associated with nuad boran, and in this unspoken way, encourage them to reprogram their patterns. Therapists, however, can only serve as guides; each individual must face himself and make the necessary changes. The motivation for personal change and growth must come from within.

Standing Thai Massage on Its Head

PAUL FOWLER

Let's talk about inversions – inversions Thai style. First, let's define them. An inversion is when the heart is higher in the air than the head. It's as simple as that. Think of the poses in Thai massage where the head is higher than the heart. Now think about what you have to do to put someone in that position. Is it easy or is it difficult? Does it take strength or energy on your part, or are you able to use gravity and alignment to make it happen? Are you doing it because you think the client expects something like that from a Thai massage, or in order to impress someone with a fancy Thai massage move? I can only answer these questions for myself. For me, most inversions take a lot of energy, and oftentimes they are difficult to perform. And sometimes, I have found myself trying to impress my client, especially when a session may seem otherwise uneventful.

All of this poses a question: Is it that our Western bodies aren't well suited to give and receive inversions comfortably? And here's another question: How often do you use inverted poses in your practice? For me, the answer is very rarely. They only rarely feel good to me as a Thai therapist, and I'm often concerned that I might injure someone. When I receive sessions in Thailand, I am rarely put into an inversion. They don't seem to be popular there. So why do we do them more often in the West?

When I analyze the poses that are in a traditional Thai massage sequence, I remove from that sequence those poses or techniques that I cannot do comfortably. After all, if it's not comfortable for me, then it probably won't be comfortable for my client. And if it's not comfortable, how can it be of help?

All the well-known teachers I've met in Thailand say the same thing over and over again. Create a practice that works for you and that works for your client. Throw out the book. Throw out your ideas. Just tune into the body and to what it needs. Take care of your body first of all. Once you do that, then you can address your clients' bodies. And if you are uncomfortable in any way when you do the practice, stop, back up, and take another look at what you are doing and why you are doing it.

Regarding inversions, suspensions, and lifts, ask yourself the following questions while you are doing them: "If I were to stay here for a longer period of time, would I be comfortable? Would my client be comfortable?" If the answer is no, then examine what you had hoped to achieve by applying that particular technique, and then see if you can achieve that result in another way – in a way that is more supported and relaxed for both you and your client.

I realize that to some of you, it may be far reaching to suggest removing all inversions from the practice of Thai massage, but the health and safety of yourself and your client is much more important than carrying out a fixed sequence that you were once taught. After years of practice, one's approach to Thai massage ultimately does not come from a teacher or a book, but from tapping into one's own wisdom, experience, and body.

Pay attention to your body when and if you put someone in an inversion, then let your body – and not your mind – be your guide. If you approach it this way, you will know exactly what to do, because you will be listening and working with compassion, sensitivity, and your own inherent wisdom.

Thai Massage on an Amputee Client

BOB HADDAD

I have given regular Thai sessions to a leg amputee for a long time, and I'd like to share my experiences with the Thai massage community about the first session we had together. The client, a sixty-year-old man, had suffered from leg pain over a period of years, and his cancer went largely misdiagnosed until it had already metastasized. His entire left leg and part of his pelvis were eventually amputated in a procedure called hemipelvectomy, and flaps of skin from his buttocks were folded over each other and grafted over the stump. When I first began to work with him, he was on chemotherapy and had begun walking on crutches. He hoped that regular Thai treatments would aid in his recovery and increase his mobility.

For our first session I wanted to get comfortable with the afflicted area and to be aware of any residual soreness or pain. A thorough visual inspection of the stump and the incision and skin graft areas helped me to feel more confident. I tried to feel where the *sen* lines were residing in the stump, and at which point each of the major lines may have been interrupted. I tried to imagine how his energy may have been affected by the trauma, and which types of Thai techniques I could use to increase energy flow to the affected area. As I thumb-pressed the stump, I realized that I could apply quite a bit of pressure to the area, and that helped me to relax, knowing I would not be hurting him.

I folded the remainder of his pant leg over the stump, I knelt at his feet, and I prayed silently for his well-being. As I rubbed my hands together and opened my eyes, suddenly I was faced with a dilemma. How should I begin my work? I couldn't palm press both feet. I couldn't even touch both of his legs at the same time. If I worked only on his remaining leg, would the energy be balanced on the other side?

After a few seconds, I decided that somehow, someway, I had to work with both of my hands. I needed to do my dance on his body, whether or not both legs existed in the physical realm. I rationalized that his energy still existed on a metaphysical level in that truncated leg, and that it needed to be addressed, not neglected. Prior to the session, I'd researched the phenomenon called "phantom pain" in amputee victims, and my client had told me about the strange sensations of tingling, pain, and itching that sometimes occurred at various points along the missing leg. I was curious and excited . . . but I was also concerned and apprehensive.

As if by natural impulse, I began to palm-press both feet – one visible and one invisible. I started with simultaneous palm pressing, but I began to alternate from left to right at one point. My usual sense of rocking and movement helped to fuel me forward. I focused on my energy, and I imagined a missing leg there in front of me, needing to be touched and healed.

As I proceeded upward, one hand on his right inner lower leg and the other hand on the floor, I had a strong sensation that something was wrong. I wasn't feeling connected to the energy on his left side. I reasoned that if his left leg were actually there in physical form, that his medial sen lines would not be lying flat on the floor; they would be about four inches above the mat and at an inward angle. I lifted my right hand off the ground, and I began to "feel" for his leg in the air, at the same height of his other calf.

My palm presses suddenly became balanced, and my shoulders fell into alignment. I was actually palm pressing in the air, sensing for his energy, and the thought of it brought a smile to my face. Only a few days earlier at a meeting with Thai massage colleagues, we were joking about making t-shirts with the words "What Would Jivaka Do?" That thought made me focus on my Jivaka altar, and gazing at his bronze image and at the photos of my teachers, I felt a validation that helped me through this unusual session.

I began to work on the phantom leg in exactly the same way as I had worked on the physical leg: when I palm-pressed the real leg, I also pressed the phantom leg. A few minutes later, as I was palm-walking up his physical leg, I felt a strong vibration midway up the medial thigh. I stopped, and I directed all my energies to that area, and I located a large energy blockage with my thumbs. The energy was very strong, and it was rapidly intermittent, sending waves of vibrations through my hands and into the ether. I felt *sen kalathari* melting under my fingers, and I eased my pressure a bit in order to be more sensitive.

As I released the pressure and focused inward, my client spoke. He had begun to feel his phantom leg come alive. It was tingling, he said, and it felt very good. There was no pain, no soreness, no itching, just a sense of presence that he hadn't felt since the amputation. As he said this aloud, his entire body immediately relaxed, and he began breathing deeply. His facial expression changed from apprehension and sadness to peacefulness and ease. Aside from the obvious physical restrictions, the treatment proceeded normally, and I felt much more at ease, knowing that his entire energetic body was being affected by our work together.

As I continue to work with him, I have felt much more confident, and he has continued to open up to the work. I have also learned how to modify my techniques, to use pillows and cushions in supportive ways, and to improvise in order to work with him more effectively. We've done assisted cobras in prone position and spinal twists with my leg draped over his stump. I've worked both sets of his back lines in side-lying position, and I've been using my feet and toes in creative ways to attend to his needs.

I am excited to be exploring *nuad boran* with this beautiful person, and to be sharing this time in our lives together. Although I am much more confident now than I was during that first session, I suspect that from time to time a recurrent thought will come to mind when I work with him: What would Jivaka do?

Thai Massage Beyond the Physical

ROBERT HENDERSON

Bob Haddad's piece about Thai massage on an amputee client brings up some very interesting points. First and foremost, it shows that as human beings we aren't limited to our physical bodies. Our levels of consciousness, awareness, and feelings exist on higher levels, and they extend far beyond the limitations of bones, organs, blood, tissue, and skin. Secondly, it shows that to use traditional Thai massage as a tool to treat another person only on the level of the physical body is to make limited use of this healing art. Anyone who has ever received a massage from a true Thai master has experienced the transformational power of traditional Thai massage and the effects it can have on our spirit, mind, emotions, energy, and physical body.

The irony of relying on *nuad boran* as a purely physical treatment is that the more we learn about what we can do, the less we may be able to achieve, since each technique or concept is only a fragment of the entire holistic order. Our higher level of consciousness is aware that we extend far beyond the physical. The limitations we place on ourselves, however, may cause conflicts that can eventually manifest as physical pain and dis-ease.

If we believe that we exist only in a physical body, blockages can form to prevent awareness of the greater truth that we are infinite beings. Apart from the pains that result from the physical body, a staggering range of burdens and discomforts have roots that lie beyond the physical. These include blaming other people for our own conditions or actions, doing things that we don't want to do or don't need to do (even eating when we're not hungry), not forgiving others, not forgiving ourselves, not living up to our true potential, being judgmental or selfish, feeling guilt, being insensitive to others, and so forth. Think for a moment. How many of us carry one or more of these burdens? Unless the Thai therapist has an understanding of these pains, of their roots and manifestations, and of how they may best be addressed, physical massage techniques may only have a limited effect. If the roots of some illnesses lie beyond the physical, then it is reasonable to believe that their treatment similarly lies beyond the pure physical application of bodywork.

I am concerned about the trend I am noticing in the world of commercial bodywork – of adopting a healing art such as traditional Thai massage, which is steeped in Buddhist spirituality, prayer, and meditation, and then stripping it of all or most of its roots, so that it can be performed as a series of physical exercises, stretches, and techniques. There is nothing wrong with the exercises and techniques on their own, of course, but to practice or teach this healing art without a Buddha-Shivago foundation is to literally take the soul out of traditional Thai massage. Often, there is little in common between what is promoted as "Thai massage" and what truly is traditional Thai healing. In many cases, Thai massage has been broken into parts, and only parts of it are being taught on a wide scale in the West and in Thailand.

My goal in writing this brief article is to nudge and encourage all Thai massage professionals to try to see beyond the physical as we work, and to touch and help heal our clients with the same extraphysical sensitivity that Bob used with his amputee client. By seeing beyond the physical, we can develop our practice into an extremely powerful healing art. If we are all created equal, then what is stopping us from becoming sensitive, intuitive, and powerful healers? Why couldn't we develop our own Thai massage practice into the transformational healing art that other great masters have proven it to be?

Glossary

aagaasathaat – The element of space in Thai medicine.

ajahn (achaan, อาจารย์) – A Thai language term that translates as "teacher." It is derived from the Pali word *ācariya*, and is a term of respect.

blood stop – See *wind gate*.

bpert lom – Thai term for "open the wind." See *wind gate*.

bucha – Thai pronunciation for *puja*. See *puja*.

chaloeysak – The "folk style" of Thai massage, which integrates use of practitioner's hands, feet, elbows, knees, and which is known and practiced on a wide scale by Thai people and Westerners.

chedi – Thai word (from Pali) for *stupa*, the Sanskrit word (literally "mound") for a Buddhist monument erected to house a relic.

dantien, tantien – Center of life force energy. Buddhist and Taoist teachers often instruct students to center the mind in the lower dantien. Known also by the Japanese word *hara*.

dhamma (dharma) – For practicing Buddhists, references to dharma (*dhamma* in Pali and in Thai) generally means the teachings of the Buddha.

din – Thai earth element.

fai – Thai fire element.

farang – A generic Thai word for a foreigner, usually a Caucasian of European ancestry, no matter what nationality they may be.

hara – Japanese term for stomach, and by extension, for the "center of being." Eastern martial arts and movement therapies emphasize moving from the hara, located slightly below the navel. It's an important center of movement and grounding in traditional Thai massage. See *dantien*.

horasaht – The division of Thai medicine that deals with divinatory sciences such as numerology, astrology, and palmistry.

jap sen – a style of Thai massage characterized by vigorous thumbing and plucking along the sen lines.

Jivaka – Jivaka Kumarabhacca, the legendary doctor who was a contemporary of the Buddha, is revered as the ancestral teacher of Thai traditional medicine. His last name is also known in Thailand as Gomalapato, Gomalapaj, and Komarapaj. See Shivago and Kumarabhacca.

Jivaka Amravana (Jivakamravana) – Jivaka's residence, medical dispensary, and mango grove in Rajgir, Bihar, India. The excavated ruins are preserved as a historical site.

kayaphapbambat – The division of traditional Thai medicine that deals with bone setting, external application of herbs, and Thai massage.

khatha (คาถา) – The Thai term (from the Pali word *gatha*) for sacred prayers and mantras. Khatha are used in Buddhist chanting, by reusi to recite magical incantations, and are also used by Thai people for protection, good luck, and business ventures.

khom – Ancient Khmer script used in Thailand for Buddhist manuscripts, prayers, and magical incantations. It is commonly used to transcribe Pali in the Buddhist liturgies of Thailand and Cambodia.

kriya – Sanskrit term for a technique or practice within a yoga discipline meant to achieve a specific result.

Kumarabhacca – Last name of Jivaka. Variations in spelling include Kumarbhaccha, Komarabhacca, and Kumar Bhaccha.

Lek Chaiya – Important Thai massage teacher of Chiang Mai who popularized the jap sen style of therapy.

lersi – See reusi.

leuad – Thai word for blood.

lom – The element of air in traditional Thai medicine; the word used to describe the energy that flows through Thai sen lines.

loving-kindness – See metta.

luk pra kob – Thai herbal compresses that are wrapped, steamed, and applied either hot or cold to a patient's body. They are often used to complement Thai massage treatments.

metta – Pali term for loving-kindness, the cultivation of which is a popular form of meditation in Theravada Buddhism.

nadi (prana nadi) – The channels through which, in Indian ayurvedic medicine, the energies of the subtle body are said to flow. They connect at special points of intensity called *chakras*.

nam (naam) – The element of water in traditional Thai medicine.

nam ob Thai – Lightly scented perfume water, often used in ceremonies and on holidays, especially Thai New Year (*Songkran*). It can be part of an offering made to monk or teacher, or as a gift to someone you hold in respect.

neti pot – A small vessel used to flush out excess mucus and debris from the nose and sinuses with a salt-water solution.

nuad boran (nuad phaen boran, นวดแผนโบราณ) – Thai name for traditional Thai massage. The accent of the first word is on the first syllable, pronounced *NU-odd*.

Old Medicine Hospital – Also known as Thai Massage School Shivagakomarpaj, it is an important seat of learning for Thai massage in northern Thailand.

Om namo – A salutation of deference and homage in Sanskrit/Pali. In Thai massage it refers to the name of the wai khru (prayer) to the Father Doctor Jivaka, which begins "Om namo Shivago."

parasympathetic state – A healing state whereby the body can make repairs, recharge, and be open to transformation.

paetayasaht – The division of traditional Thai medicine that treats the internal body.

Pali – An ancient language from India in which many of the earliest Buddhist scriptures are written. Pali is mostly studied to gain access to Buddhist scriptures, and it is frequently recited and chanted in ritual contexts.

phra – an honorific term used for nobility, monks, and Buddha images.

Pichest (Ajahn Pichest, Pichet) – Variations in spelling for Pichest Boonthumme, an important Thai massage teacher and healer.

point pressure – The process or technique of applying focused pressure, usually with thumbs and fingers, to specific therapeutic treatment points on the body.

prana – Sanskrit word for "life energy" in Indian ayurvedic medicine. Prana enters the body through the breath and is sent to every cell through the circulatory system. It is known as *qi* and *chi* in traditional Chinese medicine, and *lom* in traditional Thai medicine.

prana eggs – A visualization and meditation technique that may be helpful in strengthening an individual's energy system and minimizing interference from outside influences.

pranayama – Sanskrit word for "extension of prana." A body of knowledge based on manipulating breath through exercises and techniques that bring about physical and mental well-being, and expansion of consciousness.

puja – Pali and Sanskrit term for ceremonies and expressions of honor, worship, and devotional attention.

Putthayasaht – The division of Thai medicine that deals with Buddhism and mental health.

qigong (chi gong, chi kung) – A traditional Chinese practice of aligning breath with movement, and cultivating awareness for exercise, healing, and meditation.

ratchasamnak – The "royal style" of Thai massage, originally reserved for kings and royal courts, which uses only the therapist's hands. Therapists must also maintain distance from the receiver and work in a highly respectful manner.

reusi (ruesi, lersi) – Historically in Thailand, reusi are practitioners and custodians of ancient arts and sciences including alchemy, natural medicine, astrology, palmistry, mathematics, and music. The Thai word reusi, often spelled in Western languages as ruesi, and sometimes seen in Thailand as *lersi*, comes from the Sanskrit word *rishi*.

reusi dat ton (ruesi/ruesri datton) – A traditional Thai practice developed by reusi, of dynamic exercises involving self-stretching, breathing, specific postures, meditation, and self massage.

sak yant – Thai sacred tattoos.

saiyasaht – The division of Thai medicine that deals with shamanistic healing, spirit worship, incantations, magical tattoos, and amulets.

samatha – The dimension of Buddhist spiritual cultivation concerned with calming the mind. The Thai Forest tradition stresses the inseparability of samatha and vipassana.

sangha – The first order of Buddhist monks and nuns. Lay practitioners in the West often use the word as a collective term for all Buddhists, or for a localized spiritual Buddhist community.

savasana (shavasana) – An important passive yoga posture carried out by lying on the back and by maintaining deep awareness. It is traditionally used at the end of a yoga session, and is intended to rejuvenate the body, mind, and spirit.

sen, sen lines – Channels or pathways in the human body through which life-giving energy flows.

sip sen – (sen sip, sen sib) – The ten most commonly addressed sen lines in traditional Thai massage. Individually, they are: sumana, ittha, pingkhala, kalathari, sahatsarangsi, thawari, lawusang, ulangka, nanthakrawat, and khitchana.

Shivago (Shivaga, Shevaga, Shivaka) – variations in spelling of the name Jivaka.

songthaew – A customized covered pickup truck, with two long benches for sitting, used in Thailand as a means of public transportation. The word means "two rows."

stupa – The Sanskrit word for a mound-like structure containing Buddhist relics that is used by Buddhists as a place of meditation and prayer. See *chedi*.

thaat jao reuan – Thai medicine term used to describe the core elemental constitution of each individual.

Tipitaka (Tripitaka) – The traditional term used by different Buddhist traditions to describe their canons of scriptures.

tok sen – A northern Thai (Lanna) healing tradition whereby a wooden hammer and chisel are used to tap along sen lines and on pressure points of the body.

Vinaya Pitaka – One of three parts of Buddhist scripture that comprise the Tipitaka. It primarily deals with monastic rules for monks and nuns. The name Vinaya Pitaka (*vinayapitaka*) derives from Pali/Sanskrit and means "basket of discipline."

vipassana – The term vipassanā (from Pali) is commonly used as a synonym for a style of meditation that centers on mindfulness of breath and awareness of the impermanent nature of all things.

wai – The traditional Thai greeting, which consists of a slight bow, with the palms pressed together in prayer position. The higher the hands are held in relation to the face and the lower the bow, the more respect or reverence is shown to the receiver.

wai khru – A Thai ritual in which students express gratitude and pay respect to their teachers. Rituals may be formalized events involving a large number of people, or more intimate ceremonies involving prayers and reflection. *Wai khru* is an important rite in traditional martial arts, astrology, classical dance, music, and Thai healing arts. In traditional Thai massage, a wai khru generally includes prayers to the Buddha and to Jivaka Kumarabhacca.

wat – A monastery temple of Thailand, Laos, or Cambodia. Technically, a *wat* is a Buddhist complex with a temple, monks' quarters, a building of worship with a large image of Buddha, and an area for lessons and community events.

Wat Po (Pho) – A common name for the Wat Phra Chetuphon temple complex in Bangkok. The Thai massage school associated with Wat Po is an important seat of learning for traditional Thai massage in southern Thailand.

wind gate, wind gate opening – An ancient Thai healing technique that is sometimes referred to as "blood stop," "arterial compression," or "wind gate opening" in English, whereby arteries are temporarily compressed, and then released. The result is a sensation of heat and a rush of blood and energy through the area that was compressed. The Thai name for this technique is *bpert lom*, which translates as "open the wind."

winyaanathaat – The element of consciousness in Thai medicine.

yam khang – A traditional northern Thai healing art in which therapists use their feet to massage oil heated by fire onto the receiver's body.

Selected Bibliography

These publications were written by contributing authors or consulted by them for this book:

Anderson, Peter A. *Body Language.* New York: Alpha/Penguin, 2004.

Asokananda, (a.k.a. Harald Brust). *The Art of Traditional Thai Massage.* Bangkok, Thailand: DK Books, 1990.

— *Thai Traditional Massage for Advanced Practitioners.* Bangkok, Thailand: Editions Duang Kamol, 1996.

—*Thai Traditional Massage in The Side Position.* Bangkok, Thailand: Nai Suk's Editions, 2001.

Axtell, Roger E. *How to Read Body Language Signs and Gestures.* www.businessballs.com.

Balaskas, Kira. *Thai Yoga Massage.* Wellingborough, UK: Thorsons, 2002.

Bose, Sen & Subbarayappa. *A Concise History of Science in India.* Indian National Science Academy, India, 1971.

Brunner and Suddarth. *Textbook of Medical Surgical Nursing, 3rd Edition.* Lippincott, Williams, and Wilkins, 1975.

Bullit, John T (ed). *Vinaya Pitaka: The Basket of the Discipline.* www.accesstoinsight.org, 2010.

Calais-Germain, Blandine. *Anatomy of Breathing.* Vista, CA: Eastland Press, 2005.

Chia, Mantak. *Chi Nei Tsang: Internal Organs Chi Massage.* Chiang Mai, Thailand: Healing Tao Books, 1990.

Corsi, Enrico and Elena Fanfani. *Traditional Thai Yoga: The Postures and Healing Practices of Ruesi Dat Ton.* Rochester, VT: Healing Arts Press/Inner Traditions, 2008.

De Vito, Merrill. "Invisible Energies: Self-Protection for Practitioners." *Massage & Bodywork Magazine*, April–May 2007.

Gach, Michael Reed. *Acupressure's Potent Points.* New York: Bantam Books, 1990.

Gach, Michael Reed and Beth Ann Henning. *Acupressure for Emotional Healing.* New York: Bantam Books, 2004.

Haddad, Bob. "Care & Feeding of Your Thai Massage Practice." Teaching manual, Chapel Hill, NC, 2006.

— "Ergonomics and Breathwork in Nuad Boran." Teaching manual, Chapel Hill, NC, 2006.

— "Luk Pra Kob: Thai Herbal Compress Therapy." Teaching manual, Chapel Hill, NC, 2007.

Hartley, Gregory and Maryann Karinch. *I Can Read You Like A Book*. Pompton Plains, NJ: Career Press, 2007.

Horner, I. B. *The Book of the Discipline (Vinaya Pitaka), Vol. IV*. Oxford, UK: Pali Text Society, 2000.

Jacobsen, Nephyr. "Wai Khru" unpublished paper, USA, 2006.

Jaggi, O. P. *Scientists of Ancient India*. Delhi, India: Atma Ram, 1966.

Jarboux, Damaris. "Self-Protection Issues," unpublished paper from Therapeutic Touch class, TTI#5, USA, 2001.

Kashyap, Bhikkhu J. *Mahavagga*. Nalanda, India: Bihar Government Pali Publications Board, 1956.

Kuraishi, M. H. & A. Ghosh. *Rajgir*. Dept. of Archaeology, New Delhi, India, 1958.

Lanna Thai Massage School. "Balancing Body Exercise Program *(Luesee Dud Ton)*." Teaching manual. Chiang Mai, Thailand, 2006.

Mukhopadhyaya, G. N. *History of Indian Medicine, Vol. III*. Calcutta, India, 1923.

Muley, Gunakar. *Pracna Bharata ke Mahana Vaijñanika* (Hindi). Delhi, India.

Mulholland, Jean. *Medicine, Magic, and Evil Spirits*. Canberra: The Australian National University, 1987.

Panda, Rajaram. *A Latest Guide Book of Rajgir*. New Delhi, India: Mittal Publications, 2005.

Pease, Allan and Barbara. *The Definitive Book of Body Language*. New York: Bantam, 2004.

Pomeranz, Bruce. "Brain Opiates as They Work in Acupuncture." *New Science*. 1977.

Royal Flora Ratchaphruek. *Guidebook to the International Horticultural Exposition in Chiang Mai, Thailand*, 2007.

Salguero, C. Pierce. *A Thai Herbal: Traditional Recipes for Health and Harmony*. Forres, Scotland: Findhorn Press, 2003.

— *Traditional Thai Medicine: Buddhism, Animism, Ayurveda*. Chino Valley, AZ: Hohm Press, 2007.

Sankrityayan, Rahul. *Vinaya Pitaka* (Pali text Hindi translation). Buddha Educational Foundation, Taipei, Taiwan, 2000.

Saraswati, Swami Ambikananda. *Principles of Breathwork*. Wellingborough, UK: Thorsons, 1999.

Satchidananda, Sri Swami. *The Breath of Life: Integral Yoga Pranayama*. Yogaville, VA: Integral Yoga Publications, 1993.

Sharma, P. V. *History of Medicine in India*. New Delhi, India: INSA, 1992.

Tan, Leng T. and Margaret and Veith Ilga Tan. *Acupuncture Therapy: Current Chinese Practice*: Ambler, PA: Temple University, 1973.

Tyroler, Noam. *Thai Acupressure for Orthopedic Disorders*. Self-published. Israel, 2008.

Vidyalankar, Atridev. *Syurveda ka Bihat Itihasa* (Hindi). Lucknow, India, 1960.

Zysk, Kenneth G. "Studies in Traditional Indian Medicine in the Pali Canon: Jivaka and Ayurveda." *Journal of the International Association of Buddhist Studies* 5, 1982.

Photo and Illustration Credits

Cover: Buddha statue draped in saffron robes, Nakhon Pathom, Thailand, by
Vladimir Wrangerl/Shutterstock.com. All rights reserved.
Leading full page photo: Decorative doors at Grand Palace, Bangkok, by
Celia Barenholtz.

One: Introduction
Leading full page photo: Chedi and lotus pond at Wat Mahathat, Sukhothai by
Celia Barenholtz.
Traditional Thai Massage: An Overview: Wat Po photo by Bob Haddad; Ayurvedic
illustration public domain.
Foundations and Basic Principles of Thai Massage Therapy: Illustration courtesy
Asokananda and Editions Duang Kamol.

Two: Mastery of your Practice
Leading full page photo: Pressure point epigraph detail, Wat Po, Bangkok by
Golfx/Shutterstock.com.
The Care and Feeding of Your Thai Massage Practice: All photos courtesy
Bob Haddad; charts and forms courtesy Thai Healing Alliance International.
Using your Feet in Thai Yoga Massage: All photos courtesy Ralf Marzen.
The Sen Sip: Understanding Thai Sen Lines: Illustration courtesy of the estate of
Asokananda and Editions Duang Kamol.
Introduction to Thai Element Theory: Charts courtesy Nephyr Jacobsen.
Pregnancy and Thai Massage: all photos by Bob Haddad; illustrations public
domain, with point placement by Bob Haddad.
Considering Body Language: Photos by Robert Agriopoulos, courtesy of
Bob Haddad.
Breath and Body Mechanics in Nuad Boran: All photos by or courtesy of Bob Haddad.
The three body movement illustrations were hand drawn by Bob Murray Design
and are © Thai Healing Alliance International.
Thai Acupressure and the Wat Po Treatment Protocols: Illustrations courtesy of
J.B. Worsley and Noam Tyroler. Photo courtesy Noam Tyroler. All rights
reserved.
*Luk Pra Kob: The Art of Using Thai Herbal Compresse*s: All photos by or courtesy of
Bob Haddad. Body illustrations public domain, with point placement by
Bob Haddad.

Self-Protection Techniques for the Thai Therapist: All photos by Robert Agriopoulos; Prana eggs and sun/moon illustrations public domain, with line placement by Bob Haddad; kaya kriya illustration courtesy of the estate of Asokananda.

Three: Spiritual and Cultural Connections

Leading full page photo: Reusi convocation at Wat Sri Mahathat chedi, Suphanburi by Matthieu Duquenois.

The Art of Tok Sen: All photos by Joel Sheposh.

Memorial For Chaiyuth: All photos by Bence Ganti.

The Vinaya Pitaka: Stories about Jivaka Komarbhacca: Tibetan thangka painting public domain.

Thai Magic Amulets and Sacred Tattoos: Takrut amulet against tattooed chest by Matthieu Duquenois; Collection of Buddha tablets by Sukpaiboonwat/Shutterstock.com; tablet encased in protective silver housing, with chain by Maetisa/Shutterstock.com; tattoo on back of monk by Gina Smith/Shutterstock.com, all rights reserved; participants at Tattoo Festival by Thor Jorgen Udvang/Shutterstock.com, all rights reserved; monk applying tattoo with a metal rod by Matthieu Duquenois.

Introduction to Reusi Dat Ton: Photos and illustrations courtesy Enrico Corsi. All rights reserved.

The Reusi of Thailand: All photos by Matthieu Duquenois.

Om Namo …What? – The Thai Massage Wai Khru: Transcription of wai khru mantra by Bob Haddad.

Four: Thai Therapists Speak

Leading full page photo: Giant Buddha statue at Wat Sra Si, Sukhothai by Celia Barenholtz.

Acupuncture and Thai Massage: Same-Same but Different: Two illustrations public domain.

One Week with Pichest Boonthumme: Photo by Michelle Tupko.

Integrating General Acupressure into Traditional Thai Massage: All photos by Bob Haddad.

Pilgrimage to Rajgir: All photos by Bob Haddad, except for Venuvana, by Namit Arora. Illustration of the Jivaka Amravana compound by Bob Murray, courtesy Bob Haddad.

Interview with Asokananda: Photo of Asokananda by Bob Haddad; anterior point chart prepared by Asokananda, with handwritten notes from an earlier version.

Credits and References

Photo of Bob Haddad by Dan Crawford Photography.

Author and Contributing Writers

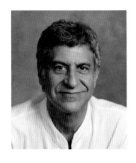

BOB HADDAD, AUTHOR AND EDITOR

Bob began his first studies in Thai massage in 1999, after having already fulfilled careers as a language teacher, musician, and world music producer. He was gradually drawn into the depths of Thai healing arts as he studied with a variety of teachers.

In his study and work in traditional Thai massage, Bob has learned that *nuad boran* is inextricably connected to Buddhist healing traditions and Thai spiritual and cultural values, and that to practice it outside of these contexts, as a mechanical form of bodywork and applied yoga therapy, will generally bring about reduced healing effects.

Bob has studied Thai massage with many teachers over the years, but he has been most influenced by Asokonanda and Ajahn Pichest Boonthumme. He has written books in several disciplines that have been published by Bilingual Press and Glencoe/McGraw Hill. In 2005, he founded Thai Healing Alliance International (THAI), a network of professionals who promote and adhere to basic standards of study and practice of traditional Thai massage. He lives and maintains a professional practice in the United States, and he teaches Thai massage workshops internationally.

Contributing Writers

KIRA BALASKAS has studied Thai massage in Thailand with Asokananda and other Thai teachers since the 1980s, and has practiced and taught yoga for many years. She co-founded the Sunshine Network, and she directs the School of Thai Yoga Massage in London, England. She maintains private practice there, and teaches workshops in the United Kingdom and internationally. She is the author of *Thai Yoga Massage* (Thorsons/Tagman, 2002).

EMILY CANIBANO has a background in education, yoga, fitness, and the healing arts. She practices Thai massage and directs Sky Yoga Studio in Naperville, Illinois, in the United States.

ENRICO CORSI studied Thai massage and *reusi dat ton* at Wat Po, and with other teachers. He directs the Accademia di Massaggio Tradizionale Thailandese in Milan, Italy, where he teaches Thai massage and reusi dat ton. Enrico returns to Thailand regularly to continue his studies. He is the author of *Traditional Thai Yoga: The Postures and Healing Practices of Ruesri Dat Ton* (Healing Arts Press, 2008).

PAUL FOWLER has studied and practiced Thai massage since 1999. He leads study groups to Thailand, and directs Blue Lotus Thai Healing Studies in Chicago, Illinois, in the United States.

MICHAEL REED GACH, PH.D is founder of the Acupressure Institute in Berkeley, California, a leading training school for Asian bodywork. He developed Acu-Yoga, a system of self-acupressure combined with yoga. He practices acupressure and Thai massage, teaches internationally, and is the author of seven books, including *Acupressure for Emotional Healing* (Bantam, 2004) and the best-selling *Acupressure's Potent Points* (Bantam, 1990).

BENCE GANTI is a psychologist who teaches workshops in Integral Flow Therapy, which combines bodywork and psychology. He practices vipassana meditation and yoga, and has studied traditional Thai massage. He was with Chaiyuth Priyasith when he passed away in Chiang Mai, and that experience had a profound impact on his life. Bence lives and practices in his native Hungary, and also in California in the United States.

ROBERT HENDERSON has studied and practiced Thai yoga massage since 2000. He studied for several years with Asokananda, Chaiyuth Priyasith, and Pichest Boonthumme, and began teaching with the Sunshine Network in 2003. Robert offers energy treatment sessions and teaches workshops throughout Europe on energy work, spiritual healing, and Thai massage. He lives in Vienna, Austria.

TIM HOLT has studied Western and Asian bodywork styles for many years. He maintains a practice in deep tissue massage, shiatsu, and Thai massage in California in the United States.

NEPHYR JACOBSEN is the founder and director of The Naga Center, a school for traditional Thai massage and Thai medicine in Portland, Oregon. With over twenty years as a massage therapist, she researches, practices, and teaches traditional Thai medicine, and spends extensive time in Thailand with her family.

CHRIS JONES has lived in Southeast Asia for many years, and is particularly interested in Thai Buddhism and culture. He is a passionate collector and researcher of Thai amulets and votive tablets, and he helps to disseminate information through his web site on Buddhist amulets.

FELICITY JOY began her training in 1989 at the Old Medicine Hospital and returns to Thailand yearly. Her main teachers are Asokananda, Chaiyuth Priyasith, Pichest Boonthumme, Super Lek, and Khun Ni. She lives in Chiang Mai and London and teaches workshops internationally.

GREG LAWRENCE explores the traditional healing arts of northern Thailand and leads groups to study with Lanna and other hill tribe healers. He lives in Australia, where he directs Inner Journeys, an organization dedicated to spiritual journeys and eco-travel adventures.

RALF MARZEN is the director of Mudita School of Thai Yoga Massage and StillPoint in London in the United Kingdom. He studied with Asokananda, Chaiyuth Priyasith, and Pichest Boonthumme, and has visited Thailand for many years. As a senior teacher in the Sunshine Network, he helps spread Asokananda's message about Thai massage as mindfulness and *metta* (loving-kindness) in action. He lives in London and Amsterdam.

GORAN MILOVANOV began learning Thai massage with Danko Lara Radic and Davor Haber. He has continued his studies with many other teachers, and in addition to Thai massage, he also practices therapeutic sports massage in Pancevo, Serbia.

GUNAKAR MULEY is a researcher and prolific author who has written and translated over thirty books in Hindi and English since 1960. His articles and essays on science, archaeology, technology, and Indian history and culture have appeared in many newspapers and magazines. He has a special interest in early Indian historical figures, including Jivaka Kumarabhaccha. He lives in Delhi, India.

DANKO LARA RADIC is a physical therapist who first studied Thai massage in Thailand. His teachers include Chongkol Setthakorn, Andrea Baglioni, Davor Haber, Pichest Boonthumme, and others. He teaches Thai massage and maintains a private practice in Belgrade, Serbia.

C. PIERCE SALGUERO, PH.D. studied History of Medicine at the Johns Hopkins School of Medicine, and specializes in Buddhist-influenced Asian medical traditions. A university professor and a practitioner and teacher of traditional Thai massage, he is the author of several books on Thai healing arts including *Encyclopedia of Thai Massage* (Findhorn Press, 2004) and *Traditional Thai Medicine: Buddhism, Animism, Ayurveda* (Hohm Press, 2007).

JOEL SHEPOSH began his study and practice of Thai massage in 1993 with Rick Gold, and has studied with many teachers in Thailand including Sompong Proparat, Bundit Sitthiwej, Jack Chaiya and Sinchai Sukparsert. He teaches workshops and practices Thai massage, herbal compress therapy and *tok sen* in Arizona, in the United States.

ERIC SPIVACK has studied in Thailand since 1996. He is a licensed acupuncturist and massage therapist and leads study groups to Thailand. He lives and practices in Seattle, Washington, in the United States.

NOAM TYROLER has studied and practiced Thai massage and Thai acupressure since 1989, and taught at Reidman College in Tel Aviv, Israel. He studied acupressure with Suchat Wonguraprasert and Guniga Piyapong at Wat Po, Bangkok, and with many others in Chiang Mai. He helps to raise awareness of Thai acupressure by teaching workshops and through his book *Thai Acupressure For Orthopedic Disorders* (self-published, 2008). He lives in Israel.

MICHELLE TUPKO began her studies with Chuck Duff and Paul Fowler. She has studied with Pichest Boonthumme, Jack Chaiya, Mor Noi, Homprang Chaleekanha, and others. She lives in Michigan in the United States.

KAREN UFER has studied nuad boran with a variety of teachers, and has been influenced by the teachings of Asokananda, Pichest Boonthumme, and Arno L'Hermitte. She lives and practices in Arizona in the United States.

TEVIJJO YOGI has studied under many different teachers within the Thai medicine tradition, and has attended the Traditional Doctor program at the Ministry of Public Health and at Wat Po. Tevijjo has apprenticed under various doctors, and was initiated into the tradition by his teachers.

Index